T0282655

Clinical Staging in Psychiatry

Clinical Staging in Psychiatry

Making Diagnosis Work for Research and Treatment

Edited by

Patrick D. McGorry
University of Melbourne

Ian B. Hickie
University of Sydney

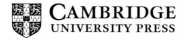

CAMBRIDGE
UNIVERSITY PRESS

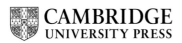
CAMBRIDGE
UNIVERSITY PRESS

Shaftesbury Road, Cambridge CB2 8EA, United Kingdom

One Liberty Plaza, 20th Floor, New York, NY 10006, USA

477 Williamstown Road, Port Melbourne, VIC 3207, Australia

314–321, 3rd Floor, Plot 3, Splendor Forum, Jasola District Centre, New Delhi – 110025, India

103 Penang Road, #05–06/07, Visioncrest Commercial, Singapore 238467

Cambridge University Press is part of Cambridge University Press & Assessment, a department of the University of Cambridge.

We share the University's mission to contribute to society through the pursuit of education, learning and research at the highest international levels of excellence.

www.cambridge.org
Information on this title: www.cambridge.org/9781108718844

DOI: 10.1017/9781139839518

First published 2019
Reprinted 2019

A catalogue record for this publication is available from the British Library

Library of Congress Cataloging-in-Publication data
Names: McGorry, Patrick D., editor. | Hickie, Ian, editor.
Title: Clinical staging in psychiatry : making diagnosis work for
    research and treatment / edited by Patrick McGorry, Ian Hickie.
Description: Cambridge, United Kingdom ; New York, NY : Cambridge
    University Press, 2019. | Includes bibliographical references.
Identifiers: LCCN 2019009292 | ISBN 9781108718844 (pbk. : alk. paper)
Subjects: | MESH: Mental Disorders–diagnosis | Disease Progression | Mental
    Disorders–classification | Risk Assessment | Mental Disorders–therapy
Classification: LCC RC473.D54 | NLM WM 141 | DDC 616.89/075–dc23
LC record available at https://lccn.loc.gov/2019009292

ISBN   978-1-108-71884-4   Paperback

....

Contents

Contributors

Kelly Allott
Orygen, The National Centre of Excellence in Youth Mental Health
The Centre for Youth Mental Health, University of Melbourne, Parkville, Australia

Mario Alvarez-Jimenez
Orygen, The National Centre of Excellence in Youth Mental Health
The Centre for Youth Mental Health, University of Melbourne, Parkville, Australia

G. Paul Amminger
Orygen, The National Centre of Excellence in Youth Mental Health
The Centre for Youth Mental Health, University of Melbourne, Parkville, Australia

Cali F. Bartholomeusz
Orygen, The National Centre of Excellence in Youth Mental Health
The Centre for Youth Mental Health, University of Melbourne, Parkville, Australia

Bernhard T. Baune
Department of Psychiatry, Melbourne School of Medicine, University of Melbourne, Melbourne, Australia
Department of Psychiatry, University of Munster, Munster, Germany

Gregor E. Berger
Psychiatric University Hospital Zurich, Department of Child and Adolescent Psychiatry, Zurich, Switzerland

Maximus Berger
James Cook University, Townsville, Australia

Joanne S. Carpenter
Youth Mental Health Team, Brain and Mind Centre, University of Sydney, Sydney, Australia

Shane Cross
Youth Mental Health Team, Brain and Mind Centre, University of Sydney, Sydney, Australia

Stijn de Vos
University of Groningen, University Medical Center Groningen, Groningen, The Netherlands

Jessica A. Hartmann
Orygen, The National Centre of Excellence in Youth Mental Health
The Centre for Youth Mental Health, University of Melbourne, Parkville, Australia

Daniel F. Hermens
Youth Mental Health Team, Brain and Mind Centre, University of Sydney, Sydney, Australia

Ian B. Hickie
Youth Mental Health Team, Brain and Mind Centre, University of Sydney, Sydney, Australia

Frank Iorfino
Youth Mental Health Team, Brain and Mind Centre, University of Sydney, Sydney, Australia

Eóin Killackey
Orygen, The National Centre of Excellence
in Youth Mental Health
The Centre for Youth Mental Health,
University of Melbourne, Parkville,
Australia

Suzie Lavoie
Orygen, The National Centre of Excellence
in Youth Mental Health
The Centre for Youth Mental Health,
University of Melbourne, Parkville, Australia

Patrick D. McGorry
Orygen, The National Centre of Excellence
in Youth Mental Health
The Centre for Youth Mental Health,
University of Melbourne, Parkville,
Australia

Cristina Mei
Orygen, The National Centre of Excellence
in Youth Mental Health
The Centre for Youth Mental Health,
University of Melbourne, Parkville,
Australia

Barnaby Nelson
Orygen, The National Centre of Excellence
in Youth Mental Health
The Centre for Youth Mental Health,
University of Melbourne, Parkville,
Australia

Christos Pantelis
Melbourne Neuropsychiatry Centre,
Department of Psychiatry, University of
Melbourne & Melbourne Health, Parkville,
Australia

Elizabeth Scott
Youth Mental Health Team, Brain and
Mind Centre, University of Sydney,
Sydney, Australia

Johanna T. W. Wigman
University of Groningen, University
Medical Center Groningen, Groningen,
The Netherlands

Foreword

Back to the Future

This volume addresses the single most important challenge facing psychiatry today, interrogating the very nature of mental disorder and its myriad forms, and offering an alternative to the orthodoxy of the binary classificatory approach that has dominated clinical practice and research methods for decades. The staging approach, essentially an attempt to blend binary and dimensional approaches to describing mental health problems, posits that, rather than being static, discrete health conditions (which imply distinct aetiologies and therapies), these problems are syndromes which overlap and develop in stages. This framing is also one of the guiding principles of the *Lancet* Commission on Global Mental Health and Sustainable Development. Ironically, perhaps, the central message to embrace the reality of the dimensional approach to mental health problems is, in fact, not dissimilar from that championed by earlier approaches to mental health which proposed just a few dimensions (such as neuroticism) to describe psychopathology.

It is now abundantly obvious that while the rush to operationalise binary diagnostic categories, despite the absence of any biological foundation, was well-intended to provide reliable tools for practitioners and to enhance the biomedical grounding of psychiatry, adopting identical approaches to classification as used in other branches of medicine was also wrong. We now know that interactions between our genes, neurodevelopmental processes, biological exposures and social environments lie at the heart of our mental health, and these are simply too complex and specific to each individual to justify categorisation into discrete diagnostic envelopes. The binary approach is exemplified by the question 'what is a case?', which, despite decades of research, has turned out to be almost impossible to define for virtually any mental disorder. This approach has also contributed to the alienation of mental health care from the community and contributed to decades of lost opportunities for uncovering the aetiology of mental health problems and their effective management. This book offers a timely, up-to-date and comprehensive overview of an alternative approach to describing, studying and managing mental health problems.

Implicit in the staging approach is the notion of a continuum from the complete absence of psychopathology to states in which phenomena are mild and often undifferentiated, to states in which clusters of phenomena begin to emerge, to an 'end stage' when they become severe and chronic. Across this continuum, there is a high degree of correlation with social functioning, with psychopathology and social functioning interacting in bidirectional pathways across the spectrum of severity. While the current state of knowledge presents many unresolved challenges, some of which I note later, the staging approach represents the most promising framework for describing psychopathology as it tries to bridge the binary and dimensional approaches in a manner that is intuitive and well aligned with diverse perspectives on mental health problems. From a clinical and public health perspective, whose practitioners are the primary audience for this book, the staging approach points to the opportunity to shift the care of those with mild, early-stage problems to low-intensity interventions, such as digitally delivered guided self-care and community health worker-delivered psychological and social interventions. This is not only an efficient way to reserve expensive mental health specialist services for those individuals who are at the more severe end of the continuum, but it is simultaneously also more empowering to the large proportion of individuals with milder conditions who can recover and stay well without the need for a diagnosis through interventions that may be accessed through diverse, affordable delivery platforms. The staged approach also offers a mechanistic foundation for the growing body of evidence in support of transdiagnostic interventions.

But, despite this enthusiasm, there is still much which requires clarification, not least the continuing need to define what constitutes the boundaries of each stage and how these can be assessed in routine health care settings so that the clinical decisions implicit in the stepped care approach can be made reliably. Relatedly, a more fundamental question is what constitutes the phenomena that should be the focus of description in staged models; for example, how 'deep' should our phenotyping go beyond reported phenomena such as specific symptoms of mental health problems, to cognitive phenotypes such as impulsivity, or what are the valid clusters of phenomena, and to what extent should these also capture social and somatic phenomena? In this context, the alignment of the staging approach with other frameworks, in particular research domain criteria (RDoC) and network theories, which have challenged the binary disease model, is necessary going forward.

Assuming we will be able to address these questions of operationalising our mental health outcomes, then staging models can also be applied to testing precision medicine approaches to treatment selection. Such approaches must not only address the question of identifying which clinical intervention works for whom but, equally important, it must also identify who does not need any intervention and who will not respond to any known intervention. And we need to clarify the relationship of the staging approach from a life course perspective (i.e. the emergence of mental health phenomena in a graduated manner across the early years of life) with staging from a clinical perspective (i.e. the graduated appearance of phenomena from milder to more severe forms of psychopathology). In any event, a graduated approach emphasising efforts to reverse distress, or at the least to slow its progression, the hallmark of prevention, remains the imperative for health care.

The staging approach has the unique potential to unite the divergent frameworks for the description of mental health adopted by neuroscientists (who study endophenotypes or biological processes which are dimensional), communities (who reject being labelled with diagnoses, in particular when their cognitive and emotional experiences are understood as an indivisible extension of social suffering or spiritual unease), practitioners (who, more often than not, struggle to neatly pigeon-hole a patient into a diagnostic box) and policy makers (who are left staggered by the vast numbers of people with a 'diagnosis' rather than the number of people with mental health problems that need clinical interventions). In short, the staging approach is compatible with neuroscientific observations, explanatory models in the general population, clinician experiences and policy-maker expectations. No other approach comes close to the goal of achieving such a consensus.

Vikram Patel

The Pershing Square Professor of Global Health and Wellcome Trust Principal Research Fellow, Department of Global Health and Social Medicine, Harvard Medical School

Professor, Department of Global Health and Population, Harvard TH Chan School of Public Health, Co-Founder and Member of Managing Committee, Sangath Adjunct Professor, Public Health Foundation of India

Boston, November 2018

Acknowledgements

The editors acknowledge the pioneers of the original staging idea in clinical medicine and its early application to psychiatry by Giovanni Fava in anxiety and mood disorders. The search for a diagnostic approach that works in the complex and contested world of psychiatry and mental health is challenging, but a hugely worthwhile endeavour and we pay respect to and value the painstaking and creative efforts of all our colleagues – past, present and emerging – to create, evolve and build a better system for the benefit of people with mental ill-health everywhere. The editors would also like to acknowledge the endless support and patience of their families, the creative insights and contributions of their colleagues and patients and the scholarly work of the contributors to this volume. Finally, we wish to thank Cambridge University Press for their patience, professionalism and support in bringing this volume to completion and to the wider world.

Chapter

1

Diagnosis without Borders
A Pluripotential Approach to Preventive Intervention in Emerging Mental Disorders

Patrick D. McGorry

Diagnosis in medicine has been seen as an essential process in choosing appropriate treatment and predicting the future course of the illness, and providing a sense of clarity and relief to patients that their illness is legitimate and understood. In many fields of medicine the diagnostic process has evolved in complexity over the past few decades from a predominantly clinical process based on a careful case history and physical examination to a blend which places a great deal of weight on investigations aimed at staging and stratifying or personalising treatment in a more precise manner. The term *precision medicine* (National Research Council, 2011) has been coined to reflect this aspiration and growing reality. New technology has boosted the power and precision of diagnosis, though it has reduced reliance on high-level clinical skill and expertise, which commands less respect (Moffitt, 2016).

By contrast, in psychiatry, attitudes to diagnosis remain ambivalent and polarised, and its value is continuously questioned both in professional circles and in the public arena (Greenberg, 2013; McGorry, 2013). Recent revisions to international diagnostic systems for psychiatry have reignited this deep ambivalence, which reflects Cartesian tensions between the extremes of 'mindless' and 'brainless' psychiatry (Dominguez et al., 2011). New life has been injected into an enduring culture war (Angell, 2011) in which victories are elusive or pyrrhic. As this storm subsides we risk entering a new period of stasis in which old ideas are recycled (Jablensky, 2016) and admittedly erudite yet ultimately frustrating metaphysical analyses are presented (Kendler, 2016). Other equally erudite reviews (Stephan et al., 2016a; 2016b) pose all the key questions but provide few answers. How can we move beyond such static, even defeatist, mindsets to the heuristic? Is there a more productive pathway? Several possibilities have been advanced (Borsboom, 2017; Cuthbert & Insel, 2010; Kotov et al., 2018; McGorry et al., 2006). But first let us consider what is the fundamental purpose of diagnosis.

The Nature and Purpose of Diagnosis

Robert Kendell (1975a) pointed out four decades ago that human beings possess three sets of characteristics. The first set of characteristics is more or less universal and is shared with all other human beings, such as having essential organs like the brain, possessing the ability to think and reflect, and being able to breathe. The second set is unique to that individual, such as their fingerprints, dental records, particular skin blemishes and personal life experiences. The third set of characteristics is those that are shared with some but not other human beings. Only the latter group is of use for the purposes of classification and therefore for diagnosis, which is a specific form of classification.

In purely medical diagnosis, there are now layers and subsets within this third domain. For example, some people with breast cancer share this characteristic with each other, but not with those who do not have breast cancer. However, they can be further subgrouped according to the stage of the illness in that they share certain features linked to stage (notably extension or spread of the disease) with some breast cancer sufferers and not with others. Further profiling, subcategorisation or *stratification* (Trusheim et al., 2007), as it is known, can be carried out using specific genotyping and use of other biomarkers. This increasing precision means that the treatment options can be personalised in quite a fine-grained manner (Collins & Varmus, 2015). However, we still do not approach the reductio ad absurdum that treatment may ultimately be uniquely different for every individual. There are still groupings, albeit much smaller than before, and the treatment sequence according to stage is also especially important.

In psychiatry, in the light of the mind–body split as created by Cartesian dualism, many are prepared to ask the question: does diagnosis really apply at all? Impressed by the great diversity of human experience and the uniqueness of the individual, which manifests at the level of the person and character, they argue that even stratification is insufficient and that *every* individual's mental health care must be unique and personalised. This is an argument that could apply most clearly to psychological forms of therapy, and it is true that the critique of the value of diagnosis in psychiatry is usually advanced by proponents of psychological therapies as the sole or dominant form of treatment. Psychoanalysis arguably represents the most extreme form of this perspective. However, taken to such an extreme, this implies that no knowledge or evidence derived from the care of other people could ever be used in the care of each new or distinct individual. This means starting anew with every new patient as a brand new learning experience. However, even in the domain of personality and character, there are subgroups and dimensions of commonality. Yet the fact is that we do all have some unique personal characteristics and experiences, we all feel a level of uniqueness as human beings as well as a sense of commonality and kindred spirit, and we would like to be related to, with this uniqueness understood and accepted. These unique aspects can be critical in personalising therapy and, for this reason, psychiatry is the field within medicine where personalised medicine is already achievable.

These considerations do not mean that psychiatric diagnosis is necessarily fundamentally different from medical diagnosis but that we need to pay more attention to not only stratifying the treatment as best we can by stage and subgroup, but also having an element in every patient of uniquely and individually tailored care. Indeed, while it is especially important in psychiatry, this may well be necessary in patients with physical diseases too if we can see beyond the mind–body split.

> The deeper we delve into the nature of mental illness, the clearer it becomes that cherished distinctions between diagnostic categories might be partly illusory.
>
> (Stephan et al., 2016a)

The other substantial difference between medical and psychiatric diagnosis is arguably maturational, in that the latter is still largely syndromal or, worse, still 'polythetic', made up of a collection of clinical features assembled by committees or based on historical sources. Traditional views (Jablensky, 2012; 2016) require there to be points of rarity between syndromes which are seen as being composed of sets of clinical features cohering in a limited number of patterns with 'points of rarity' typically seen between them. However, in real life this is the exception rather than the rule, especially as syndromes emerge. In the formation of syndromes it is apparent that some symptoms create risk for others. The analogy with clouds was one used by Robert Kendell, and indeed symptoms ebb and flow, cohere and dissipate in just that manner. Boundaries between such phenotypic expressions are indistinct, overlapping and unclear. The concept of comorbidity is a natural extension or corollary of this scenario. In physical disease, there are genuinely comorbid pathophysiological processes such as diabetes and ischaemic heart disease which coexist, with one often acting as a risk factor for the other. In psychiatry, it is far from clear that when syndromal co-occurrence occurs that this indicates comorbidity of the same type. The underlying biology may be the same or different. We are not able to be at all clear about this. Stephan et al. (2016a) contend that the dysfunctional brain appears to be quite limited in the number of major syndromal patterns it can create.

The final issue is that while diagnosis in its applied sense as providing a guide to treatment selection and outcome may be useful across the board in mental health, it may struggle more for acceptance beyond the traditional core of mental disorders, notably psychoses and severe mood disorders (Kendell, 1975b). When applied to the border zones of common mental disorders, anxiety, depression, personality dysfunction and crisis responses, the personal uniqueness argument gives the impression at least of having more strength, at least as a major influence on the problems, the value of specific biological treatments is less clear, and the boundaries of normality and need for care from mental health professionals more contested by the public, governments and sections of the mental health field (Frances, 2013). While there are valid debates to be had here, the dichotomy between low and high prevalence or common mental disorders is false, and has been unhelpfully used to ration access to quality mental health care in a way that would be quite unacceptable in physical medicine; for example, deserving low prevalence or 'genuine' cases of serious mental illness versus the less deserving 'worried well', including subthreshold cases where much treatable chronic distress and disability resides. On the other hand, with the revolution in 'awareness' in high-income country settings, this scenario is changing, and it is the common mental disorders that are gaining better acceptance and access to care, while the more severe and persistent mental disorders are increasingly neglected (Demytte-naere et al., 2004; Wang et al., 2002). In order to step back from this familiar vortex, which confuses so many, and fascinates and oddly gratifies some, it is crucial to seek some practical solutions.

Diagnosis: Classification with Utility

Diagnosis is essentially *classification with utility* (Kendell & Jablensky, 2003). The aim is to characterise the clinical phenotype in a condensed or shorthand way that helps to distinguish those who are ill and in need of health care from those who are not, and genuinely enhance the selection of treatment and prediction of outcome. Medicine is a pragmatic field, utility in medicine is the ultimate test, and this utilitarian definition is necessary and sufficient to justify the central role of diagnosis in clinical practice. If an underlying pathophysiology or biosignature can be closely linked, then that is welcome added value. Yet much of current psychiatric diagnosis has low utility and such biosignatures remain elusive, or are transdiagnostic. This is part of the reason for its weak and ambivalent support for diagnosis among many mental health clinicians as well as the wider world. Nor do the current diagnostic systems appear to have optimally assisted the search for disorder-specific pathophysiological mechanisms and biological and cognitive markers;

indeed they may well have obscured such progress. Hence, many researchers are seeking other heuristic frameworks (Cuthbert & Insel, 2010; Kendler et al., 2011; Kotov et al., 2018; McGorry et al., 2010). The latter can be divergent from and fail to meet clinical needs.

Other problems that have been highlighted by critics include continuing poor reliability, despite the advent of operational criteria, potentially harmful effects of the more stigmatising diagnoses, the inevitably bureaucratic and political nature of the international classification industry, the retention of time-honoured diagnostic categories past their use-by date, while at the same time poorly validated new categories have mushroomed (i.e. from 182 disorders in DSM-II to 265 in DSM-III and 297 in DSM-4), and poor predictive value for consumption of health care resources (Rutledge & Osler, 1998). To this could be added a failure to clearly define the earliest clinical stages of emerging mental disorders as has been done in other medical illnesses. This has hampered preventive psychiatry and the capacity for early diagnosis. A consequent lack of confidence in, even suspicion of, early diagnosis, combined with stigma and a failure to invest in mental health care to scale, has helped to embed late diagnosis, inadequate quality of care and consequently poorer outcomes across the world, which seem inevitable through the lens of the 'clinician's illusion', and which further entrench stigma and therapeutic nihilism, and reinforce the dichotomy between the high-prevalence or common mental disorders (often derided as overlapping with the 'worried well'). With new versions of the DSM and ICD, we can expect little more than incremental and desultory change, increasingly buffeted by the forces of public opinion, politics and ideology (Ahuja & McGorry, 2012; Boseley, 2012; Carey, 2012; Frances, 2010). We are faced with some stark choices. These are: a resigned acceptance of the status quo and a retreat into another round of introspection (Jablensky, 2016; Kendler, 2016); a revival of earlier attempts to develop a system based on quantitative nosology (Kotov et al., 2018); and the design of innovative and heuristic new approaches (Cuthbert & Insel, 2010; McGorry et al., 2007). A creative leap is desperately required, but is it within reach or merely a mirage, or another false dawn?

Mental Ill-Health Starts Well before Traditional Diagnosis

Mental ill-health has to start somewhere. Eaton et al. (1995) described how what we call symptoms arise either from *intensification* of subjective experiences or behaviours that have been present for some time or from *acquisition* of new experiences or behaviours, or most commonly a combination of both. Daily human experience involves periodic and sometimes intense and mercurial changes in affect and salience in response to the social environment. When these become more prominent, they can be discerned as subclinical 'microphenotypes', which wax and wane, interact sequentially or become confluent, and may mature or stabilise towards pure or hybrid 'macrophenotypes' (van Os & Linscott, 2012). This process is undeniably fluid and dimensional, and several (but not endless) dimensions of psychopathology can be readily identified, such as aberrant salience and affective dysregulation. Categories could be arbitrarily imposed within such dimensions, but the notion of the syndrome, in which various elemental symptoms somewhat predictably cohere but also impact on each other over time (Kendler et al., 2011), is an important construct to retain. In real people, and these phenomena can be best observed in young people in transition to adulthood when the force of incidence of mental ill-health surges to a peak (McGorry et al., 2011; Paus et al., 2008), several dimensions of psychopathology emerge sequentially and concurrently in an interactive and dynamic way, ebbing and flowing. Persistence and severity (perceived distress) are key dimensions setting the threshold for need for care (Dominguez et al., 2011), irrespective of the specific constellation of features. An initial or provisional diagnosis merely represents a categorical decision that there is a need for care on the basis of severity and persistence of distress with or without clear-cut impairment, though this has also involved a recognition of this need for care and help-seeking by the person or someone close to them. This is a minimalistic approach that does not overextend specific diagnosis, which is usually not necessary to offer initial and non-specific forms of intervention. We know it is challenging to rigidly define the boundary between 'normality' and mental disorder and need for care. But how critical or feasible is it to create such a precise definition? Could it even be self-defeating? And could we tolerate a 'grey area' or fuzziness, with soft and flexible entry (and exit) and personal choice as key features of a new primary care culture? One variable is the person's level of tolerance of suffering, which is highly variable in relation to both physical and mental symptoms. Unlike in physical medicine, where even asymptomatic 'normal' people have no problem accessing preventive health care of many kinds, financial forces, an exaggerated fear of stigma and labelling, and perhaps also of poor-quality care, tend to oppose this tolerance and flexibility in mental health.

The debate over whether a *clinical high risk, ultra-high risk* or *attenuated psychosis syndrome* (CHR, UHR or APS – a constellation of low-grade psychotic experiences in help-seeking and distressed individuals that research indicates represents a precursor syndrome of first-episode psychosis) should be included in the DSM-5 brought all of these issues to the fore (Carpenter & van Os, 2011; Fusar-Poli & Yung, 2012; Woods et al., 2010). It also showed that while this concept was a genuine advance, its key value may be prototypical; there is a bigger fish to fry, namely a broader transdiagnostic precursor stage (McGorry et al., 2018). The classical patterns of psychopathology that are represented in the major psychiatric disorders, such as schizophrenia, major depression, borderline personality disorder, anorexia nervosa and bipolar disorder, are late-stage concepts, largely derived from late nineteenth- and early twentieth-century tertiary care settings. Advances in psychiatric epidemiology have revealed widespread subdiagnostic and relatively non-specific expression of mental ill-health in the general population; some of this is transient or intermittent, some persistent, but most of it justifies a need for care, and there is substantial cumulative public health impact (Judd et al., 2002; Linscott & van Os, 2013). A key question is how these phenomena should link with and shape diagnostic classification. All major psychiatric disorders have early clinical stages or 'prodromes' during which sustained distress and disability embed and care is needed, yet this occurs well before traditional diagnostic 'clarity' is achieved (McGorry et al., 2006). Primary care physicians know this only too well and find the DSM and ICD relatively unhelpful. They are finding the greater flexibility of new transdiagnostic staging-based models liberating. Recent work suggests that persistence of psychotic experiences with associated distress in the general population begins to approach the level of risk for sustained psychotic disorder as seen in enriched clinical APS samples (Kaymaz et al., 2012; van Os & Linscott, 2012).

The UHR criteria for psychosis, developed by our group over 20 years ago (Yung & McGorry, 1996; Yung et al., 1998), do have a strong valence for psychosis as an outcome, yet even with this as the primary target, other targets were hit, and a substantial proportion of patients manifest other syndromal outcomes, mainly mood and anxiety, much but not all of which had been expressed prior to the emergence of psychotic symptoms. This indicated that introducing a single prodromal or early clinical phenotype (APS) within one of the diagnostic silos in an otherwise relatively unchanged DSM-5, without reference to other diagnostic streams, would produce an asymmetry that could obscure the wider issue and undermine wider reform. The current UHR or APS criteria were clearly not the last word on the issue, and ultimately this is the reason that we support the decision (made for other reasons) to not include the definition in the main clinical section of the DSM-5. Most psychosis researchers believe the predictive power of these UHR criteria should be enhanced using additional clinical predictors and key biomarkers; however, this may be a very challenging task in isolation, given the syndromal nature of the exit syndrome of interest and the overlap and comorbidity that is inevitable. Alternatively, we can take a broader transdiagnostic view, as suggested originally by Cuijpers (2003), who stressed the value of including multiple outcome targets or exit syndromes, particularly when each of these individually is of relatively low incidence. This makes a virtue of necessity, and particularly when the emerging syndromes we are seeking to define are somewhat elusive, overlapping and unfold sequentially. Traditionally, this has been handled with hierarchical models with organic and psychotic syndromes 'trumping' more common syndromes regarded as less specific and lower in the hierarchy. Another response to this issue is the clinical staging model, which allows predictors and preventive treatment for multiple specific exit syndromes to be studied in parallel and allows the possibility that risk factors and treatment strategies alike may be common or cross-diagnostic (McGorry et al., 2007). This certainly reflects the behaviour of clinicians and may help to account for 'off label' broad-spectrum use of both drug and psychosocial treatments. This is generally seen as a vice, rather than a case of clinical reality exposing the fiction created by the wishful thinking of an excessively reductionist biological psychiatry, and cemented by the FDA and the pharmaceutical industry, that an array of poorly validated and differentiated syndromes can be equated with diseases.

Are Early Clinical Phenotypes Pluripotential?

This discussion and the logic of Cuijpers (2003) suggests the notion of pluripotentiality of the early clinical phenotypes of mental disorders and the value of expanding the UHR operational definition with subthreshold features and risk markers for several non-psychotic exit syndromes to define a broad-spectrum ultra-high-risk or pluripotential state. Such a definition might be expected to result in greater enrichment of the sample for progression to one or more of several forms of sustained, recurrent mental disorder of at least moderate severity. It might then be feasible to identify from within a less specific and undifferentiated cohort of distressed and help-seeking young people the enriched subset at greatly enhanced risk of serious mental illness, and would pave the way for sophisticated sequential treatment trials to be conducted in due course. The sequences of evolving syndromes may be linear, consistent with a hierarchical model, or much more variable, with homotypic, heterotypic and mixed patterns of evolution. Other approaches have sought to capture and design natural structures and pathways within a closed system of psychopathology (the Hierarchical Taxonomy of Psychopathology (HiTOP) and network analysis – see Chapters 3 and 4). HiTOP attempts to cross-sectionally provide a hierarchical dimensional approach to psychiatric classification (Kotov et al., 2018), whereas network theory conceptualises mental health as a system in which the interplay between symptoms underpins disorder onset (Borsboom, 2017). Alternatively, the 'p factor' approach proposes that a general psychopathology factor underlies a range of disorders, representing lesser to greater severity of psychopathology (Caspi et al., 2014). Although these approaches may facilitate the mapping of mental disorders, their clinical utility remains unclear, particularly in guiding treatment planning.

Nonetheless, these raise a fundamental question of whether static quantitative nosology alone is capable of defining a system in which the natural structure of symptoms and syndromes can be utilised by clinicians to make treatment decisions. Furthermore, what is the relationship of the 'p factor' to subordinate components of the array of syndromes and symptoms? Is the 'p factor' a representation of pluripotentiality? Similarly, while network analysis allows longitudinal patterns to be captured, to what extent are symptom dynamics and influences the major determinants of emergence of fully fledged and stable syndromes and disorders?

Careful longitudinal studies from initial onset of symptoms and with broad entry criteria are needed to distinguish between a pluripotential model and one that is more hierarchical and deterministic. Concepts and tools such as the 'p factor', hierarchy staging and quantitative nosology are all of potential value and could be utilised in the creation of a more definitive model, which can only be validated through its utility. Using biomarkers or biosignatures to assess risk of progression or remission, to subtype within stages and further refine treatment would introduce 'profiling' and a more personalised or stratified approach. Ultimately, it may be that sophisticated sequential intervention studies stratified using biomarkers are needed to uncover early specificity behind a deceptively pluripotential screen. Alternatively, there may be some quasi-universal interventions which benefit all or most patients.

Clinical Staging May Be More Important than Prematurely Specific Syndromal Diagnosis

There is a natural tension between overtreatment and inhibiting the capacity for resilience and coping, and undertreatment, which is fuelled in psychiatry by poor awareness, stigma and limited access to care. To a large extent this is a false dichotomy, which along with stigma itself can be overcome by *normalising* approaches to early intervention, which include 'soft entry' to assessment and care in a welcoming and optimistic culture and setting. Crisis theory is one key framework that illustrates this point and allows normal responses to severe adverse life events to receive a safe and proportional therapeutic response event, even though the distress and impairment is understandable and mostly self-limited. Relief of distress and early and sustained care for the subgroup who turn out to not make a speedy recovery is fully justifiable. In the same way, early forms of therapeutic intervention in mental health care can generally have a light initial touch, with elements such as support, information, exercise and e-health as their mainstay. The clinical staging model in psychiatry (described in Chapter 2) adapted from general medicine ensures that interventions are proportional to both need and the risk of 'extension' of the clinical phenotype and its consequences (McGorry et al., 2006). It recognises that persistent and multiple 'microphenotypes' of disturbance can justify a need for care on their immediate merits *as well as risk* for progression to more familiar 'macrophenotypes'; however, it also recognises the need for blending dimensional and categorical models. Staging moves outside the current diagnostic boundaries to include the full spectrum of disorder, and while highly congruent with notions of an extended phenotype for individual disorders, which involves continuity with the healthy population, it places strong diagnostic emphasis on where a person sits in the evolution of the clinical phenotype. A staging perspective explicitly recognises that this is a moving feast, and that there is homotypic and heterotypic continuity as well as discontinuity and remission. The goal of staging is to improve *diagnostic utility* in relation to treatment selection and evaluation. We regard this as preeminent in diagnosis and this contrasts so far with other new developments in diagnosis (Borsboom, 2017; Cuthbert & Insel, 2010; Kotov et al., 2018). Traditionally, the nexus between diagnosis and prognosis has been used as a criterion for judging utility. In our view, in psychiatry, this has been overemphasised and exaggerated, with frequent negative, even iatrogenic, consequences. Blending, and even embedding, prognosis within diagnosis led to the creation of the schizophrenia concept, which had the effect of extinguishing hope for recovery from generations of patients. Staging also has a longer-term heuristic goal of facilitating linkages between biological and cognitive markers and clinical phenotypes agnostically rather than diagnostically, though this may not be relevant to all mental health conditions.

Staging Aims to Enhance Treatment Selection, Safety and Success

So when would it make sense to move beyond a general diagnosis of 'mental ill-health' or the notion of a 'p factor'? This has to do with the specificity and safety of the range of psychosocial and biological treatments, and remains to be defined by further clinical research. It also has to do with the success or otherwise of simpler and more generic early-stage interventions. The principle could be that we should allow no more specificity in the diagnostic term or label than is necessary to guide treatment selection. We might start to see some of this specificity emerge with the advent of clearer, more stable and sustained, or severe syndromes or macrophenotypes such as psychosis, mania, depression, anxiety, addiction and the borderline syndrome, either alone or, more typically, in 'comorbid' blends. Network analysis, which maps the pathways of risk and flow of symptom patterns, might provide avenues for intervention targeting pivotal symptoms which increase risk for progression, such as insomnia or rumination. While the 'p factor' might conceal therapeutic targets, deploying a hierarchical lens beyond the top level (Reininghaus et al., 2013; 2016; 2018) similarly might guide therapeutic strategies. Alternatively, such treatment specificity might be determined by other variables. On the psychosocial side, it might be a question of matching different forms of psychotherapy to personal styles, temperaments and preferences, or practical needs. Biologically, there may be underlying endophenotypes or mechanisms which mean a response to a particular biotherapy will be positive and these mechanisms may very well manifest pleiotropy, meaning that the clinical phenotype varies for any single disturbed biomarker or mechanism. As concluded in this book (Chapter 14), it is obvious that new transdiagnostic clinical trials and other research designs are required to determine the value of staging and these related ideas.

Conclusion

Diagnosis that works for the patient, the family, the clinician and the researcher is definitely possible but it needs to be relatively simple, though multilayered. The current approach to revisions of the existing diagnostic manuals, rooted as they are in the psychiatry of traditional tertiary care, will not reinvent diagnosis. Nor will a stale and stalled introspection on the theme of diagnosis and its discontents, or a simple recycling of quantitative nosology from a static and purely psychopathological perspective. The field needs testable new models which are parsimonious enough to work in the clinic and yet complex enough to support more personalised and sequential treatment selection. Clinical staging, a novel initiative that links the tertiary care perspective to the modern and more inclusive population-based and primary care context, may be best suited to take up the challenge of modernising the diagnosis of mental disorders from first principles. It could certainly be enhanced by quantitative nosology, network analysis and biomarkers as potent research and design tools. The most important benefit to be gained is better utility and a freer pathway to the holy grail of validity. This should moderate the ever-increasing generation (and occasional extinction) of diagnostic categories, by allowing the timing, and mode and extent of progression of illness, to anchor the diagnostic process, and forge a stronger link to treatment decisions sensitive to risk–benefit considerations and patient choice. Formal recognition of what is already tacitly accepted should follow: namely, that relative syndrome specificity is a later-stage marker of progression, severity and poorer outcome of illness, and that much is to be gained by acknowledging the need for proportional, and yet possibly pre-emptive, care in the earlier, relatively non-specific, stages of illness.

A crucial step in constructing such a novel diagnostic strategy is to operationally define the early clinical phenotypes, which require intervention in their own right, but also connote risk for later stages and more elaborated syndromes, which are likely to be multiply comorbid and more persistent, recurrent and disabling. The early clinical phenotypes may be initially truly pluripotential, or there may be early hints or warning signs, emerging symptom relationships and biosignatures suggesting particular sequences, patterns and outcomes. Treatments may also be characterised by cross-diagnostic effectiveness and preventive influence, and at the same time, have specificity for certain aspects as well. These considered conjectures require a more heuristic approach to the early course and treatment of mental disorders.

References

Ahuja, A., & McGorry, P. (2012, 23 March). Diagnostic disorder and how to help its recovery. *Australian Financial Review*.

Angell, M. (2011, 14 July). The illusions of psychiatry. *New York Review of Books*.

Borsboom, D. (2017). A network theory of mental disorders. *World Psychiatry, 16*(1), 5–13.

Boseley, S. (2012, 9 February). Psychologists fear US manual will widen mental illness diagnosis: mental disorders listed in publication that should not exist, warn UK experts. *Guardian*.

Carey, B. (2012, 19 January). New definition of autism will exclude many, study suggests. *New York Times*.

Carpenter, W. T., & van Os, J. (2011). Should attenuated psychosis syndrome be a DSM-5 diagnosis? *American Journal of Psychiatry, 168*(5), 460–463.

Caspi, A., Houts, R. M., Belsky, D. W., Goldman-Mellor, S. J., Harrington, H., Israel, S., . . . Poulton, R. (2014). The p factor: one general psychopathology factor in the structure of psychiatric disorders? *Clinical Psychological Science, 2*(2), 119–137.

Collins, F. S., & Varmus, H. (2015). A new initiative on precision medicine. *New England Journal of Medicine, 372*(9), 793–795.

Cuijpers, P. (2003). Examining the effects of prevention programs on the incidence of new cases of mental disorders: the lack of statistical power. *American Journal of Psychiatry, 160*(8), 1385–1391.

Cuthbert, B. N., & Insel, T. R. (2010). Toward new approaches to psychotic disorders: the NIMH Research Domain Criteria project. *Schizophrenia Bulletin, 36*(6), 1061–1062.

Demyttenaere, K., Bruffaerts, R., Posada-Villa, J., Gasquet, I., Kovess, V., Lepine, J. P., . . . Zaslavsky, A. M. (2004). Prevalence, severity, and unmet need for treatment of mental disorders in the World Health Organization World Mental Health Surveys. *JAMA,* **291** (21), 2581–2590.

Dominguez, M. D., Wichers, M., Lieb, R., Wittchen, H. U., & van Os, J. (2011). Evidence that onset of clinical psychosis is an outcome of progressively more persistent subclinical psychotic experiences: an 8-year cohort study. *Schizophrenia Bulletin,* 37(1), 84–93.

Eaton, W. W., Badawi, M., & Melton, B. (1995). Prodromes and precursors: epidemiologic data for primary prevention of disorders with slow onset. *American Journal of Psychiatry,* **152**(7), 967–972.

Frances, A. (2010, 14 August). Good grief. *New York Times.*

Frances, A. (2013). *Saving normal: an insider's revolt against out-of-control psychiatric diagnosis, DSM-5, big pharma, and the medicalization of ordinary life.* New York: William Morrow.

Fusar-Poli, P., & Yung, A. R. (2012). Should attenuated psychosis syndrome be included in DSM-5? *Lancet,* **379**(9816), 591–592.

Greenberg, G. (2013). *The book of woe: the DSM and the unmaking of psychiatry.* New York: Blue Rider Press.

Jablensky, A. (2012). Prototypes, syndromes and dimensions of psychopathology: an open agenda for research. *World Psychiatry,* **11**(1), 22–23.

Jablensky, A. (2016). Psychiatric classifications: validity and utility. *World Psychiatry,* **15**(1), 26–31.

Judd, L. L., Schettler, P. J., & Akiskal, H. S. (2002). The prevalence, clinical relevance, and public health significance of subthreshold depressions. *Psychiatric Clinics of North America,* **25**(4), 685–698.

Kaymaz, N., Drukker, M., Lieb, R., Wittchen, H. U., Werbeloff, N., Weiser, M., . . . van Os, J. (2012). Do subthreshold psychotic experiences predict clinical outcomes in unselected non-help-seeking population-based samples? A systematic review and meta-analysis, enriched with new results. *Psychological Medicine,* **42**(11), 2239–2253.

Kendell, R. E. (1975a). *The role of diagnosis in psychiatry.* Oxford: Blackwell.

Kendell, R. E. (1975b). The concept of disease and its implications for psychiatry. *British Journal of Psychiatry,* **127**, 305–315.

Kendell, R. E., & Jablensky, A. (2003). Distinguishing between the validity and utility of psychiatric diagnoses. *American Journal of Psychiatry,* **160**(1), 4–12.

Kendler, K. S. (2016). The nature of psychiatric disorders. *World Psychiatry,* **15**(1), 5–12.

Kendler, K. S., Zachar, P., & Craver, C. (2011). What kinds of things are psychiatric disorders? *Psychological Medicine,* **41**(6), 1143–1150.

Kotov, R., Krueger, R. F., & Watson, D. (2018). A paradigm shift in psychiatric classification: the Hierarchical Taxonomy Of Psychopathology (HiTOP). *World Psychiatry,* **17**(1), 24–25.

Linscott, R. J., & van Os, J. (2013). An updated and conservative systematic review and meta-analysis of epidemiological evidence on psychotic experiences in children and adults: on the pathway from proneness to persistence to dimensional expression across mental disorders. *Psychological Medicine,* **43** (6), 1133–1149.

McGorry, P. D. (2013). The next stage for diagnosis: validity through utility. *World Psychiatry,* **12**(3), 213–215.

McGorry, P. D., Hartmann, J. A., Spooner, R., & Nelson, B. (2018). Beyond the 'at risk mental state' concept: transitioning to transdiagnostic psychiatry. *World Psychiatry,* **17**(2), 133–142.

McGorry, P. D., Hickie, I. B., Yung, A. R., Pantelis, C., & Jackson, H. J. (2006). Clinical staging of psychiatric disorders: a heuristic framework for choosing earlier, safe and more effective interventions. *Australian and New Zealand Journal of Psychiatry,* **40**(8), 616–622.

McGorry, P. D., Nelson, B., Goldstone, S., & Yung, A. R. (2010). Clinical staging: a heuristic and practical strategy for new research and better health and social outcomes for psychotic and related mood disorders. *Canadian Journal of Psychiatry,* **55** (8), 486–497.

McGorry, P. D., Purcell, R., Goldstone, S., & Amminger, G. P. (2011). Age of onset and timing of treatment for mental and substance use disorders: implications for preventive intervention strategies and models of care. *Current Opinion in Psychiatry, 24*(4), 301–306.

McGorry, P. D., Purcell, R., Hickie, I. B., Yung, A. R., Pantelis, C., & Jackson, H. J. (2007). Clinical staging: a heuristic model for psychiatry and youth mental health. *Medical Journal of Australia, 187*(7 Suppl.), S40–S42.

Moffitt, P. (2016). *My way* (2nd ed.). Newcastle, NSW: Principal Print.

National Research Council. (2011). *Toward precision medicine: building a knowledge network for biomedical research and a new taxonomy of disease*. Washington, DC: National Academies Press.

Paus, T., Keshavan, M., & Giedd, J. N. (2008). Why do many psychiatric disorders emerge during adolescence? *Nature Reviews Neuroscience, 9*(12), 947–957.

Reininghaus, U., Böhnke, J. R., Chavez-Baldini, U., Gibbons, R., Ivleva, E., Clementz, B. A., . . . Tamminga, C. A. (2018). Transdiagnostic dimensions of psychosis in the Bipolar-Schizophrenia Network on Intermediate Phenotypes (B-SNIP). *World Psychiatry, 18*(1), 67–76.

Reininghaus, U., Böhnke, J. R., Hosang, G., Farmer, A., Burns, T., McGuffin, P., & Bentall, R. P. (2016). Evaluation of the validity and utility of a transdiagnostic psychosis dimension encompassing schizophrenia and bipolar disorder. *British Journal of Psychiatry, 209*(2), 107–113.

Reininghaus, U., Priebe, S., & Bentall, R. P. (2013). Testing the psychopathology of psychosis: evidence for a general psychosis dimension. *Schizophrenia Bulletin, 39*(4), 884–895.

Rutledge, R., & Osler, T. (1998). The ICD-9-based illness severity score: a new model that outperforms both DRG and APR-DRG as predictors of survival and resource utilization. *Journal of Trauma, 45*(4), 791–799.

Stephan, K. E., Bach, D. R., Fletcher, P. C., Flint, J., Frank, M. J., Friston, K. J., . . . Breakspear, M. (2016a). Charting the landscape of priority problems in psychiatry, part 1: classification and diagnosis. *Lancet Psychiatry, 3*(1), 77–83.

Stephan, K. E., Binder, E. B., Breakspear, M., Dayan, P., Johnstone, E. C., Meyer-Lindenberg, A., . . . Friston, K. J. (2016b). Charting the landscape of priority problems in psychiatry, part 2: pathogenesis and aetiology. *Lancet Psychiatry, 3*(1), 84–90.

Trusheim, M. R., Berndt, E. R., & Douglas, F. L. (2007). Stratified medicine: strategic and economic implications of combining drugs and clinical biomarkers. *Nature Reviews Drug Discovery, 6*(4), 287–293.

van Os, J., & Linscott, R. J. (2012). Introduction: the extended psychosis phenotype – relationship with schizophrenia and with ultrahigh risk status for psychosis. *Schizophrenia Bulletin, 38*(2), 227–230.

Wang, P. S., Demler, O., & Kessler, R. C. (2002). Adequacy of treatment for serious mental illness in the United States. *American Journal of Public Health, 92*(1), 92–98.

Woods, S. W., Walsh, B. C., Saksa, J. R., & McGlashan, T. H. (2010). The case for including Attenuated Psychotic Symptoms Syndrome in DSM-5 as a psychosis risk syndrome. *Schizophrenia Research, 123*(2–3), 199–207.

Yung, A. R., & McGorry, P. D. (1996). The initial prodrome in psychosis: descriptive and qualitative aspects. *Australian and New Zealand Journal of Psychiatry, 30*(5), 587–599.

Yung, A. R., Phillips, L. J., McGorry, P. D., McFarlane, C. A., Francey, S., Harrigan, S., . . . Jackson, H. J. (1998). Prediction of psychosis: a step towards indicated prevention of schizophrenia. *British Journal of Psychiatry, 172*(33), 14–20.

Chapter

2

Clinical Staging and Its Potential to Enhance Mental Health Care

Cristina Mei, Patrick D. McGorry and Ian B. Hickie

Introduction

Over the last two decades, application of the clinical staging model in mental health has been advanced to improve diagnosis, intervention, prediction of illness trajectory and, ultimately, outcomes. While clinical diagnosis remains the cornerstone for selecting appropriately targeted interventions and predicting long-term outcomes, diagnosis in mental health care has historically been very limited in its focus, utilising concepts largely based on characteristics of chronic or persistent phases of illness. Critically, this can lead to inappropriate treatment choices for individuals with earlier-stage presentations who do not meet full diagnostic criteria or sufficient severity (e.g. use of medications when simpler psychological or behavioural options are sufficient) (McGorry, 2013). The clinical staging model offers a substantive advance for mental health care as it goes beyond traditional fixed categories to incorporate a stepwise continuum to guide much more appropriate treatment planning and prognosis. In this chapter, an overview of this advanced type of clinical staging is provided.

Clinical Staging: An Overview

Clinical staging has wide application in other areas of medicine (e.g. cancer, arthritis and diabetes) as it promotes appropriate matching of stage of illness with treatment options. In essence, the model assumes that various 'clinical' stages of an illness lie along a spectrum of illness trajectory, with progressive movement of a variable proportion of cases (not all) over time to poorer functional outcomes. At any clinical presentation, a person's current state is mapped onto that spectrum to guide treatment selection and predict potential pathways of illness progression or remission. A fundamental goal is to prioritise earlier intervention with the aim of slowing or arresting movement along that continuum and promoting remission. Within oncology, clinical staging has been used to delineate the stage or progression of the lesion (buttressed by objective markers, e.g. biopsy, biomarker and imaging studies) and to determine the best course of management to maximise survival and quality of life. Here, it has long proved to be an important clinical development prior to the more recent discovery of a small number of highly personalised or very specific (genetically based) tumour markers. In various forms of arthritis, clinical staging has emphasised the need to greatly reduce the severity and duration of inflammation early in the course of illness, not simply to reduce pain, but also to protect the underlying joints from further destruction.

As detailed in Chapter 1, clinical staging is fundamentally a more refined form of diagnosis, given its emphasis on detailed understanding of the consequences of illness progression rather than relying simply on static diagnostic descriptors. The model differentiates early clinical presentations from those seen during later or chronic phases of the illness. This then enables interventions to be targeted towards the specific stage of the illness rather than it being tailored to an overarching diagnostic category (e.g. breast cancer) that does not consider symptom severity or the potential evolution of the illness. Thus, individuals at an early illness stage may receive a different management approach from someone at a more advanced stage, with the underlying premise that interventions delivered earlier during the illness course are more successful, cost-effective and safer than those implemented at later stages (McGorry et al., 2006).

Clinical Staging in Mental Health Care

Limitations of Current Diagnostic Systems

Clinical staging is recognised increasingly as a promising framework to realise the goal of personalised care and predictive tools in mental health (Insel, 2007). Traditionally, clinical management for mental disorders has been hampered by the reliance on diagnostic systems that list cross-sectional features (rather than longitudinal syndromal trajectories) typically reported by individuals who have well-established and often long-standing disorders (McGorry et al., 2007). Consequently, these lists contain an admixture of features that have developed both early and late in the course of these conditions. The main virtue and purpose of these operationalised systems when they were developed was to remove the serious lack of reliability of psychiatric diagnosis which meant that the same concepts were variably applied in different centres and parts of the world. In research studies, the objective of consistency and reliability could be achieved. However, in routine clinical practice, reliability remained poor (Regier et al., 2013), and their validity and clinical utility remains poorly established (Kendell & Jablensky, 2003). Consequently, their fundamental clinical purpose, namely supporting the capacity to select appropriate and efficacious interventions for individuals, remains under constant challenge (Greenberg, 2013).

This widespread and publicly promoted critique of contemporary clinical practice is most acute in the arena of early intervention. By their nature, new early-intervention strategies for the major anxiety, mood and psychotic disorders have at their heart a need to recognise the importance of subthreshold, mixed, comorbid and frequently changing clinical presentations in young people. While often 'indeterminate' from a classical 'single' or 'discrete disorder' perspective, these syndromes are already associated with significant functional impairment, risk of self-harm or suicidal thoughts and behaviours, comorbid substance misuse and high risk for physical ill-health (Rickwood et al., 2014; 2015; Scott, E. M. et al., 2012a; 2012b). Most importantly, a significant sub-proportion already manifest or are at risk, short and longer term, of more significant functional impairment (Cross et al., 2014).

Our current diagnostic systems embed duration criteria and longitudinal perspectives in inconsistent and, at times, dysfunctional ways. They fail to recognise the ebbs and flows of both symptom sets and functional impairment associated with the common mental disorders, and to capture the tendency for subgroups to recur, persist or progress to more severe symptom sets and related functional impairment. Clinical features of the early phases of illness are not distinguished from those that develop later – either as a consequence of underlying illness progression, resulting psychological or social impairment, secondary comorbidity or adverse consequences of active treatment. Continuing and precise demarcation of symptom sets by phases of illness course is crucial, given that individuals at different stages of mental disorders show diverse responses to treatment (i.e. those at earlier stages often show more responsive and favourable outcomes than individuals at later illness stages).

Clinically, the staging concept proposes the potential value of stage-specific interventions, emphasising not only differential needs in terms of acute treatment efficacy, but also the need to employ differential secondary prevention and clinical versus psychosocial recovery strategies at different phases of illness (Berk et al., 2011; Hegelstad et al., 2012; Kessler & Price, 1993; Scott et al., 2006). The field is most complex with regard to which interventions are safest and most effective for young people who present for care with subthreshold symptoms but accompanying functional impairment and risk of self-harm (Cross et al., 2014). Simplistic notions, often derived from the arbitrary application of current thresholds for assigning a specific diagnosis, propose that these young people have no need for care and that there is no need to develop relevant health service systems to meet their needs. This has been oddly justified by the fact that some of these features, such as deliberate self-harm, subside after a considerable period of time, assuming the patient survives; however, the functional impacts persist for much longer, even for decades (Patton et al., 2014). However, there remains a major lack of relevant longitudinal cohort or clinical intervention studies to guide best clinical practice, or health service developments, to best meet these needs.

Another major failing of current diagnostic systems based on phenomena experienced by those with late-stage or chronic forms of mental disorder is that they have not substantially facilitated research into the mechanisms, or objective markers, underpinning the longitudinal course of common mental disorders (McGorry & van Os, 2013). Highly personalised and phase-dependent treatment selection will ultimately depend on our capacity to utilise such objective markers, as well as psychosocial experiences, such as bullying and abuse, in clinical practice.

Application of Clinical Staging to Mental Health Care

Clinical staging offers a practical yet scientific way forward to bridge current gaps in linking common diagnostic models to more personalised and effective intervention, prognosis, neurobiological markers and psychosocial outcomes (Hickie et al., 2013a; McGorry et al., 2007). Inherently, clinical staging is applicable to disorders whose clinical phenotypes are known to change in relation to course of illness, with specific relevance to conditions that have at least a moderate propensity (though not inevitable) to progress to more severe or impairing clinical conditions. In oncology, the progression from isolated or undetected tumours to widespread disease is common. In inflammatory arthritis, the progression from joint inflammation to progressive joint destruction is characteristic.

Our working assumption is that similar concepts are relevant for anxiety, mood, personality, eating, substance use and psychotic disorders. The last three decades of epidemiological research in mental health have emphasised the extent to which some childhood risk states are followed by adolescent-onset disorders and the extent to which rather non-specific adolescent-onset disorders (commonly underpinned by shared anxiety/depressive phenomena) progress (at least in subpopulations) to adult-type major mood (depressive and bipolar) or psychotic disorders (Kim-Cohen et al., 2003; Merikangas et al., 2010; Patton et al., 2014). Adaptation of clinical staging, limited to affective disorders, was proposed in the early 1990s by Fava and Kellner (1993), who argued that the model was superior to widely used diagnostic criteria due to its focus on characterising mental illness according to its severity, progression and features. Drawing largely on the experience from the early psychosis field from the early 1990s, the last decade has seen extensive development and refinement of the model so that it can be more widely used (i.e. transdiagnostically) in individuals who develop psychotic and major affective syndromes and well beyond (Hickie et al., 2013b; McGorry et al., 2006; 2010; 2014). This new phase of development of clinical staging is especially pertinent to adolescent and young adult populations, where the onset of adult-type mental disorders is most likely to occur (Kessler et al., 2005).

Consequent to this new phase of clinical staging studies, the concept has been recognised as also being potentially suitable for a very wide range of mental disorders, including schizophrenia, anxiety, affective, eating, personality and substance misuse (McGorry et al., 2007). Typically, current diagnostic approaches still operate within narrow 'disorder-specific' boundaries, which cannot accommodate the 'comorbidity' and overlap that is the everyday reality for clinicians. That is, they employ a retrospective view, working backwards from cohorts of individuals who have developed 'full-threshold' or 'dominant' disorders (e.g. bipolar disorder, schizophrenia, anorexia nervosa) to characterise the earliest clinical phase.

By contrast, the specific clinical staging model developed by McGorry, Hickie and colleagues includes a collection of syndromes within a single 'transdiagnostic' model (specifying one non-clinical and four relevant clinical stages, and linked substages) (Figure 2.1; Hickie et al., 2013a; McGorry et al., 2006). Symptom specificity, severity, persistence and disability are used to define advancing stages of mental disorder. That is, early clinical stages are characterised by phenotypes that are milder in symptom severity,

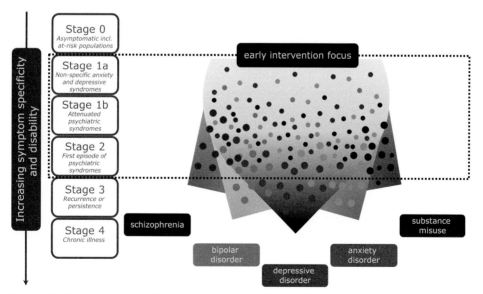

Figure 2.1 Clinical staging model depicting the progression of mental illness whereby early clinical phenotypes are broad and non-specific, with clearer syndromes emerging in more advanced stages, coinciding with increased disability. Reprinted from *The Lancet*, Vol. 381, McGorry, P. & van Os, J., Redeeming diagnosis in psychiatry: timing versus specificity, 343–345, Copyright 2013, with permission from Elsevier. *A black and white version of this figure will appear in some formats. For the colour version, please refer to the plate section.*

lack specific or fully formed syndromal features (e.g. the full manic or psychotic syndrome) and are associated with less impairment, while later stages are characterised by more severe symptom sets, more specific features, functional impairment, greater degrees of stable comorbidity or clear evidence of syndromal stability, persistence or recurrence (Cross et al., 2014; Hickie et al., 2013a).

The goal for the model is to progress from simple clinical staging to develop an evidence-based clinicopathological framework, whereby each syndromal stage (described in the following section) is complemented by comprehensive psychological, neurobiological and clinical phenotyping. This will then form the substantive basis for highly personalised and stage-specific intervention selection, secondary prevention, recovery-oriented practice and prediction of illness trajectory (Table 2.1; Hickie et al., 2013a; McGorry et al., 2006).

While clinical staging models do assume that at least some substantive subgroups of individuals are at high risk of progression of illness, it conversely acknowledges the inherent heterogeneity of illness course within mental health populations. From its outset, this model has clearly stated that it does not assume that all young people who present for care will progress to later stages (Hickie et al., 2013a). A central function of any clinical model is, first, to ameliorate the immediate impacts and short-term risks that are apparent at illness onset or initial presentation for care. The second inherent function is then to reduce the risk of progression to later stages, greater impairment, or secondary comorbidity through the implementation of early effective treatments targeting those specific neurobiological or psychosocial factors that are evident in early illness phases (McGorry et al., 2014). The clear goals of targeted and successful early management are, therefore, both to reduce current symptoms and impairment and also to alter illness trajectories (e.g. prevention of full-threshold disorders in those who present with subthreshold syndromes), which may result in full remission (McGorry et al., 2007). Positive treatment outcomes (e.g. reduction in symptoms, reduced disability, reduced risk of suicidal thoughts or behaviours) are attainable at any stage, although it is recognised that the likelihood of full remission or complete recovery reduces with advancing illness stage (McGorry et al., 2014). In comparison, stepped care is essentially reactive and tackles the more modest goal of reducing symptoms and impairment at any given stage (National Mental Health Commission, 2014). Pre-emptive or staged care (implied by the adoption of a clinical staging model) is more ambitious and seeks to reduce the risk of progression to more advanced stages of severity and impairment (see Chapter 13 for further discussion).

Stages of the Model

This transdiagnostic model clearly delineates various phases across the spectrum from being asymptomatic but at-risk, through various early, but not necessarily progressive, phases of experiencing symptoms and seeking health care, to later persistent, recurrent of enduring syndromes, as summarised below (Hickie et al., 2013a; McGorry et al., 2006). Here, arbitrary cut-points are imposed on dimensional phenomena for the purpose of seeking better clinical utility for treatment decisions and for clearer understanding of the neurobiology. While consistent with universal prevention approaches (Stage 0), and selective prevention (high-risk groups such as children of parents with serious mental illness; also Stage 0), the clinical staging model really comes into its own when an early clinical phenotype has emerged and some level of distress and/or impairment is present. It extends the clinical mandate to reach forward in time from late-stage and severe forms of mental

Table 2.1 Clinical staging model for psychiatric disorders

Stage	Definition and presentation	Target populations for recruitment	Potential interventions[a]	Indicative biological and endophenotypic markers
Stage 0 *Asymptomatic including at-risk populations*	Increased risk of psychiatric symptoms; no current symptoms Not seeking health care	• First-degree young relatives (12–25 years) of probands	• Enhanced mental health literacy • Family and drug education • Brief cognitive skills training	• Trait marker candidates and endophenotypes (e.g. smooth pursuit eye movements, P50, niacin sensitivity, mismatch negativity, olfactory deficits)
Stage 1a *Non-specific anxiety and depressive syndromes*	Non-specific, mild to moderate symptoms; mild functional change or decline; normal cognitive profile (or potential developmental deficit) GAF/SOFAS > 70–100 QIDS 0–11	• Screening of youth populations • Referral by primary care physician, school counsellor, family or self	• Formal mental health literacy • Supportive counselling, problem-solving • Family psychoeducation • Exercise • Substance misuse reduction	• Normal brain cortical volumes or potential developmental abnormalities • Reduced total sleep time or phase delays
Stage 1b *Attenuated psychiatric syndromes*	Ultra-high risk: moderate but subthreshold symptoms; moderate neurocognitive changes (attention, learning, memory, executive functioning); moderate to severe functional decline GAF/SOFAS 60–70 QIDS 11–20 YMRS >9	• Referral by educational or welfare agencies, primary care physician, ED, drug/alcohol services, family or self	• Family psychoeducation • Cognitive behavioural therapy • Cognitive remediation and social cognition interventions • Psycho and neuroprotective interventions (e.g. cognitive dissonance) • Neuroprotective agents • Substance misuse reduction • Internet interventions	• Mild grey matter loss (prefrontal cortex, temporal lobe, cerebellum or mesencephalon) • Increased grey matter (frontal and ventral striatal areas) • Prolonged sleep times, phase delay • Impaired olfactory identification • Frontal MMN disturbance; reduced parietal P3 • Pro-inflammatory cytokine elevation

17

Table 2.1 (cont.)

Stage	Definition and presentation	Target populations for recruitment	Potential interventions[a]	Indicative biological and endophenotypic markers
Stage 2 *First episode of psychiatric syndromes*	First episode of full-threshold disorder; significant neurocognitive changes (learning, processing speed, executive functioning); major functional impacts GAF/SOFAS 40–60 QIDS >20 YMRS >15	• Referral by primary care physician, ED, welfare or specialist care agencies, drug/alcohol services, family or self	• Family-based interventions, psychoeducation • Cognitive behavioural therapy • Substance misuse reduction • Guided self-care • Atypical antipsychotics • Antidepressants or mood stabilisers • Lithium • Vocational rehabilitation	• Continue with markers of illness state, trait and progression • Significant grey matter loss (reduced hippocampal, temporal and dorsal prefrontal cortex volume) • Phase delay in circadian rhythm; daytime fatigue and/or sleepiness • Impaired olfactory identification • Frontal MMN impairment; reduced parietal P3 • HPA axis dysfunction: hypercortisolaemia and reduced responsiveness to feedback • Pro-inflammatory cytokine elevation, reduced markers of cell-mediated immunity

Stage	Clinical features	Service	Treatment	Markers
Stage 3 *Recurrence or persistence of psychiatric syndromes*	Incomplete remission from first episode of care (12 months after entry to care and at least 3 months of treatment); recurrence of discrete disorder after period of recovery; deterioration in neuropsychological and functional abilities; moderate to severe cognitive deficits (including social cognition) GAF/SOFAS <40	• Primary and specialist care services	• As per Stage 2, with emphasis on: – medical and psychosocial strategies to achieve remission – relapse prevention and strategies for warning signs – long-term stabilisation	• Continue with markers of illness state, trait and progression • Reduced hippocampal volume • Frontal and temporal MMN impairment; reduced frontal and parietal P3
Stage 4 *Chronic illness*	Severe, persistent or unremitting illness; severe neuropsychological deterioration; marked decline in functioning GAF/SOFAS <30	• Specialised care services	• As per Stage 3, with emphasis on clozapine, other tertiary treatments, social participation, quality of life, vocational rehabilitation	• Continue with markers of illness state, trait and progression • Reduced hippocampal volume, enlarged ventricles • Frontal and temporal MMN impairment; reduced and delayed frontal and parietal P3 • Neuroadaptation: altered reward habit learning

ED: emergency department; GAF: global assessment of functioning; HPA: hypothalamic–pituitary–adrenal; MMN: mismatch negativity; SOFAS: Social and Occupational Functioning Assessment Scale; QIDS: Quick Inventory of Depressive Symptomatology; YMRS: Youth Mania Rating Scale.

[a] Although most interventions can be applied across traditional mental disorder diagnoses, some drug treatments may be limited to specific populations (e.g. clozapine for schizophrenia).

Adapted from: McGorry, P. D., Hickie, I. B., Yung, A. R., Pantelis, C., & Jackson, H. J. Clinical staging of psychiatric disorders: a heuristic framework for choosing earlier, safer and more effective interventions, *Australian and New Zealand Journal of Psychiatry* Vol. 40, pp. 616–622. Copyright © 2006 (The Royal Australian and New Zealand College of Psychiatrists). Reprinted by permission of SAGE Publications.
Other sources: Hickie et al., 2013a; Treasure et al., 2015.

ill-health. Most traditional, poorly designed and resourced services for young people only provide care to those with well-established disorders, and largely exclude those with certain diagnostic labels (e.g. borderline personality disorder), non-specific symptom sets (e.g. subthreshold anxiety and depression), certain patterns of comorbidity (e.g. concurrent alcohol or substance misuse) or coexisting service patterns (e.g. engagement with criminal justice systems). That is, those services with a more restricted focus may only be operating with a narrow part of the whole spectrum (e.g. largely being focused on the later Stages 3 and 4).

Clinical staging in mental health is applicable to *all* health care presentations. It is not limited to those with early presentations of disorders (though that is where the maximum preventive value is focused). Unfortunately, many young people (as in oncology and other inflammatory disorders) present for the first time to our service environments at the final stage (Stage 4: chronic illness) or with a full-threshold syndrome and substantive impairment following an earlier course of desultory or otherwise unsuccessful treatment (Stage 3) (McGorry et al., 2006). Another important feature of traditional systems when making clinical decisions regarding staging and access to care is, when faced with uncertainty, to stage 'down' not 'up'. This means that many young people who already meet DSM or ICD criteria for various anxiety, mood or psychotic syndromes are incorrectly classified as Stage 1b rather than Stage 2 and are excluded from the health system. Enhanced primary care models, notably headspace (Rickwood et al., 2014), seek to correct this mistake (see Chapter 13 for further discussion).

Another key assumption of clinical staging models is that once a person has reached a certain stage of illness (very specifically in our model, Stage 2), one cannot move backwards. By analogy, once you have had a diagnosis of early breast cancer and been treated you may well achieve full remission and have no further progression or recurrence – *but* you never return to that population group who was at risk but had never had a specific clinical diagnosis or episode of clinical care. At all stages, full remission, functional recovery and prevention of recurrence remain key goals. However, it is our working assumption that it is very likely that quite different strategies will be required at each different major stage (1 vs 2 vs 3+) to achieve these goals.

Stage 0: Asymptomatic Including At-Risk Populations

Individuals who are asymptomatic and are not presenting for health care but are part of a clearly defined at-risk group can be classified at the first stage of the model (e.g. first-degree adolescent siblings of individuals with bipolar disorder or schizophrenia, children with neurodevelopmental disorders, low birthweight or gestation, children or adolescents exposed to trauma, adolescent-onset substance misuse). That is, this stage is designed for cohort studies that seek to recruit populations considered at risk for adolescent-onset psychotic or severe mood disorders (Hickie et al., 2013a; McGorry et al., 2014). This stage is *not* used in clinical cohort studies, since by definition those who present (or would be eligible) for health care, independent of the presence of other risk factors, are already at least at clinical Stage 1a. Interventions for those in these at-risk cohort studies are targeted towards modifying risk factors (e.g. cessation of illicit drug use) or active use of other strategies (e.g. sleep–wake cycle stabilisation, cognitive behavioural skills) designed to prevent the onset of anxiety, mood, psychotic or other mental disorders.

Stage 1: Non-specific Syndromes with Variable Degrees of Impairment

Stage 1 includes those early phases of illness associated with health care seeking. In this phase, clinical features are typically a mix of anxiety and depressive symptoms, with the episodic presence of hypomanic-like, psychotic-like experiences or other 'warning signs' of more specific syndromes. The working assumption for Stage 1 disorders is that the syndromes identified at this point along the illness spectrum have not yet reached a stage of development that is at very high probability or inevitability of progression to more severe or persistent disorders, although the phenotype may include suicide ideation (Scott et al., 2012b) and coping mechanisms such as self-harm or substance use. In many of the clinical, longitudinal and neurobiological studies we have conducted, we have evaluated the validity of an arbitrary cut-point between Stage 1 (essentially early presentations that are assumed to be non-progressive) and Stage 2 disorders (essentially severe, impairing and typically recurring or persistent disorders, although progression to later stages is not inevitable). For Stage 1 disorders, therefore, treatment options emphasise the need to relieve distressing symptoms, reduce risk of self-harm or suicidal behaviours and prevent the later development of comorbidity (both substance misuse and physical ill-health) or progression to Stage 2 disorders.

For clinical purposes, we have divided Stage 1 of the model into two sections. This is based on the likelihood that the earliest stage (1a) with minimal impairment is most likely to benefit from basic psychological and social interventions with a relatively low need to employ specific medical strategies, whereas the next stage (1b), although assumed to be not necessarily progressive either, is more frequently associated with functional impairment and more severe mood disturbance, comorbidity or other associated warning signs and symptoms that require more specific and prolonged psychological and medical/drug interventions. Consequently, in our various clinical intervention and neurobiological studies we have also tested the validity of this distinction (Cross et al., 2016; Hickie et al., 2013a; Scott et al., 2016).

The distinction between Stage 1 and Stage 2 disorders does not equate with the thresholds used by other international classification systems (e.g. DSM-4 or -5, ICD-10) to differentiate subthreshold from threshold disorders. That is, many cases that we classify as Stage 1a may actually meet other international criteria for specific anxiety or neurodevelopmental disorders. Additionally, most Stage 1b disorders will meet international criteria for anxiety or major depressive disorders. Further, at least some of these people will meet emerging operational criteria for bipolar mood or psychotic spectrum disorders.

Stage 1a: Non-specific Anxiety and Depressive Syndromes, Presenting for Care

By definition, therefore, Stage 1a consists of help-seeking individuals, typically adolescents or young adults, who present with non-specific symptoms (e.g. admixtures of anxiety and depression), without significant or persisting impacts on social, educational or occupational performance and without major comorbidities. Neuropsychological deficits may be present, typically as a consequence of earlier neurodevelopmental factors or, if due to the current disorder, are typically only mild in severity.

Stage 1b: Attenuated Psychiatric and Comorbid Syndromes

By definition, individuals at Stage 1b show significantly increased symptom severity, specificity, comorbidity and functional impairment compared to those at Stage 1a (Hickie et al., 2013a). At Stage 1b, most young people present with attenuated major mood or psychotic-like syndromes with increased specificity and severity of anxiety, depressive, hypomanic, psychotic or mixed (e.g. anxiety and depression) symptoms. Other treatment-relevant subthreshold clinical features, such as disordered eating, body image disturbance, substance misuse and subthreshold borderline features may be present as 'warning signs' of full-threshold phenotypes beyond mood and psychotic disorders. Individuals may also meet the criteria for some broad DSM or ICD diagnoses which define full-threshold in a liberal way. However, in our system they have not yet exhibited the more severe and persistent features consistent with key treatment decisions, such as the commencement of potent psychotropic medications (Hickie et al., 2013a). The attenuated Stage 1b syndromes are typically associated with moderate to severe functional impairment, accumulating comorbidity and intermediate, even if episodic rather than pre-existing or persistent, neuropsychological deficits (Hamilton et al., 2011; Hermens et al., 2013; Hickie et al., 2013a).

Stage 2: Specific Psychiatric or Comorbid Syndromes, First Clinical Presentation

By definition, Stage 2 signifies that an individual has presented for care above our threshold for a fully developed syndrome characterised by severe and specific major mood, psychotic or comorbid features and major functional impairment. While the threshold for this distinction has so far been defined according to when a substantial change in treatment approach is currently warranted (e.g. the commencement of antipsychotic medication for psychosis or antidepressant medication for depression), it is also hypothesised that the individual may have crossed a key neurobiological threshold and is, consequently, at very high risk of persistence or recurrence of that disorder (Hickie et al., 2013a). That is, individuals present with clear and sustained moderate to severe features of psychotic, manic or depressive, borderline or eating disorders. Comorbidity of such syndromes is common so that clinical presentations still do not necessarily fit with conventional diagnostic criteria for stand-alone anxiety, depressive, manic or psychotic syndromes. The thresholds for different comorbid dimensions may not align perfectly with each other in the same patient. At this point along the illness spectrum or trajectory, individuals typically present with significant neuropsychological impairment (based on pre-existing risk or persisting dysfunction).

Hence, for Stage 2, the notion of 'transitions' from an early stage to one that has a need for more intensive and specific treatment and has a greater propensity to persist is a key concept, although persistence is by no means inevitable. In our studies, such transitions are often seen in terms of progression from (a) Stage 1b major depressive disorders to severe and persisting depressive (often psychotic-like) disorders; (b) Stage 1b major depressive disorders, or brief comorbid hypomanic episodes, to episodic manic episodes or other bipolar phenotypes; (c) Stage 1b depressive or attenuated psychotic or hypomanic syndromes to 'first-episode' affective or non-affective psychosis; (d) severe but brief anxiety, mood or psychotic syndromes that persist and are then associated with marked deterioration in social function or accumulating comorbidity; (e) progression from Stage 1b depressive and subthreshold borderline traits to full-threshold borderline syndrome, complicated often by substance misuse, as are many of the other transitions to Stage 2; or (f) transition from Stage 1b depressive and subthreshold eating disorder to fully fledged anorexia nervosa or other similar phenotype.

The determination of Stage 2 disorders, therefore, typically occurs in one of two ways: (1) by determination at first clinical presentation and on the basis of current clinical phenotype and past (treated or untreated) history; or (2) following longitudinal assessment where progression from Stage 1 (a or b) to Stage 2 has been formally documented by the same clinical service. In the latter situation, the young person may well have received treatment during the Stage 1 period. However, the pattern of response to treatment does *not* play a role in the determination of clinical stage, though the manifest need for an escalation to a more potent intervention, based on progression of the phenotype, may very well do so. That is, non-response to particular psychosocial treatments per se is not a reason to re-categorise a person from Stage 1b to Stage 2. People can remain in Stage 1b for long periods, with the key issue here being whether a change in treatment is required (e.g. when to commence antipsychotic or antidepressant medication).

Stage 3: Recurrence or Persistence of Psychiatric Syndromes

Stage 3 disorders include those individuals with clear syndromes, usually with significant functional impairment and clear (past history or longitudinal) evidence of illness progression (as demonstrated by incomplete remission, recurrence or persistence over 12 months). A very important distinction needs to be made between Stage 3 and those who are often in Stage 1b but also have persisting or recurrent difficulties. The clear distinction is that a young person can only reach Stage 3 after having clearly progressed through Stage 2 first. When there is doubt about whether the syndrome was severe enough to justify assigning Stage 2 status, even when that syndrome has persisted or recurred, then it should still be classed as Stage 1b. The difference may seem arbitrary but is a matter of intensity and the threshold reached for symptoms.

Therefore, Stage 3 is assigned to individuals who have clearly experienced Stage 2 syndromes and then experienced: (1) incomplete remission or persistence from discrete disorders at 12 months after initial service contact; (2) recurrence of discrete disorder after a period of complete remission lasting for at least three months; or (3) multiple relapses. Individuals in Stage 3 typically demonstrate a plateauing or further deterioration in functional outcomes and significant (pre-existing, concurrent or worsening) neuropsychological function.

Stage 4: Chronic Illness

Individuals with chronically debilitating and unremitting illness are classified at this final stage of the model. By definition, individuals must have passed through Stage 2, have received relevant services for at least two years and have a persistent illness without a clear period of complete remission (lasting at least three months). It is possible to bypass Stage 3 and progress directly from Stage 2 to Stage 4. Typically individuals in Stage 4 experience severe functional and (pre-existing, concurrent or worsening) neuropsychological impairment.

Frequency of Mental Illness at Each Stage

Across select Australian headspace centres that provide early intervention mental health services to individuals aged 12–25 years, the proportion of clients assigned to each stage at presentation varies. This is likely to reflect differences in service location, collocated service partnerships and the range of clinical health and psychosocial services offered (Cross et al.,

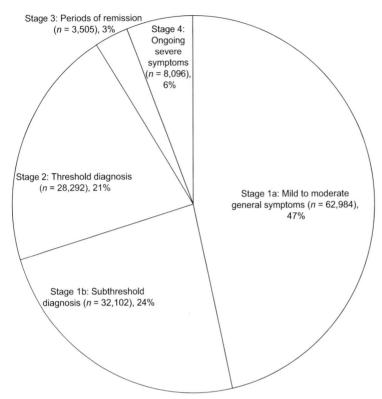

Stage 3: Periods of remission
(n = 3,505), 3%

Stage 4:
Ongoing
severe
symptoms
(n = 8,096),
6%

Stage 2: Threshold diagnosis
(n = 28,292), 21%

Stage 1a: Mild to moderate
general symptoms (n = 62,984),
47%

Stage 1b: Subthreshold
diagnosis (n = 32,102), 24%

Figure 2.2 Stage allocation of headspace clients (n = 134,979) at first presentation for mental health services between April 2013 and March 2017.

2014). For clinical services, the prevalence ranges from 24 to 40 per cent for Stage 1a and 24 to 52 per cent for Stage 1b. As these services are largely clinic-based, with a focus on early intervention, and do not provide acute or emergency care or significant outreach services, the prevalence of later stages are lower, including 9–21 per cent for Stage 2 and 7–30 per cent for Stage 3+ (Hamilton et al., 2011; Purcell et al., 2015; Scott et al., 2012a).

At a national level, large-scale pooled data from Australian headspace centres highlight key differences in the proportion of clients assigned to each stage at presentation (Figure 2.2). Of the 134,979 clients accessing mental health services over a four-year period (between April 2013 and March 2017), nearly three-quarters were classified below Stage 2, underscoring the need for adequate resources targeting these early phases. Those in Stages 2–4, while legitimately entering this portal, require but frequently do not gain access to specialised mental health care due to under-resourcing of such services. The independent evaluation of headspace confirmed that such patients do not respond as well to what is on offer in the headspace system since they require a greater level of intensity and specialisation of care (Hilferty et al., 2015). This must now be seriously addressed (McGorry, 2017).

With regard to longitudinal transition rates, a key clinical concept for predicting illness trajectories, it is estimated that 15 per cent of young people accessing mental health services progress to a later stage over a 12-month period despite access to interventions (unpublished data). One could speculate that this might well be much higher if no treatment were available, though definitive studies have not yet been carried out and will now be difficult. Stage-to-stage transition rates suggest that 11–22 per cent of patients at Stage 1a with non-specific symptoms progress to Stage 1b (attenuated syndromes); 8–19 per cent progress from Stage 1b to Stage 2 (first episode); and 22–33 per cent progress from Stage 2 to a later stage (Cross et al., 2017; Hickie et al., 2013a; unpublished data). Of note, transitioning from Stage 1b to Stage 2 is most likely to be seen within the first 12 months of initial contact with services and this may occur despite intensive clinical care (Hickie et al., 2013a). In psychosis, the first three years are the peak period of risk; however, some transitions can occur up to ten years later (Nelson et al., 2013).

While few studies have used a transdiagnostic approach to examine predictors of transition from at-risk states or attenuated syndromes (Stage 1b) to first episode (Stage 2), recent evidence has revealed three key factors predicting this progression: not in education, employment or training (NEET) status, increased negative psychological symptoms at baseline and being female (Cross et al., 2017). Further, preliminary findings suggest that progression to any later stage is predicted by a range of factors, including younger age, higher levels of psychological distress, reduced social function at service entry and greater neuropsychological impairment (unpublished data).

Reliability and Validity of the Clinical Staging Framework in Mental Health

To date, a range of clinical and early longitudinal studies, utilising a staging approach and based largely in early intervention youth services, have provided preliminary evidence regarding the model's reliability and validity. Inter-rater reliability of the proposed staging model has been investigated by examining the degree of concordance between sub-syndromal or attenuated states (i.e. Stages 1a and 1b) against more established disorders (i.e. Stages 2–4) (Hickie et al., 2013a). Ratings were made for 49 subjects (from a subset of 209 individuals aged 12 to 30 years seeking services for anxiety, depressive and/or psychotic symptoms). Stage allocation ratings were completed by the treating clinician and two consensus raters, all experienced clinical and research psychiatrists or psychologists. The level of concordance was very acceptable (kappa = 0.72, $p < 0.001$), with 90 per cent agreement between raters achieved (Hickie et al., 2013a).

With regard to validity, evidence of the model's construct validity is supported by studies demonstrating the progression of disability by later stage, as proposed by the model (Hamilton et al., 2011; Scott et al., 2012a). In an early study of self-reported disability in 330 help-seeking patients aged 12–25 years with affective and anxiety disorders who were classified clinically between Stages 1a and 3+, psychological distress, social and occupational functioning, and disability all worsened with advancing illness progression (Hamilton et al., 2011). Notably, individuals at Stage 2 reported significantly higher levels of psychological distress and disability than those at Stages 1a and 1b (Hamilton et al., 2011). In the next large Sydney-based cohort of 1260 young people (12–25 years) with diagnoses ranging across anxiety, depression, bipolar and psychosis, levels of psychological distress, reduced functioning and disability were again higher for individuals at later stages of illness (Scott et al., 2012a).

In an independent sample ($n = 802$) with anxiety, depressive and psychotic symptoms recruited subsequently for a longitudinal study, illness severity and functioning (measured by the Social and Occupational Functioning Assessment Scale; SOFAS) significantly decreased stepwise across Stages 1a, 1b and 2+ (Purcell et al., 2015). This stepwise trend was not observed in relation to psychological distress, where Stage 1b and Stage 2 states were comparable. Significant differences were, however, observed between Stages 1a and 1b, and Stages 1a and 2 (Purcell et al., 2015). Analysis of large-scale data across headspace centres (n = 133,464) also reveals a significant association between clinical Stages 1–4 and SOFAS ratings ($p < 0.001$), albeit a small effect size (0.11). Post-hoc testing revealed that SOFAS mean scores significantly differed across all stages.

Increasingly, we are focusing on longitudinal studies of those receiving care – linking initial clinical stage not only with clinical course (with the focus on 'clinical transitions') but also on functional outcomes. Preliminary analyses of Sydney-based data indicate the extent to which those entering care at earlier stages not only have better functioning initially but run more benign courses over both short and longer time frames (Cross et al., 2016; see Chapter 5 for further details). The resolution of the relative impact of prior functional deficits (i.e. neurodevelopmentally driven deficits prior to the adolescent onset of anxious, depressive, manic, psychotic or other symptoms), other comorbidities (notably alcohol and other substance misuse) and illness-driven deficits is a major feature of this ongoing prospective work. Such knowledge is critical to the evaluation of the likely impacts of stage-specific and early intervention strategies. The clinical staging model shows promising potential to strengthen service provision, with youth mental health clinicians recognising its clinical utility, alongside traditional diagnostic categories, to improve service attributes (Hamilton et al., 2017).

In addition, a range of neurobiological and neuropsychological studies have also provided preliminary evidence supporting the model's validity. For example, neuroimaging and circadian studies have revealed key differences between early attenuated syndromes and later established disorders (Lagopoulos et al., 2012; Naismith et al., 2012). Stage of illness has further been linked to (1) neurocognitive deficits (e.g. poorer outcomes in psychotic syndromes relative to attenuated states); (2) enlarged pituitary gland and increased cortisol secretion (e.g. predictors of transition from at-risk to psychosis); (3) inflammation (e.g. pro- and anti-inflammatory levels differentially altered during early- and late-stage bipolar disorder); and (4) fatty acids (e.g. their potential involvement in the progression of major mood and psychotic disorders) (McGorry et al., 2014). See Section 2 of this book for further discussion on neurobiological and cognitive markers.

In summary, the majority of these clinical, longitudinal and neurobiological findings lend support to the construct validity of the clinical staging model and strongly suggest the importance of early intervention to prevent illness progression.

Transdiagnostic versus Disorder-Specific Staging Approaches

The clinical staging model thus far described recommends a transdiagnostic framework for common mental disorders. That is, it does not rest on the segregated, categorical and static approach of our common international diagnostic systems. This is consistent with ongoing debates regarding the utility of classic diagnostic models as compared with alternatives such as the NIMH-promoted 'agnostic' Research Domain Criteria (RDoC; Cuthbert & Insel, 2013). The proposed clinical staging model advocates a 'lumping' approach largely because it is most useful for providing health care to young people early in the course of their disorders, when undifferentiated clinical phenotypes for psychotic and mood disorders are the typical presentations. As illness advances over time, and as typically seen in mid-life, these disorders may progressively be split, subtyped or stratified into more conventional diagnostic categories (despite the likelihood that they are also comorbid). Whether even by that period these categories are useful remains an open question, one that could be answered from a utility perspective (McGorry et al., 2006).

While there appear to be substantial benefits to this approach (as discussed further in this chapter), it is always difficult to challenge the status quo, and there is debate regarding the utility of a universal framework as opposed to disorder-specific models (i.e. separate models for anxiety, bipolar disorder, schizophrenia, etc.). Proponents of the disorder-specific models are typically framing their research questions in relation to a specific aspect of each proposed disorder. For example, neurobiological or neuroimaging studies for bipolar disorder now utilise recruitment of pre-illness onset 'high-risk' relatives of probands with pure bipolar disorder only. These studies are predicated on the contestable assumption that it may be possible to use this methodology to identify some objective marker, so far highly elusive, that is actually specific to bipolar disorder and not shared with the other common mood or psychotic disorders. Additionally, some argue that not all common mood or psychotic disorders are amenable to a broad staging approach given their heterogeneous pattern of progression (Duffy et al., 2017). Consequently, these proponents prefer to promote more conventional single-disorder staging models (Cosci & Fava, 2013; Duffy, 2014).

We contend that the value of discrete single-disorder staging models and their critique of a transdiagnostic approach are as questionable as these diagnostic concepts themselves. The early symptoms of common mood or psychotic disorders, especially in young individuals, lack specificity, are unstable longitudinally and are typically comorbid in their patterns. In these circumstances, it would appear that a transdiagnostic approach is much more consistent with the available cross-sectional and longitudinal epidemiology (McGorry & Nelson, 2016; McGorry et al., 2008; Scott et al., 2013). Inevitably, single-disorder models will fail to include early presentations that are expressed by mixed and fluid symptomatology, overlap discrete syndromal boundaries, or do not meet criteria for an established disorder (Cross et al., 2014; Hickie et al., 2013a). Owing to the generic or non-specific phenotypes seen in earlier illness stages, interventions directed towards these early phases would not substantially differ across single-disorder models (Cross et al., 2014). This approach is also consistent with data demonstrating the shared genetic basis of mental disorders, the array of common environmental risk factors, and the extent of shared neurobiological and neuropsychological correlates (Anttila et al., 2018; Lichtenstein et al., 2009; Tsuang et al., 2004). Finally, the ubiquity of comorbidity across the late stages of all disorders also supports a transdiagnostic and 'lumping' stance.

Rather than focusing research, and perhaps more importantly population-based or individual clinical interventions, on putative unique risk factors and biomarkers associated with single disorders, the proposed transdiagnostic model allows for the incorporation of shared genetic and environmental factors that can be therapeutically targeted across a broad range of individuals (Hickie et al., 2013b). Further, we would propose that discovery-focused research that is inclusive of earlier broader phenotypes – as a consequence of the power of comparisons with 'positive' illness controls – is more likely to unravel the complex pathophysiology (meaning both shared and unique pathways) of the major mental disorders (McGorry, 2010).

Clinical and Research Implications of Clinical Staging

In the above sections, we have highlighted the premise of clinical staging and its use in modern mental health care. The model offers the field numerous potential clinical and research benefits, described below. In particular, as mental health care moves towards both pre-emptive and more precise and personalised medicine (Insel, 2007; Scott et al., 2012c), the distinct stages outlined within the model provide a framework for evaluating interventions that both prevent mental illness onset and alter its progressive course. With better characterisation of biomarkers and mechanisms linked to stage as well as syndrome, the potential for genuine personalised medicine is greatly enhanced.

Clinical Benefits

Ultimately, clinical staging aims to promote optimal health outcomes by preventing the onset and evolution of mental illness in at-risk or affected populations through early intervention (McGorry et al., 2008). Reducing progression to later stages of major mental disorders may diminish the need for ongoing treatment, potentially lessening the significant burden of mental illness at an individual, societal, health system and economic level. To achieve this intended goal and to offer a more personalised management approach, identification of key risk factors (e.g. biological, personal, social, environmental) underlying the persistence of mental illness and progression to each stage is needed to inform the development of both general and specific, and preventive and targeted, interventions (McGorry et al., 2006; 2010). This will not only strengthen treatment selection but also the timing of therapy delivery, with safer, simpler, briefer and more effective treatments being offered to much larger numbers of people during earlier stages (McGorry et al., 2006).

For example, non-specific psychological interventions and other approaches such as self-help, digital health, physical activity and suicide prevention for individuals at Stages 1a and 1b may well be most relevant (Hetrick et al., 2008; Hickie et al., 2013a). However, to enhance therapeutic selection, it first needs to be determined whether these current interventions are also effective in reducing progression to later stages, including preventing a first episode of Stage 2 disorders in at-risk populations, preventing progression (and reducing severity) following a first episode and decreasing the risk of recurrence (McGorry et al., 2010). It is worthwhile re-emphasising the subtle but important distinction between the currently popular yet reactive notion of 'stepped care' in which treatment failure at each step permits graduation to the next step and the pre-emptive, preventively oriented and appropriately 'staged' care. In the latter case, which is more congruent with the orientation of clinical staging and best understood in oncology, more risk can be accepted in the interests of reducing the risk of progression to the next stage. What is at the heart of this is a balance between undertreatment (a hallmark of much mental health care globally) and overtreatment, which can result in a different set of negative outcomes. This balance may be best informed by data from sophisticated or sequential clinical trials utilising early-stage and genuinely transdiagnostic cohorts (Nelson et al., 2018).

Another notable benefit of the clinical staging model is its potential inclusion in clinical practice guidelines that promote higher quality and equity of care. Of note, the clinical utility of the model has already been recognised by its inclusion in guidelines for the management of schizophrenia and related disorders where the framework facilitated development of recommendations for assessment, treatment selection and timing, and ongoing clinical care (Early Psychosis Guidelines Writing Group and EPPIC National Support

Program, 2016; Galletly et al., 2016; McGorry et al., 2005). This approach of embedding staging into clinical practice guidelines demonstrates the utility of the model, though there is a real risk that it will remain constrained within existing diagnostic silos.

Research Benefits

To capitalise on the clinical benefits proposed by the model, further longitudinal research is needed investigating the clinical and neurobiological correlates of diverse mental illness trajectories (McGorry et al., 2014). As it stands, traditional diagnostic classifications are likely to be inadequate to integrate future insights into brain- and gene-based discoveries in mental health (Hickie et al., 2013b; Kendell & Jablensky, 2003). An advantage of the clinical staging model is that it provides the necessary framework for future research evaluating pathophysiology and biomarkers for each stage that are then linked to innovative neurobiological and psychosocial treatments (see Chapters 11 and 12 for further discussion on intervention). Importantly, identification of objective biomarkers linked to both stage and differential illness trajectory would validate mental disorder diagnoses (McGorry, 2013).

Currently, a variety of biomarkers associated with various mental disorders (in general or with some specificity) have been identified (McGorry et al., 2014). These include neural (Chapter 6), cognitive (Chapter 7), inflammatory (Chapter 8) and electro-encephalographic technologies (Chapter 10). For instance, neuroimaging research has suggested stage-specific findings (within single-disorder cohorts) for psychosis (Bartholomeusz et al., 2017) and bipolar disorder (Frank et al., 2015), although not for depression (Dohm et al., 2017). To facilitate the development of targeted and personalised interventions, further biomarker research is required, particularly investigating (1) the relationship between markers (e.g. gene–environment interactions); (2) their influence on mental illness progression and transition across stages; and (3) whether markers of syndrome specificity, disease and vulnerability can be discerned (McGorry et al., 2008; 2014). These findings will likely have the greatest utility during the early stages of the model to guide therapeutic selection and predict both treatment response and progression to clearer phenotypes (Banati & Hickie, 2009). That is, further biomarker research will provide the much-needed data to develop predictive tools for mental illness onset, progression, persistence, reoccurrence and recovery, strengthening a staging model based purely on clinical phenotypes (McGorry et al., 2014).

Conclusion

The advent of clinical staging in mental health care may create a new pathway to a personalised and preventive approach to clinical management. With its focus on the continuum of mental illness and underlying differential trajectories of illness progression that are not well captured by current categorical diagnostic practice, the model addresses the key limitations of traditional diagnostic categorical systems. It has greater clinical potential than the superficially similar RDoC approach, in that it superimposes categories over a dimensional approach that mesh with treatment decisions and potentially changing neurobiological states. RDoC has no such utility-based features and is a purely research-focused tool. The staging model provides a useful heuristic framework to guide and support early intervention and research, at both the level of individual clinical practice and broader youth-focused health systems development. At its heart, it proposes that effective, safe and timely stage-specific treatments can be implemented to inhibit and retard illness onset and progression. It also enables biomarkers to be analysed according not only to syndrome but also stage. While clinical staging has clear and immediate potential benefits, further research investigating risk and protective factors and treatment outcomes across different stages, and the creation of tools that clinicians can routinely use will determine the ultimate utility and value of the model.

References

Anttila, V., Bulik-Sullivan, B., Finucane, H. K., Walters, R. K., Bras, J., Duncan, L., . . . Neale, B. M. (2018). Analysis of shared heritability in common disorders of the brain. *Science*, **360**(6395), eaap8757.

Banati, R., & Hickie, I. B. (2009). Therapeutic signposts: using biomarkers to guide better treatment of schizophrenia and other psychotic disorders. *Medical Journal of Australia*, **190**(4), S26–S32.

Bartholomeusz, C. F., Cropley, V. L., Wannan, C., Di Biase, M., McGorry, P. D., & Pantelis, C. (2017). Structural neuroimaging across early-stage psychosis: aberrations in neurobiological trajectories and implications for the staging model. *Australian and New Zealand Journal of Psychiatry*, **51**(5), 455–476.

Berk, M., Brnabic, A., Dodd, S., Kelin, K., Tohen, M., Malhi, G. S., . . . McGorry, P. D. (2011). Does stage of illness impact treatment response in bipolar disorder? Empirical treatment data and their implication for the staging model and early intervention. *Bipolar Disorders*, **13**(1), 87–98.

Cosci, F., & Fava, G. A. (2013). Staging of mental disorders: systematic review. *Psychotherapy and Psychosomatics*, **82**(1), 20–34.

Cross, S. P., Hermens, D. F., & Hickie, I. B. (2016). Treatment patterns and short-term outcomes in an early intervention youth mental health service. *Early Intervention in Psychiatry*, **10**(1), 88–97.

Cross, S. P., Hermens, D. F., Scott, E. M., Ottavio, A., McGorry, P. D., & Hickie, I. B. (2014). A clinical staging model for early intervention youth mental health services. *Psychiatric Services*, **65**(7), 939–943.

Cross, S. P., Scott, J., & Hickie, I. B. (2017). Predicting early transition from sub-syndromal presentations to major mental disorders. *British Journal of Psychiatry Open*, **3**(5), 223–227.

Cuthbert, B. N., & Insel, T. R. (2013). Toward the future of psychiatric diagnosis: the seven pillars of RDoC. *BMC Medicine*, **11**, 126.

Dohm, K., Redlich, R., Zwitserlood, P., & Dannlowski, U. (2017). Trajectories of major depression disorders: a systematic review of longitudinal neuroimaging findings. *Australian and New Zealand Journal of Psychiatry*, **51**(5), 441–454.

Duffy, A. (2014). Toward a comprehensive clinical staging model for bipolar disorder: integrating the evidence. *Canadian Journal of Psychiatry*, **59**(12), 659–666.

Duffy, A., Malhi, G. S., & Grof, P. (2017). Do the trajectories of bipolar disorder and schizophrenia follow a universal staging model? *Canadian Journal of Psychiatry*, **62**(2), 115–122.

Early Psychosis Guidelines Writing Group and EPPIC National Support Program. (2016). *Australian clinical guidelines for early psychosis* (2nd ed.). Melbourne: Orygen, The National Centre of Excellence in Youth Mental Health.

Fava, G. A., & Kellner, R. (1993). Staging: a neglected dimension in psychiatric classification. *Acta Psychiatrica Scandinavica*, **87**(4), 225–230.

Frank, E., Nimgaonkar, V. L., Phillips, M. L., & Kupfer, D. J. (2015). All the world's a (clinical) stage: rethinking bipolar disorder from a longitudinal perspective. *Molecular Psychiatry*, **20**(1), 23–31.

Galletly, C., Castle, D., Dark, F., Humberstone, V., Jablensky, A., Killackey, E., . . . Tran, N. (2016). Royal Australian and New Zealand College of Psychiatrists clinical practice guidelines for the management of schizophrenia and related disorders. *Australian and New Zealand Journal of Psychiatry*, **50**(5), 410–472.

Greenberg, G. (2013). *The book of woe: the DSM and the unmaking of psychiatry*. New York: Blue Rider Press.

Hamilton, B. A., Naismith, S. L., Scott, E. M., Purcell, S., & Hickie, I. B. (2011). Disability is already pronounced in young people with early stages of affective disorders: data from an early intervention service. *Journal of Affective Disorders*, **131**(1), 84–91.

Hamilton, M. P., Hetrick, S. E., Mihalopoulos, C., Baker, D., Browne, V., Chanen, A. M., . . . McGorry, P. D. (2017). Targeting mental health care attributes by diagnosis and clinical stage: the views of youth mental health clinicians. *Medical Journal of Australia*, **207**(10), 19–26.

Hegelstad, W. T. V., Larsen, T. K., Auestad, B., Evensen, J., Haahr, U., Joa, I., . . . McGlashan, T. (2012). Long-term follow-up of the TIPS early detection in psychosis study: effects on 10-year outcome. *American Journal of Psychiatry*, **169**(4), 374–380.

Hermens, D. F., Naismith, S. L., Lagopoulos, J., Lee, R. S., Guastella, A. J., Scott, E. M., & Hickie, I. B. (2013). Neuropsychological profile according to the clinical stage of young persons presenting for mental health care. *BMC Psychology*, **1**(1), 8.

Hetrick, S. E., Parker, A. G., Hickie, I. B., Purcell, R., Yung, A. R., & McGorry, P. D. (2008). Early identification and intervention in depressive disorders: towards a clinical staging model. *Psychotherapy and Psychosomatics*, **77**(5), 263–270.

Hickie, I. B., Scott, E. M., Hermens, D. F., Naismith, S. L., Guastella, A. J., Kaur, M., . . . McGorry, P. D. (2013a). Applying clinical staging to young people who present for mental health care. *Early Intervention in Psychiatry*, **7**(1), 31–43.

Hickie, I. B., Scott, J., Hermens, D. F., Scott, E. M., Naismith, S. L., Guastella, A. J., . . . McGorry, P. D. (2013b). Clinical classification in mental health at the cross-roads: which direction next? *BMC Medicine*, **11**(1), 125.

Hilferty, F., Cassells, R., Muir, K., Duncan, A., Christensen, D., Mitrou, F., . . . Katz, I. (2015). *Is headspace making a difference to young people's lives? Final report of the independent evaluation of the headspace program*. Sydney: Social Policy Research Centre, UNSW Australia.

Insel, T. R. (2007). The arrival of preemptive psychiatry. *Early Intervention in Psychiatry*, **1**(1), 5–6.

Kendell, R., & Jablensky, A. (2003). Distinguishing between the validity and utility of psychiatric diagnoses. *American Journal of Psychiatry*, **160**(1), 4–12.

Kessler, R. C., Berglund, P., Demler, O., Jin, R., Merikangas, K. R., & Walters, E. E. (2005). Lifetime prevalence and age-of-onset distributions of DSM-IV disorders in the National Comorbidity Survey Replication. *Archives of General Psychiatry*, **62**(6), 593–602.

Kessler, R. C., & Price, R. H. (1993). Primary prevention of secondary disorders: a proposal and agenda. *American Journal of Community Psychology*, **21**(5), 607–633.

Kim-Cohen, J., Caspi, A., Moffitt, T. E., Harrington, H., Milne, B. J., & Poulton, R. (2003). Prior juvenile diagnoses in adults with mental disorder: developmental follow-back of a prospective-longitudinal cohort. *Archives of General Psychiatry*, **60**(7), 709–717.

Lagopoulos, J., Hermens, D. F., Naismith, S. L., Scott, E. M., & Hickie, I. B. (2012). Frontal lobe changes occur early in the course of affective disorders in young people. *BMC Psychiatry*, **12**(1), 4.

Lichtenstein, P., Yip, B. H., Björk, C., Pawitan, Y., Cannon, T. D., Sullivan, P. F., & Hultman, C. M. (2009). Common genetic determinants of schizophrenia and bipolar disorder in Swedish families: a population-based study. *Lancet*, **373**(9659), 234–239.

McGorry, P. D. (2010). Staging in neuropsychiatry: a heuristic model for understanding, prevention and treatment. *Neurotoxicity Research*, **18**(3–4), 244–255.

McGorry, P. D. (2013). The next stage for diagnosis: validity through utility. *World Psychiatry*, **12**(3), 213–215.

McGorry, P. D. (2017). Youth mental health: building beyond the brand. *Medical Journal of Australia*, **207**(10), 428–429.

McGorry, P. D., Hickie, I. B., Yung, A. R., Pantelis, C., & Jackson, H. J. (2006). Clinical staging of psychiatric disorders: a heuristic framework for choosing earlier, safer and more effective interventions. *Australian and New Zealand Journal of Psychiatry*, **40**(8), 616–622.

McGorry, P., Keshavan, M., Goldstone, S., Amminger, P., Allott, K., Berk, M., . . . Hickie, I. (2014). Biomarkers and clinical staging in psychiatry. *World Psychiatry*, **13** (3), 211–223.

McGorry, P., Killackey, E., Lambert, T., & Lambert M. (2005). Royal Australian and New Zealand College of Psychiatrists clinical practice guidelines for the treatment of schizophrenia and related disorders. *Australian and New Zealand Journal of Psychiatry*, **39**(1–2), 1–30.

McGorry, P. D., Killackey, E., & Yung, A. (2008). Early intervention in psychosis: concepts, evidence and future directions. *World Psychiatry*, **7**(3), 148–156.

McGorry, P., & Nelson, B. (2016). Why we need a transdiagnostic staging approach to emerging psychopathology, early diagnosis, and treatment. *JAMA Psychiatry*, **73**(3), 191–192.

McGorry, P. D., Nelson, B., Goldstone, S., & Yung, A. R. (2010). Clinical staging: a heuristic and practical strategy for new research and better health and social outcomes for psychotic and related mood disorders. *Canadian Journal of Psychiatry*, **55**(8), 486–497.

McGorry, P. D., Purcell, R., Hickie, I. B., Yung, A. R., Pantelis, C., & Jackson, H. J. (2007). Clinical staging: a heuristic model for psychiatry and youth mental health. *Medical Journal of Australia*, **187**(7), S40–S42.

McGorry, P., & van Os, J. (2013). Redeeming diagnosis in psychiatry: timing versus specificity. *Lancet*, **381**(9863), 343–345.

Merikangas, K. R., He, J. P., Burstein, M., Swanson, S. A., Avenevoli, S., Cui, L., . . . Swendsen, J. (2010). Lifetime prevalence of mental disorders in US adolescents: results from the National Comorbidity Survey Replication – Adolescent Supplement (NCS-A). *Journal of the American Academy of Child and Adolescent Psychiatry*, **49**(10), 980–989.

Naismith, S. L., Hermens, D. F., Ip, T. K., Bolitho, S., Scott, E., Rogers, N. L., & Hickie, I. B. (2012). Circadian profiles in young people during the early stages of affective disorder. *Translational Psychiatry*, **2**(5), e123.

National Mental Health Commission (NMHC). (2014). *Contributing lives, thriving communities: report of the national review of mental health programmes and services*. Canberra: NMHC.

Nelson, B., Amminger, G. P., Yuen, H. P., Wallis, N., Kerr, M. J., Dixon, L., . . . McGorry, P. D. (2018). Staged treatment in early psychosis: a sequential multiple assignment randomised trial of interventions for ultra high risk of psychosis patients. *Early Intervention in Psychiatry*, **12**(3), 292–306.

Nelson, B., Yuen, H. P., Wood, S. J., Lin, A., Spiliotacopoulos, D., Bruxner, A., . . . Yung, A. R. (2013). Long-term follow-up of a group at ultra high risk ('prodromal') for psychosis: the PACE 400 study. *JAMA Psychiatry*, **70**(8), 793–802.

Patton, G. C., Coffey, C., Romaniuk, H., Mackinnon, A., Carlin, J. B., Degenhardt, L., . . . Moran, P. (2014). The prognosis of common mental disorders in adolescents: a 14-year prospective cohort study. *Lancet*, **383** (9926), 1404–1411.

Purcell, R., Jorm, A. F., Hickie, I. B., Yung, A. R., Pantelis, C., Amminger, G. P., . . . McGorry, P. D. (2015). Demographic and clinical characteristics of young people seeking help at youth mental health services: baseline findings of the Transitions Study. *Early Intervention in Psychiatry*, **9**(6), 487–497.

Regier, D. A., Narrow, W. E., Clarke, D. E., Kraemer, H. C., Kuramoto, S. J., Kuhl, E. A., & Kupfer, D. J. (2013). DSM-5 field trials in the United States and Canada, part II: test–retest reliability of selected categorical diagnoses. *American Journal of Psychiatry*, **170**(1), 59–70.

Rickwood, D. J., Mazzer, K. R., Telford, N. R., Parker, A. G., Tanti, C. J., & McGorry, P. D. (2015). Changes in psychological distress and psychosocial functioning in young people visiting headspace centres for mental health problems. *Medical Journal of Australia*, 202(10), 537–542.

Rickwood, D. J., Telford, N. R., Parker, A. G., Tanti, C. J., & McGorry, P. D. (2014). headspace: Australia's innovation in youth mental health – who are the clients and why are they presenting? *Medical Journal of Australia*, 200(2), 108–111.

Scott, E. M., Hermens, D. F., Glozier, N., Naismith, S. L., Guastella, A. J., & Hickie, I. B. (2012a). Targeted primary care-based mental health services for young Australians. *Medical Journal of Australia*, 196(2), 136–140.

Scott, E. M., Hermens, D. F., Naismith, S. L., White, D., Whitwell, B., Guastella, A. J., . . . Hickie, I. B. (2012b). Thoughts of death or suicidal ideation are common in young people aged 12 to 30 years presenting for mental health care. *BMC Psychiatry*, 12(1), 234.

Scott, E. M., Robillard, R., Hermens, D. F., Naismith, S. L., Rogers, N. L., Ip, T. K., . . . Hickie, I. B. (2016). Dysregulated sleep–wake cycles in young people are associated with emerging stages of major mental disorders. *Early Intervention in Psychiatry*, 10(1), 63–70.

Scott, J., Hickie, I. B., & McGorry, P. (2012c). Pre-emptive psychiatric treatments: pipe dream or a realistic outcome of clinical staging models? *Neuropsychiatry*, 2(4), 263–266.

Scott, J., Leboyer, M., Hickie, I., Berk, M., Kapczinski, F., Frank, E., . . . McGorry, P. (2013). Clinical staging in psychiatry: a cross-cutting model of diagnosis with heuristic and practical value. *British Journal of Psychiatry*, 202, 243–245.

Scott, J., Paykel, E., Morriss, R., Bentall, R., Kinderman, P., Johnson, T., . . . Hayhurst, H. (2006). Cognitive-behavioural therapy for severe and recurrent bipolar disorders. *British Journal of Psychiatry*, 188(4), 313–320.

Treasure, J., Stein, D., & Maguire, S. (2015). Has the time come for a staging model to map the course of eating disorders from high risk to severe enduring illness? An examination of the evidence. *Early Intervention in Psychiatry*, 9(3), 173–184.

Tsuang, M. T., Bar, J. L., Stone, W. S., & Faraone, S. V. (2004). Gene–environment interactions in mental disorders. *World Psychiatry*, 3(2), 73–83.

Time for a Change

A More Dynamic Perspective on Psychopathology

Johanna T. W. Wigman and Stijn de Vos

Why New Perspectives Are Needed

Our view on psychopathology is changing. It is increasingly acknowledged that the way we have conceptualised psychopathology in current psychiatric diagnostic systems, such as the *Diagnostic and Statistical Manual of Mental Disorders* (DSM) (American Psychiatric Association, 2013) or *the International Statistical Classification of Diseases and Related Health Problems* (ICD-10) including the classification of mental and behavioural disorders (World Health Organization, 1993), remains a poor representation of the actual mental illness that people have to deal with. Such instruments are, without question, useful and needed in terms of clinical decision-making. However, an over-reliance on them brings the risk that, over time, these instruments are seen as more than the tools they are: they may become reified as representing the true nature of psychopathology (Frances & Widiger, 2012; Kendell & Jablensky, 2003; Kendler et al., 2011; Kupfer et al., 2008), instead of being practical aids in the diagnostic and clinical process. This brings the risk of these man-made diagnoses eventually becoming the guiding principles of, for example, the organisation of health care, insurance structures, research agendas and even policy-making (Hyman, 2010).

One of the consequences of the prominent role of diagnostic systems such as the DSM is that mental health research is often performed to conform to its classifications. For example, individuals with one diagnosis (say, major depressive disorder) are compared with individuals with another diagnosis (say, schizophrenia) or with healthy controls on certain characteristics (say, cognitive impairment). However, this practice has several drawbacks. Patients with mental health problems often do not fit snugly into one diagnostic category. Instead, individuals often report symptoms that may belong to multiple disorders. In fact, having more than one mental health disorder is the rule rather than the exception (Kessler et al., 2005b; 2011). In addition, patients with the same diagnosis can show large differences in terms of clinical presentation, aetiology, course and outcome (Fried, 2015; Fried & Nesse, 2014). Also, many (biological, cognitive, social and psychological) risk factors that are currently known as risk factors for psychopathological problems are quite non-specific, increasing risk for multiple mental disorders (Breetvelt et al., 2010; Hill et al., 2009; Kendell & Jablensky, 2003; Kessler et al., 1985; 2010; Weiser et al., 2005). Finally, the diagnoses in our current classification system have so far not led to more accurate prediction of course and outcome of early expressions of psychopathology (Fusar-Poli et al., 2012; Keshavan et al., 2011; Lin et al., 2012), regardless of extensive research effort. Taking a longitudinal perspective, it is seen that especially the *development* of mental illness often involves the crossing of diagnostic borders (Keshavan et al., 2011; Kessler et al., 2011; McGrath et al., 2016; Scott et al., 2013). For example, early psychotic symptoms have been shown to predict later psychotic disorders (Chapman et al., 1994; Dominguez et al., 2010;

Poulton et al., 2000; Rössler et al., 2007) but also other, non-psychotic disorders (McGrath et al., 2016; Rössler et al., 2011; Werbeloff et al., 2012). Vice versa, psychotic disorders have been predicted by other, non-psychotic precursors (McGrath et al., 2016; Tien & Eaton, 1992; Yung et al., 2004).

Another important drawback of current classification systems is that diagnoses are primarily based on clinical presentations of adults, who often present 'end state' levels of symptomatology (i.e. the most severe end of the full spectrum of psychopathological severity) (McGorry, 2011; McGorry et al., 2006). Thus, the clinical pictures listed in our classification systems are based on a quite narrow range of psychopathological expression and do not do justice to the fact that mental disorders often gradually evolve and exist rather as a continuum of severity than as an 'all-or-nothing' phenomenon (Johns & van Os, 2001). In line with this argument is the notion that diagnoses are often based on cross-sectionally assessed information. However, it can be disputed whether this gives the optimal representation of mental illness (Bystritsky et al., 2012; McGorry, 2011). Psychopathology does not exist according to separate, static labels; rather, subtle signs, symptoms and even diagnoses can change over time in much more complex ways (Paulus & Braff, 2003). Bystritsky et al. (2012) present the appealing analogy of current diagnostic systems as taking a photograph (i.e. momentary snapshot) of mental illness, whereas psychopathology acts rather as a movie, with multiple variables interacting over time. Taken together, these observations suggest that the current classification system of mental health problems, although useful in clinical practice, may not be an optimal starting point for research on psychopathology and its development.

New Ideas

In the past decades, new ways of thinking about psychopathology have been gaining momentum and our insights into its nature are changing rapidly. Several of the developments that have been very influential for our thinking about mental illness are discussed below. It is important to keep in mind that most of these developments are not so much meant as a radically alternative paradigm to current diagnostic systems, but rather as complementary approaches.

From Dichotomies to Continua

Over the past decades it has been increasingly recognised that psychopathology is often expressed dimensionally, rather than existing as 'all-or-nothing' phenomena (Krueger & Markon, 2011; Krueger & Piasecki, 2002). In the case of psychosis, this has led to the development of the hypothesis of a psychosis continuum (Johns & van Os, 2001). This idea conceptualises psychosis as a continuum of severity, ranging from (mild expression of) liability at the level of the general population, through subclinical expression, to full-blown clinical psychopathology at the clinical end of the spectrum. The notion of a psychosis continuum is supported by multiple lines of research (Fleming et al., 2014; Johns & van Os, 2001; Linscott & van Os, 2013; Shevlin et al., 2007; van Os et al., 2009). First, research supports the notion of phenomenological continuity between clinical and subclinical psychotic phenomena. The prevalence of subclinical psychotic experiences is much higher in the general population than the prevalence of psychotic disorder, with estimates of prevalence of psychotic experiences varying from 10 to 30 per cent (McGrath et al., 2015; Nuevo et al., 2012; van Os et al., 2009). This suggests that psychotic phenomena can exist outside the clinical range. Furthermore, the underlying factorial structure of both clinical and subclinical psychosis has been shown to be comparable (Johns & van Os, 2001; Krabbendam et al., 2004; Rossi & Daneluzzo, 2002; Stefanis et al., 2002; Vollema & Hoijtink, 2000). Also, similar factors have been shown to be relevant along the full spectrum of the extended psychosis phenotype, such as younger age (Kelleher et al., 2012a; Verdoux et al., 1998) and gender (Maric et al., 2003; Verdoux & van Os, 2002), and risk factors such as urbanicity, trauma, cannabis use and neuroticism (Myin-Germeys et al., 2003; van Os et al., 2005). Taken together, these studies suggest that psychosis indeed may exist as one, extended phenotype that captures both subclinical and clinical expression. Second, there is evidence for longitudinal continuity of the extended psychosis continuum. It has been suggested that psychotic symptoms are more likely to gradually evolve than to arise suddenly (Shevlin et al., 2007). Longitudinal studies have shown that early, subclinical psychotic phenomena are a risk factor for the development of clinical psychotic states (Chapman et al., 1994; Dominguez et al., 2010; Hanssen et al., 2005; Poulton et al., 2000; Rössler et al., 2007). Evidence for a dimensional expression of psychopathology has been reported for multiple other domains besides psychosis (Widiger & Clark, 2000; Widiger & Samuel, 2005), including depression (Kendler & Gardner Jr, 1998), mania (Angst et al., 2003) and personality (Haslam et al., 2012).

Thus, the transition from mentally healthy to mentally ill, in general, may be gradual rather than sudden. In addition, the demarcations between mental disorders that are listed as separate disorders are also less clear-cut than our classification systems imply. In fact, comorbidity of mental disorders (i.e. the co-presence of more than one disorder in the same patient at the same time) is one of the most notorious criticisms of our current diagnostic classification systems. In the field of mental illness, comorbidity seems to be the rule rather than the exception (Kessler et al., 2011; Krueger & Markon, 2006; 2011), with more than 50 per cent of patients meeting criteria for multiple mental disorders (Kessler et al., 2011). Estimates of the actual level of comorbidity can vary widely across studies and across the different disorders, with, for example, almost 80 per cent of patients with non-affective psychotic disorder (Kessler et al., 2005b) and around 50 per cent of patients with schizophrenia (Buckley et al., 2009) meeting criteria for additional mental disorders. Around half of individuals at clinical high risk for psychosis also meet criteria for other non-psychotic disorders (Rutigliano et al., 2016). These high levels of comorbidity raise concerns regarding the adequacy of the classifications of mental disorders. In addition, previous studies on the patterns of co-occurrence of symptoms did not find evidence for the existence of actual boundaries (or 'zones of rarity') between separate mental disorders (Kendell & Jablensky, 2003) or between mental health and mental illness (Pickles & Angold, 2003). These studies also suggest that psychopathology may be dimensional in nature rather than categorical.

The question of whether to take a categorical or dimensional approach towards psychopathology is an important and fundamental one to ask. However, it should also be kept in mind that it is perhaps not always the most *relevant* to ask. Pickles and Angold (2003) suggest that the central question to ask ourselves is, rather, '*Under what circumstances* does it make sense to regard psychopathology as being scalar and *under what circumstances* does it make sense to regard psychopathology as being categorical?' Thus, the most useful approach depends on the context of the question asked. They also remark that, in the end, all clinical decisions on whether to treat or not are categorical, even when based on dimensional assessment of severity and impact (Pickles & Angold, 2003). Although there is still ongoing debate on whether a dimensional approach can actually improve our diagnostic process (e.g. Phillips, 2016), the dimensionality of psychopathology is acknowledged in the latest version of the DSM-5 (Krueger & Markon, 2011) and, in the field of psychosis, a dimensional approach has been suggested to be of (complementary) value in terms of diagnosis (Rosenman et al., 2003; van Os et al., 1999).

From Diagnosis-Specific to Cross-Diagnostic Systems

Symptom expression is not diagnosis-specific. Rather, several symptoms can be present in the context of multiple disorders; for example, 'feeling agitated' can be part of a clinical picture of mania, psychosis, anxiety or behavioural disorders. Especially psychotic symptoms have been suggested to have a transdiagnostic nature (van Os & Reininghaus, 2016) and to act as an 'index of severity' (Kelleher et al., 2012b; 2012c). One reason for this is that psychotic symptoms have also been found to be present in the context of other mental disorders (e.g. Altman et al., 1997; Kelleher et al., 2012b; 2014; Perlis et al., 2011; Wigman et al., 2012; Yung et al., 2006). It seems, thus, that psychiatric symptoms do not adhere to the diagnostic boundaries that we have set them. In addition, no biomarkers or genetic effects have been found so far that uniquely define one specific mental disorder (Kendell & Jablensky, 2003; Kendler, 2005a; Weiser et al., 2005) and most studies that have tried to identify clear boundaries between two related disorders or between a disorder and normality have failed (Kendell & Jablensky, 2003). Also, substantial overlap is found between multiple mental disorders when it comes to risk factors (e.g. trauma) or endophenotypes (e.g. cognitive or social impairments) (Weiser et al., 2005). All these findings challenge our practice to approach mental disorders as separate, unique and independent entities. Instead, the awareness that a transdiagnostic approach may be much more fruitful is increasingly acknowledged.

The recent concept of the Research Domain Criteria (RDoC) (www.nimh.nih.gov/research-priorities/rdoc; Insel, 2014; Insel et al., 2010) is an attempt to encourage researchers to examine psychopathology based on cross-diagnostic behavioural dimensions and neurobiological measures, specifically encouraging them to move outside traditional diagnostic boundaries. The RDoC initiative, developed not as a diagnostic system but specifically as a research framework (Insel, 2014), works with a matrix of constructs. The current matrix consists of rows, representing five domains: negative and positive valence systems, cognitive systems, systems for social processes and arousal/regulatory systems (each consisting of multiple subsystems), and columns representing the level of examination – for example, genes, molecules, circuits, physiology or behaviour. Although the RDoC project is certainly a serious attempt to move the field forward, it also faces critical questions. For example, although it facilitates a transdiagnostic approach, it does not incorporate the developmental aspect of psychopathology (Insel, 2014). Another issue with the framework is that it focuses largely on the brain, leaving out consciousness and subjective experience, by which it risks a 'psychiatry without psyche' (Parnas, 2014). As it is still a relatively new initiative, the clinical utility of the project still has to prove itself.

From Static to Developmental Thinking

Another alternative paradigm towards mental health that acknowledges the cross-diagnostic expression of symptoms, differences in severity as well as the developmental nature of psychopathology is the clinical staging model (McGorry et al., 2006). The clinical staging model offers an alternative, more refined form of diagnosis of mental disorders. Instead of producing a single diagnosis, as is common in conventional diagnostic practice, it rather defines the *extent of progression* of disease at a particular time point, focusing rather on where a person can be placed along the continuum of illness severity than on the mere presence or absence of a specific disorder. Thus, the clinical staging model captures the dimensionality of psychopathology in terms of both time and severity, while imposing a categorical structure in a way that adds utility and depth to the diagnostic process. In the context of clinical staging, initial clinical phenomena are assumed to be milder, sub-syndromal and less specific than those that accompany illness extension, progression and chronicity. The model can be used to better match clinical need to adequate treatment, so that individuals in earlier (milder) phases of illness will (1) receive simpler and more benign interventions and (2) be more responsive to these interventions and thus have better prognosis compared to individuals in later stages (McGorry et al., 2006; 2007). The clinical staging model encourages us to take a more developmental approach and to think about psychopathology as something that gradually evolves, may wax and wane and that may have different presentations in terms of symptom pattern and severity across the unfolding course. In this way, it acknowledges the dynamic nature of psychopathology. This is especially essential for the conceptualisation of mental illness in young people, as psycho-pathology often emerges for the first time during adolescence or young adulthood (Kessler et al., 2005a). To improve mental health care, it is important to acknowledge this dynamic nature and adapt clinical care to it. The latter needs to be sequential, proportional and stepwise in terms of dose and complexity.

In addition, the clinical staging model facilitates a transdiagnostic approach (McGorry & van Os, 2013; Scott et al., 2013). Although initially developed in the context of psychosis, clinical staging of other mental disorders has also been investigated in, for example, depression (Hetrick et al., 2008) and bipolar disorder (Vieta et al., 2011). However, developing clinical staging models for each disorder separately is not the ultimate goal. Rather, research on clinical staging is increasingly moving towards the idea of one pluripo-tential, transdiagnostic approach (McGorry & Nelson, 2016), in which it is acknowledged that the development of psychopathology can take many (cross-diagnostic) paths, and that individuals can differ strongly in the ways that their mental health problems develop and change (Keshavan et al., 2011).

From Reductionism to Complexity

Our views on the fundamental nature of psychopathology itself are also changing. Psycho-pathology is complex and we are still only exploring the full depth and width of its complexity (Maj, 2016). Even considering only the level of phenomenology, psychopath-ology is a very heterogeneous concept. Psychopathological symptoms can vary immensely and along multiple dimensions: at the level of the symptom, at the level of the individual and at the level of time (development). These three axes together are modelled in Cattell's data cube (Figure 3.1). The integration of these three dimensions gives rise to endless combin-ations of symptom structures (De Vos et al., 2015; Wardenaar & De Jonge, 2013). Often in research, only one 'slice' is studied – for example, when using factor analytical techniques to explore symptom patterns across persons or examining the development of one particular symptom within persons over time. It is understandable that not all dimensions are always included, given the complexity of the data this would require and the statistics to analyse it.

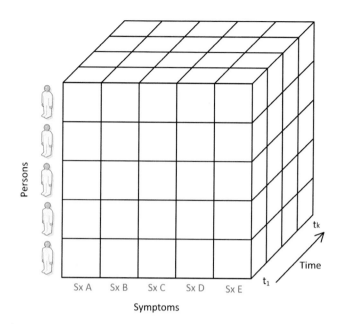

Figure 3.1 Cattell's data cube.

However, we should keep in mind that selectively focusing on some dimensions while ignoring others inevitably can lead to a more reductionist view than would be optimal.

To complicate matters even further, the emergence and development of mental illness does not only take place at the phenomenological level of symptoms. Psychiatric disorders are nowadays commonly considered to be multifactorial in aetiology, with many interactions between processes at the biological, psychological as well as social levels (Kendell & Jablensky, 2003; Kendler, 2005b; Kendler et al., 2011), calling for likewise multi-level interventions. Ultimately, this asks for 'explanatory pluralism', as advocated by Kendler (2005b): the idea that explanations for phenomena can be found at different levels. Ultimately, these different levels should be integrated, which should lead to a fuller, better understanding of complex phenomena, such as mental illness. Several studies already have shown that there are connections between actors at very different levels – for example, the experience of trauma affecting brain functioning (Buckholtz & Meyer-Lindenberg, 2012).

In science, a reductionist approach is often taken, which means that constructs are systematically disassembled into parts and these components are studied individually. However, a better understanding of the individual pieces does not always lead to a better understanding of the whole picture. This paradigm may be too simple and unrealistic to be able to account for naturally occurring phenomena, which are often complex in nature (Barabási, 2012). This may well be the case for mental illness. However, research approaches have so far struggled to employ statistical approaches that are able to capture this complexity (Paulus & Braff, 2003). We have often focused on the individual 'pieces', e.g. the psychopathological symptoms, and how they should be clustered into diagnostic categories, or on only one level of psychopathological expression (e.g. only on the symptom level, or on the level of brain activity) (Yang & Tsai, 2013). However, to really take a step further in understanding mental illness, we need to acknowledge its complexity, and allow for this complexity in our models of it (Maj, 2016).

Attempts have been made to apply complex theories, often coming from the field of physics or computer science, to the field of psychiatry (e.g. Freeman, 1992; Odgers et al., 2009; Paulus & Braff, 2003). For example, the applicability of non-linear dynamic systems theory has been explored in the field of mental health, as this may be especially suitable to explain the complex periodicity of the course of mental health issues, including phase transitions between episodes, recovery and relapse (Hosenfeld et al., 2015; van de Leemput et al., 2014; Vinogradov et al., 1992) and, in general, the full scope of behaviours, thoughts and emotions that are involved in mental illness (e.g. Odgers et al., 2009; Wichers et al., 2015). In the field of psychosis, and in particular schizophrenia, complex (non-linear) dynamic system hypotheses have been examined for example with regard to brain activity (e.g. Breakspear, 2006; Keshavan et al., 2004; Loh et al., 2007), symptomatology (e.g. Tschacher et al., 1997) and behavioural patterns (e.g. Paulus et al., 1996).

It has been proposed that mental illness may represent a loss of complexity of biological, mental and behavioural functioning (Bystritsky et al., 2012; Huber et al., 2004; Milton & Black, 1995; Yang & Tsai, 2013). This hypothesis states that the human mind and human behaviour are complex, and that it is precisely this complex nature that makes us able to adapt adequately to the world around us. When this complexity is disturbed, mental illness can arise at multiple levels. One example of complexity at the biological level is the finding that physiological processes such as heart rate variability are more variable (and so more complex) in healthy individuals than in patients with mental illness (Shaffer et al., 2014; Yang & Tsai, 2013). Another example is skin conductance, which has also been found to be less variable in both frequency and amplitude in patients with schizophrenia (Nilsson et al., 2015). So, in this sense, more rigid or 'ordered' systems can be considered as less complex and, thus, less healthy (Yang & Tsai, 2013).

However, complexity does not only refer to the *degree* of variability; the concept of complexity also encompasses the *amount of information* that is conveyed. In other words, behaviour can be random (implying lots of variability) but still be non-informative; random behaviour could also be described as less complex behaviour (Yang & Tsai, 2013). From this perspective, healthy behaviour (at levels of, e.g. biology or psychology) is complex, and behaviour that is either random or rigid is non-healthy or pathological. Yang and colleagues illustrate this with examples of the unpredictable behaviour of people with psychosis as illustrative of randomness and the stereotyped behaviour of individuals with obsessive-compulsive disorder as illustrative of ordered (rigid) behaviour. Figure 3.2 provides a visual illustration of random, complex and ordered behaviour, inspired by the elegant example provided by Yang and Tsai (2013) in their paper.

Technological advances have only recently provided us with one necessary aspect to really dive deep into complexity data (Eyre et al., 2016; Torous & Baker, 2016). Large studies, online assessments and, more recently, data collection through smart phones or technological applications such as sensors (e.g. movement, glucose levels or ECG) enable us now to collect the huge amounts of data on psychological, physiological and biological

A. Random	B. Complex	C. Order
Gegje igjgespo	Is this the real life	All we hear is
Prokw jwlif oewn	Is this just fantasy	Radio ga ga
Njgol we keoe gn	Caught in a landslide	Radio goo goo
Egefw wleo egekl	No escape from reality	Radio ga ga
Eee ot olwl woi	Open your eyes	All we hear is
Trpow irt rooairz	Look up to the skies and see	Redio ga ga

Figure 3.2 Examples of random, complex and ordered behaviour.

levels that are necessary for the analysis of complex systems (Barabási, 2012). One of the fields that is currently flourishing in the area of complexity research and gaining influence in the field of human (mental) disorders (Barabási et al., 2011; Borsboom & Cramer, 2013) is that of network theory.

Network Theory

Network theory 'aims to understand the origins and characteristics of networks that hold together the components in various complex systems' (Newman, 2010). It is especially well suited to study the way that individual components of a more complex system are linked to each other. Examples of such systems are the internet, social societies and the human brain. It enables the study of individual parts of the network as well as the interactions between these parts. This, in turn, enables the search for patterns within these interactions that may be informative for the behaviour of the total system. Concepts from network theory are being applied to several levels of the study of human behaviour, such as at the level of genetics, brain connectivity and social networks (Barabási, 2012; Buckholtz & Meyer-Lindenberg, 2012). Currently, there is much interest in the application of network theory to the phenomenology of mental illness, i.e. to the manifestation of psychopathological symptoms. Further below, network studies in psychopathology will be discussed; first, some basic concepts from the network approach will be explained.

A network (in mathematical literature also known as a 'graph') basically consists of a collection of nodes (also called vertices) and links (also called edges or arcs). The nodes represent variables of interest (e.g. questionnaire items), and the edges between them represent some measure of dependency or association (e.g. partial correlations). In networks of psychopathology, nodes represent experiences/emotions/symptoms and edges represent associations between these symptoms. The edges can be directed (implying unidirectional effects) or undirected (implying bidirectional effects), represented respectively as an arrow or plain line. Edges can be either unweighted (indicating mere presence or absence of association) or have weights representing the strength of the association (Figure 3.3). Also, edges can be positive or negative, indicating a positive or negative association between two nodes. Together, nodes and edges allow activation of one node to spread to other nodes; this concept is known as contamination, a central concept in network theory. A network view on psychopathology offers a different perspective on psychiatric symptoms and may help us to understand the emergence, development and continuation of phenomena of mental illness. There are two main types of networks that are discussed later in this chapter: networks that model cross-sectional data and networks that model time-series data (also known as dynamic graphical models).

The main advantage of graphical models over other regular analytic techniques such as linear regression (Koller et al., 2007) is the estimation of complex relationships in a collection of multiple random variables. Another advantage is the availability of concepts and tools from graph theory that allow us to analyse estimated networks in various ways. As such, graphical modelling provides information on aspects of individual nodes (symptoms) as well as on the full graph (the system of all symptoms together). Another advantage of graphical models is their flexibility. Other statistical models may be represented by a network model, or can be shown to be equivalent to one. For instance, a latent variable model can be viewed as a specific kind of network (one in which the 'latent node' is not measurable, and the other nodes are locally independent). Other examples include the close relation between multivariate vector autoregressive (VAR) models used in multivariate

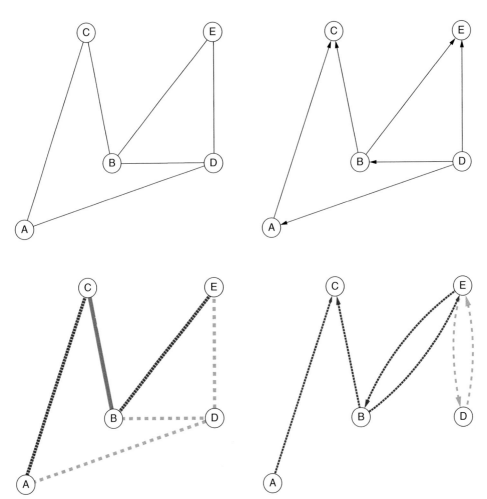

Figure 3.3 Simple examples of networks. Undirected and directed (top row, left to right); unweighted and weighted (bottom row, left to right).

time-series analysis and dynamic networks (Bringmann et al., 2013) and between network models and log-linear models (Lauritzen, 1996). There are many software resources for network analyses and visualisation, e.g. the R packages igraph (http://igraph.org/r) and qgraph (Epskamp et al., 2011). Many graphical models exist (for extensive discussion, see Lauritzen, 1996) that differ in the estimation method and other modelling properties. Once the structure of a network has been estimated, local as well as global aspects of this network can be inspected further.

Local Patterns: Aspects of Individual Nodes in the Network

At the level of individual nodes, not all nodes in a network are equally important in terms of influence on its structure or its dynamic characteristics. To investigate which nodes are important (i.e. have a more central role) in the network, we can look at the property of *node centrality*. Various notions of node centrality exist, expressed in different centrality indices

(Costantini et al., 2015; Opsahl et al., 2010). Centrality indices can help to make predictions about behaviour of the network, e.g. regarding the spread of information through the network (Costantini et al., 2015). In an unweighted, undirected network, the *degree* of a node counts the number of edges incident to that node. In a directed network, we differentiate between in-degree and out-degree, counting the number of incoming and outgoing edges, respectively. When the edges have weights, the degree also accounts for the strength of the edges by summing the absolute value of the weights. Here, degree is also known as *strength*. Degree and strength are indicators of local influence. Every node in a network has a degree, so a network can be characterised by looking at its degree sequence. When this distribution follows certain patterns, this can provide us with information on the behaviour of the full system (see below). Another notion of node centrality is *betweenness*. Betweenness centrality of a node is the number of shortest paths between any two other nodes that pass through that particular node. A node with high betweenness centrality lies on many shortest paths between other nodes in the network, acting as a kind of 'hub' (i.e. a node with a degree greatly exceeding the average degree). Thus, betweenness gives an idea of the influence of a node at a larger distance. *Closeness* is another index of centrality and serves as an indicator of more global influence. Closeness is defined as the inverse of farness, which in turn is defined as the sum of distances to all other nodes.

The different centrality indices are illustrated in Figure 3.4. In Figure 3.4a, a network is shown with 15 nodes. The degree, betweenness centrality and closeness centrality of these nodes are plotted in Figure 3.4b. It can be seen that node 1 is the most central node, because it has the highest scores on all three measures.

An example of other properties of interest besides centrality indices is that of local clustering, expressed in a local *clustering coefficient*. This node property is defined as the

(a)

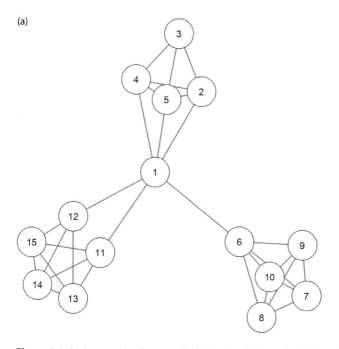

Figure 3.4 (a) An example of a network of 15 nodes. (b) Centrality indices of the nodes in the network of (a).

(b)

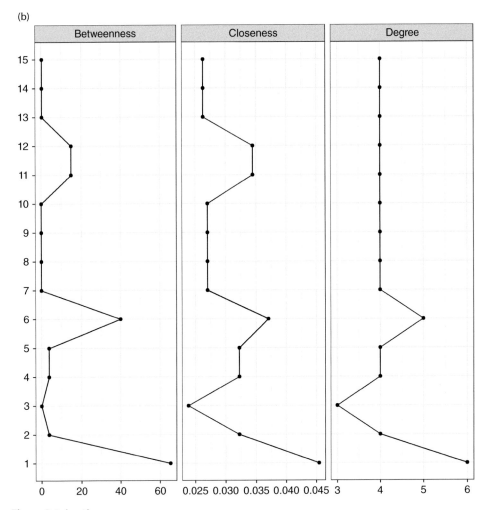

Figure 3.4 *(cont.)*

number of connections among the neighbouring nodes of a focal node over the maximum possible number of these connections. A node has a high local clustering coefficient if most of its neighbours are also connected (Costantini et al., 2015; Watts & Strogatz, 1998). Figure 3.5 shows a network visualisation of the correlation structure of the 'Big 5' dataset that is freely available in R. This dataset contains information on the Big-5 personality traits measured in 500 first-year psychology students. Correlations lower than 0.35 were not displayed. It can be seen that the amount of clustering is much higher in the 'neuroticism' subscale than in the 'openness' subscale.

Global Patterns: Aspects of the Full Network

In addition to examining individual nodes, information can also be deduced from the full network. In contrast to local clustering, the concept of transitivity refers to a global clustering coefficient. This measure considers, for the whole network, the tendency for

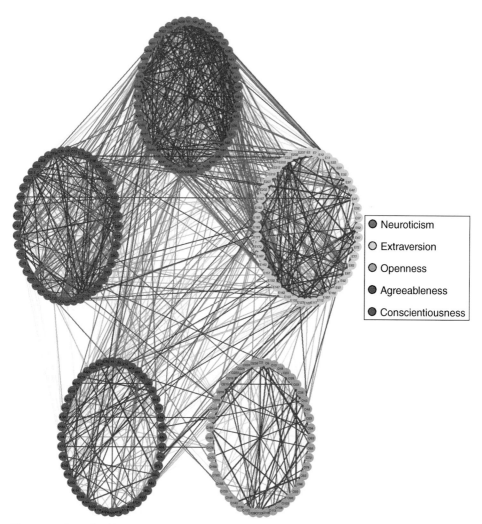

Figure 3.5 Example of high and low levels of clustering. *A black and white version of this figure will appear in some formats. For the colour version, please refer to the plate section.*

two nodes that share a neighbour to be connected themselves (Costantini et al., 2015). If this were true for all the nodes in a network, the network would consist of triangles only. The higher the clustering coefficient, the denser a network is and hence this number is a sort of summary of the overall connectedness of a network. As is the case for local clustering coefficients (i.e. cluster coefficients that concern individual nodes), there exist various global clustering coefficients for different types of networks (directed, undirected, etc.).

When investigating a full network, the distribution of connections within this network might be of interest: some nodes in a network may be more connected than others. One important network characteristic that is related to this is that of a *small world* topology (Borsboom et al., 2011; Goekoop & Goekoop, 2014; Milgram, 1967; Watts & Strogatz, 1998). This 'small world' characteristic refers to the tendency to have both a high clustering coefficient and a short average path length (Costantini et al., 2015; Watts & Strogatz, 1998).

This structure allows information to move quickly through the network. This is also the basis for the 'six degrees of separation' (Milgram, 1967) principle, the property of any two nodes in a network to be able to reach each other within six connections (or steps) to other nodes. In a small world network, the connections are not evenly distributed across all nodes: some nodes have many connections and others few. These highly connected nodes, the *hubs*, allow information to move quickly through a network. Depending on their position in the network, nodes can vary in their importance for the flow of information through a network. The tools of network theory allow for the investigation of the specific role of individual nodes in the larger context of the full network (Goekoop & Goekoop, 2014).

If the ratio of the distributions of connections across nodes follows a certain pattern, the network is said to be 'scale-free' (Barabási et al., 1999). In this case, the distribution of the connections in the network follows a *power law* distribution. This distribution is based on the mathematical formulation $f(x) = ax^k$ and has the property that scaling the input of the function results in a proportional scaling of the relationship itself. This is used to identify power law relationships: if a number of points follow a power law relation then the log–log plot of x and $f(x)$ should roughly show a straight line. It is also referred to as the '80/20 rule', meaning that (roughly) 80 per cent of the edges are connected to only 20 per cent of the nodes (Barabási, 2010). A good example of such a network is the World Wide Web, where many webpages only have a few links connected to them (e.g. a website on the specific shade of blue in the skin of a parrot fish) and some webpages have many links connected to them (e.g. Google).

Also, the study of a full network allows us to look for subgraphs within the network. In that case, we look for groups of nodes (also known as *communities*) that have a strong interdependency. In general, communities are thought of as groups of nodes that share few edges between them (i.e. between the different communities) and can be connected through hubs. Several methods for finding communities exist. One of these (Girvan & Newman, 2002) uses the concept of betweenness applied to edges. The betweenness of an edge is the number of shortest paths between other nodes that traverse it. The Girvan–Newman algorithm uses this idea to find communities by identifying those edges that have a high betweenness: edges that connect communities will have a higher betweenness than others. Figure 3.6 shows a plot of a network in which node colours are given according to which community a node belongs to. In this example, the Girvan–Newman algorithm was used to detect communities. The algorithm thus (1) calculates the betweenness of all existing edges in the network; (2) removes the edge with the highest betweenness; (3) recalculates the betweenness of all remaining edges in the network; and (4) repeats steps 1–3 until no edges remain. The bold edges are highlighted to illustrate the difference between bridge- and non-bridge nodes: edges 4–6 and 1–6 act as a bridge between the blue and green communities, whereas nodes 2 and 5 are non-bridge symptoms.

A Network Perspective on Psychopathology

The rise of the network paradigm in the field of mental health is an exciting new development. One of the pros of the network approach is that it might be better equipped to model the complex nature of psychopathology than are other paradigms. Another attractive aspect of a network approach to psychopathology is that it offers an alternative to the currently dominant medical model of mental illness. Instead, a network approach to mental illness offers a different view and allows us to circumvent the use of the diagnoses that are so heavily criticised in our current diagnostic classification systems.

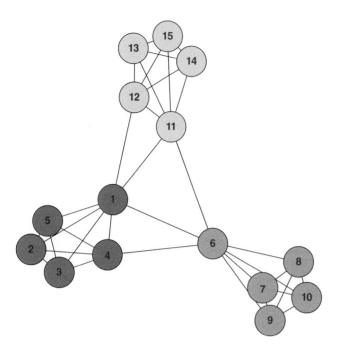

Figure 3.6 An example of a network with communities and bridge symptoms. *A black and white version of this figure will appear in some formats. For the colour version, please refer to the plate section.*

The medical disease model assumes that symptoms which patients experience can be traced back to a reasonably small set of underlying, unobservable disorders (Borsboom, 2017; Borsboom & Cramer, 2013). Thus, this model assumes that the nature of mental disorders is analogous to the nature of, say, the flu, where the symptoms of fever, muscle ache and sneezing are all caused by one virus. With regard to mental illness, the medical model assumes that symptoms of, for example, low mood, loss of interest and concentration problems are all caused by one underlying construct, being in this case depression. There has been extensive debate on the question of whether this model is the best model to explain mental illness (Borsboom et al., 2011; Fried, 2015; Kendell & Jablensky, 2003; Kendler et al., 2011; Schmittmann et al., 2013). One of the main criticisms is that the underlying constructs that are hypothesised to *cause* the different symptoms (e.g. major depressive disorder, schizophrenia) are unobservable (latent) and that, so far, research is struggling to find evidence for their existence (Kapur et al., 2012). Another is that the medical model assumes that the symptoms that flow from a disorder are independent of each other, as all variance that is shared between the symptoms is explained by this latent construct. However, this assumption is also seriously questioned (Borsboom & Cramer, 2013; McNally, 2016).

The network approach is one of the paradigms that offer alternative views. One of the important aspects of a network approach to psychopathology is that it circumvents the need for hypothesised underlying latent constructs. The network paradigm proposes that we conceptualise psychopathology as a network of symptoms, rather than as a set of independent symptoms that all flow from one underlying construct (e.g. schizophrenia or depression). This implies that change in one symptom can cause a change in another (Schmittmann et al., 2013). From a network point of view, symptoms are not reflective of latent underlying mental disorders, but constitutive of them (McNally, 2016). An episode of (any) mental disorder, then, occurs when a certain number of nodes is activated for a sufficient amount of time and recovery is characterised by deactivation of the symptoms and disappearance of the links between them (McNally, 2016).

One of the key points of the network approach is that it assumes that symptoms can actively and directly influence each other; in other words, one symptom can cause another symptom, without their association being explained by an underlying disorder. For example, hearing voices can directly lead to feelings of paranoia; this is very different from a latent construct model, where an underlying construct of psychosis is assumed to cause both, but the symptoms themselves are unrelated. Rather than being seen as underlying explanatory concepts that cause symptoms, mental disorders are hypothesised to be inseparable from their symptoms and are rather *represented as* sets of symptoms, whose interactions are represented as a network (Borsboom & Cramer, 2013; Kendler et al., 2011).

Another problematic assumption of the medical model is its implicit assumptions of equal roles for all symptoms and, thus, the idea that all symptoms are then more or less interchangeable (Boschloo et al., 2015; Fried, 2015). However, this assumption can be questioned. Item response theory (IRT) analyses on, for example, depression have shown that not all symptoms are equally likely to occur and that not all symptoms are equally pathological in nature (e.g. feeling blue is much more common and of less severity than feeling suicidal) (Wanders et al., 2015; Wardenaar et al., 2010). The notion of differential roles of symptoms is further supported by the fact that known risk factors for mental disorder are differentially associated with individual symptoms of the same domain. For example, Fried et al. (2015) found that psychomotor problems and interest loss were most responsive to increase of life stress, whereas suicidal ideation and sleep problems were less sensitive to an increase in life stress. Also, Bentall et al. (2012) report differential associations between childhood trauma and psychotic symptoms, as they found that childhood sexual abuse was associated with hallucinations, whereas institutional care was associated with paranoid beliefs (Bentall et al., 2014).

A network approach to psychopathology allows us to address both issues: it allows us to circumvent the need for assuming underlying latent constructs and encourages us to approach mental disorders as systems in which each symptom can influence other symptoms. An important additional advantage of investigating the role of individual symptoms is that no valuable information is lost by the act of simply summing up all item scores, assuming equal contributions for each symptom.

A network approach to psychopathology advocates that we should conceptualise mental illness as a complex system (Freeman, 1992; Paulus & Braff, 2003) and thus treat it accordingly. This requires analyses that incorporate the multiple ways that symptoms can interconnect and the ways that these interconnections can change over time. It acknowledges the observation that psychopathological symptoms are often not static, but can wax and wane over time, and may 'emerge or morph' into other symptoms over time within one individual (Bystritsky et al., 2012; Paulus & Braff, 2003). The network approach is already being applied at several other levels in the study of human experiences, for example at the level of the brain (Bystritsky et al., 2012) or social interactions (Lazer et al., 2009; Smith & Christakis, 2008) and is now blossoming in the area of symptom phenomenology. Networks of psychopathological symptoms or experiences have been investigated in several psychopathological domains (McNally, 2016), such as depression (van Borkulo et al., 2014; 2015), trauma and post-traumatic stress symptoms (McNally et al., 2015) and psychosis (Isvoranu et al., 2016; Vinogradov et al., 1992). Often, multiple domains are investigated simultaneously, precisely because the overlap between different domains is of particular interest from a network point of view (Borsboom et al., 2011; Boschloo et al., 2015; 2016; Goekoop & Goekoop, 2014; Wigman et al., 2017). Two aspects of networks that are relevant to explore are (1) network structure and (2) network dynamics (Schmittmann et al., 2013).

Cross-Sectional Symptom Networks: Investigating the Structure of Networks

Recent empirical work has shown that psychopathology can be meaningfully mapped as a network of symptoms. Virtually all cross-sectional studies on psychopathology report that the individual symptoms or experiences are closely interrelated and that the general structure of symptom networks is highly connected (e.g. Borsboom & Cramer, 2013; Boschloo et al., 2015; 2016; Goekoop & Goekoop, 2014). This high connectivity that is commonly found is neither random nor meaningless. Individual symptoms often differ strongly in the way they are connected to other symptoms. For example, they can differ in the number and strength of their connections to other symptoms. Symptoms are almost without exception found to be connected into clusters that often strongly resemble syndromes that we know from diagnostic systems such as the DSM. For example, Goekoop and Goekoop (2014) mapped a network of a comprehensive array of psychiatric symptoms and found that all of these symptoms were connected. However, not all of these connections were evenly distributed across all symptoms. The symptoms were clustered into several densely interacting symptom collections, or 'clusters'. These clusters strongly resemble existing syndromes such as depression, mania, anxiety or psychosis. Similarly, Boschloo et al. (2015) report that the 120 psychiatric symptoms coming from 12 major DSM-4 diagnoses that they mapped into a network structure cluster together largely according to their original grouping into diagnoses. The often reported high global connectedness of symptoms can be interpreted as evidence against a potential categorical nature of psychopathology. However, as the clusters that are found within the overall network also so strongly resemble known diagnostic constructs, it seems that the answer to the question of which approach is the 'best' is again not so black-and-white but rather a matter of 'to what extent'.

As is also often reported in research, there is frequent overlap between these syndromes that individual symptoms cluster into. One of the most commonly reported overlaps between mental disorders is that between anxiety and depression (Mineka et al., 1998). The network approach may offer an explanation for this phenomenon (Cramer et al., 2010; Schmittmann et al., 2013). Cramer et al. (2010) have mapped a network of symptoms of depression and generalised anxiety. They found that both depression and anxiety have unique symptoms but also that some symptoms are shared: these symptoms, such as fatigue or loss of concentration, can be present in both depression and anxiety. These symptoms are said to function as so-called *bridge symptoms*. These bridge symptoms form the connecting link between two or more symptom clusters (Borsboom et al., 2011; Goekoop & Goekoop, 2014) and show that the boundaries between these clusters are neither discrete nor diffuse. These bridge symptoms may be largely responsible for the spreading of information through the network and thus may play a crucial role with regard to comorbidity. Bridge symptoms have been found to show higher node centrality (Goekoop & Goekoop, 2014), which means that bridge symptoms were (1) easier to reach for other symptoms (i.e.

when other symptoms are 'activated', the chances that a bridge symptom also gets activated increases and this, in turn, increases the risk of co-activating other clusters as well); and (2) more easily influence other symptoms in the network. This underlines their importance in the structure of the network.

Thus, a network perspective shifts our attention from the level of mental disorders to the level of individual symptoms. An important advantage of this is that it allows us to examine the individual role of symptoms (Boschloo et al., 2015; Fried, 2015; Goekoop & Goekoop, 2014). Currently, we often examine psychopathology by looking at sum scores of, for example, a list assessing psychopathological symptoms and correlating this to another sum score. This, however, may lead to loss of substantial and relevant information as not all individual symptoms may be identical in their role or impact regarding mental health problems (Fried & Nesse, 2015). First, symptoms may contribute differently to mental illness if they act as bridge symptoms or as 'core' symptoms in a cluster (Goekoop & Goekoop, 2014). Boschloo et al. (2015) report that the clusters of symptoms they found were connected through specific symptoms. This could indicate whether an individual symptom has a more local (mostly within its cluster) or a more global (in terms of explaining comorbidity by acting as a connecting node between multiple clusters) role in the clinical presentation of a particular patient. Second, not all symptoms may contribute equally to a certain symptom dimension (Fried, 2015; Fried & Nesse, 2015). Some symptoms may function as a 'driving' force – for example when a symptom has a high outgoing strength. On the other hand, when a certain node has a high incoming strength, for example suicidal ideation, the activation of other nodes that are connected to this node may alert a clinician to the potential presence of this severe node (Goekoop & Goekoop 2014). Also, as mentioned above, different symptoms have been linked to different risk factors. These differential associations also underline the need for acknowledging and investigating the specific role of individual symptoms.

The fact that the relative contribution of individual symptoms can be assessed (e.g. identifying certain symptoms as hubs within a symptom network) also gives new perspectives regarding intervention (Goekoop & Goekoop, 2014; Wigman et al., 2017). Targeting specific symptoms in treatment may influence the dynamics of all other symptoms, as the network model assumes direct influence between individual nodes. Hubs and bridge symptoms in particular may be ideal for targeted intervention, because they have such central positions in a network. If activation of a hub is reversed or diminished, the 'spread' of activation throughout the network is disrupted and contamination of other symptoms may be lessened. If a bridge symptom can be deactivated, the risk of comorbidity may decrease. The opportunity that a network perspective offers to focus on the role of individual nodes gives rise to the possibility to manipulate selective nodes to drive an entire symptom network into a desired state (Goekoop & Goekoop, 2014).

Besides gaining insight in the architecture of a general symptom network, other questions that may be investigated pertain to the comparison of symptom networks between different groups. For example, van Borkulo et al. (2015) have compared the networks of depressive symptoms between patients who recovered from their depressive disorders and patients who did not. They found that the symptom network of patients who later recover was more strongly connected than that of patients who do not later recover. Wigman et al. (2017) compared the network of subclinical psychotic experiences and feelings of depression, anxiety and stress in adolescents of whom some heard voices as a child and some did not. They also found that the connections between these subclinical experiences differed between the two groups. For example, they found more connections between subclinical positive psychotic experiences in adolescents who heard voices as a child compared to those that did not. Also, even though there were some links in the network of the adolescents who did not hear voices previously that involved positive psychotic experiences, these experiences were of less severity (e.g. feeling that people are not what they seem) than the experiences that were involved in the network of adolescents that did hear voices previously (e.g. feeling under the control of an external force). Thus, the comparison of symptom networks of different subgroups may offer interesting insights into the developmental mechanisms of mental illness.

Symptom Networks Over Time: Investigating the Dynamics of Networks

Apart from lessons about the *structure* of networks of psychopathological symptoms, the network approach in addition brings our attention to the *dynamics between* the symptoms. The underlying idea here is that important information can be extracted from the way symptoms relate to each other. It could, for example, help us to understand how one symptom may cause another and this could give vital insights into the development of psychopathology and the mechanisms that may be at work. This, in turn, could provide important clues for intervention. To investigate networks of psychopathological symptoms or experiences over time, a particular type of data is necessary, namely time-series data, where the same symptom is repeatedly assessed in the same individual. In the case of psychopathology, this is often done by collecting data using diaries. Here, participants are asked to report daily on their emotions, feelings and symptoms for an extended time period. The number of assessments per day can vary (e.g. 1–10 times per day) as well as the number of days that the diary is kept. These types of data allow us to investigate dynamics between symptoms at the group level, but also, importantly, allow us to map individual pathways of the development of mental illness. This last step is an essential one towards personalised medicine.

As is the case with cross-sectional networks, the way that psychopathological symptoms or experiences interact can be compared across groups of individuals. For example, Wigman et al. (2015) compared networks of momentary mental states across three subgroups of healthy controls, individuals with a psychotic disorder and individuals with a depressive disorder. They found that the mental state networks of individuals with a depressive disorder were more strongly connected than mental state networks of the other two groups. Also, there was a positive feedback loop of positive mental states in the healthy controls that was less articulate in both groups with a mental disorder. Another domain of interest to study in dynamic networks is that of spread of activation through a network. Dynamics of a symptom network can be triggered (in other words, a network can receive 'shock') by internal or external factors. For example, an external stressor may trigger feelings of anxiety, which in turn may lead to concentration problems, which in turn could lead to feelings of shame or guilt. In such a fashion, activation of one node leads to a whole cascade of activation of other nodes (psychopathological emotions and symptoms), which could cumulate in feedback loops or downward spirals, leading from bad to worse (Wichers, 2014). The dynamic associations between nodes in a network are likely to be influenced by multiple factors. These factors could be internal (e.g. genetic liability, learned cognitive patterns) or external (e.g. a traumatic event). For example, Kramer et al. (2014) investigated the moment-to-moment dynamics between negative affect and paranoia prospectively in daily life in female twins from the general population. They found that the participant's sensitivity to stress moderated the amplitude of increase in paranoia that co-occurred with an increase of negative affect. In addition, a higher level of current depressive symptoms was associated with the persistence of momentary paranoid feelings. The exact way that the dynamics between symptoms can develop or change in a network can be investigated with actual data or by means of simulations. Simulations can be used to explore the different pathways of symptom activation and to explore the potential spread of activation through a network. Eventually, this could be used to compare different potential treatments. If a symptom network of a certain patient is known, it could be investigated which symptom would be most effective to treat. If treatment of, say, feelings of worthlessness proves to be the most influential in bringing the total system into a negative spiral (due to its high centrality), it may be productive to focus on this specific symptom than on, say, concentration problems.

Investigating networks of groups of individuals provides us with important information on the general patterns of dynamics between symptoms in mental illness. This is a useful strategy to get general insights in how psychopathology may work in a certain group of individuals, i.e. at the group level (Borsboom & Cramer, 2013). However, it does not necessarily provide us with insights into how and why mental illness emerges or develops within a certain patient (Borsboom & Cramer, 2013; Bringmann et al., 2013; Wichers, 2014). Indeed, the exact dynamic interactions between symptoms are very likely to differ strongly between individuals (Hamaker, 2012; Rosmalen et al., 2012). For example, hearing voices may lead to anxiety in one person but it may lead to paranoia in another. Individuals can differ, among others, in the nodes (symptoms) that are involved in their personal networks, in the strength of their connections or in the general architecture of their network (the relative positions and contributions of all nodes in their network). To investigate the developmental dynamics of individual persons and compare these, we need the complete 'data cube' (see Figure 3.1). In other words, we need to integrate the three dimensions of psychopathology, by studying the development (time dimension) of symptoms (symptoms dimension) across patients (person dimension) (de Vos et al., 2015; Wardenaar & De Jonge, 2013). Only the study of individual mechanisms will contribute to the development of personalised medicine, in which both the diagnostic process and the treatment that is offered is matched as closely as possible to the needs of a mental health care user (McGorry, 2013; Ozomaro et al., 2013).

One interesting example of the type of information that the dynamics of an individual symptom network can offer is the unique study of one mental health care user who kept a diary of momentary mental states up to ten times a day over a period of 239 days (Wichers & Groot, 2016). This man, aged 57 years, had a history of multiple depressive episodes. After using antidepressants for 8.5 years, he started with a gradual discontinuation of his antidepressant medication and monitored his mental states during this period. About halfway, the level of depressive symptoms strongly increased again. His diary data show that prior to this sudden increase, the associations between mental states increased both in number and strength. This suggests that a relapse could be anticipated by certain 'early warning signals' and that these signals could be used to alert both clinic and patient to an increased risk for relapse. A visualisation of the continuous changes in the structure of the dynamic network of the mental states can be found on the website www.dropbox.com/s/nppjlnpu8a7k6n8/DepressionTheMovie10%20%281%29.avi?dl=0.

Networks and Clinical Staging

Exciting new opportunities arise when we think about combining the concepts of clinical staging and network theory. This is a very new area and it should be kept in mind that most ideas put forward in this section are speculative. The network approach does not offer a definitive answer to the questions of what psychopathology exactly is, how it emerges and develops and how it should be treated. However, it does offer us many new avenues to examine psychopathology. These new insights might help us to move the field forward.

One opportunity is to compare the structure as well as the dynamics of psychopathological symptoms along their developmental pathway. For example, looking at the structure of symptoms in different stages of illness could help us to better understand the *nature* of the problems that arise in that specific phase. This information would be lost if we only work with sum scores of certain questionnaires or interviews on a certain psychopathological domain. A focus on sum scores will tell us only that overall severity may increase with progressing stages of mental illness, as expressed by higher sum scores. A network approach, in contrast, can tell us more about the nature of the problems that individuals face and how this changes with illness progression. For example, in earlier phases of mental illness, feelings of insecurity, uncertainty or shame may play a more central role in the clinical picture. With increasing stage of illness, feelings of hopelessness or worthlessness may become much more central to the experience of an individual. Thus, symptoms can differ in centrality and may need different types of treatment. Moreover, these differences may change with increasing illness severity. Identifying the most central symptoms in each stage could help early intervention, as intervening on these highly influential symptoms may prevent the development of an episode/relapse (McNally, 2016). More generally, it would suggest that the overall treatment of symptoms of the same domain could differ across stages, as the relative contribution of each symptom may change during the course of illness. The relative importance of each symptom in a symptom network can be assessed, among others, by looking at the centrality measures of all symptoms. One question of interest for future research may be whether these centrality measures can be used as predictors of course and outcome of psychopathology and whether this may lead to better predictions than estimations based on sum scores of actual symptoms. Mapping the interrelations between individual symptoms for each stage of illness and comparing those could teach us about how the nature of psychopathology changes. However, it still informs us only about the patterns at the group level. Within each group, it is very likely that the individual symptom dynamics for individual patients also differ strongly. These individual pathways can only be explored by examining the necessary time-series data on individual experiences over time. Analysing these individual patterns can add a personalised component to more general patterns that apply to a (sub)group. Thus, it is likely that we should aim for a combination of both staging and profiling in the future.

One hypothesis that is put forward by the network approach is that the network of psychopathological symptoms will become more connected with increasing psychopathological severity (Borsboom & Cramer, 2013; Pe et al., 2015; van Borkulo et al., 2015). A logical hypothesis then would be to propose that the connections between symptoms will become stronger with increasing clinical stage. In this case, symptoms would be more strongly and stably connected in the more severe stages. Different symptoms could play different roles in predicting treatment response and outcome in the different clinical stages. Some first evidence for this idea is emerging. For example, van Borkulo et al. (2015) found more connected symptom networks at baseline in patients who did not recover later compared to those of patients who did recover later. Boschloo and colleagues have performed two network studies: in one study, they mapped a network of clinical symptoms (Boschloo et al., 2015), and in another, they mapped subclinical psychopathological experiences in adolescents (Boschloo et al., 2016). They found stronger within-cluster connections in the network of clinical symptoms than in the network of subclinical experiences. These two studies together might offer support for the hypothesis that more severe psychopathological expression comes with stronger connections. Additional support comes from a study done by Wigman et al. (2013), who compared the networks of momentary mental states over time across four subgroups from the general population with increasing levels of psychopathological severity. This study suggested that the associations between mental states over time indeed become stronger with increasing psychopathological severity. However, as later follow-up work pointed out, it cannot be ruled out that this effect is due to the fact that the variances of momentary mental states also increase with increasing severity (Terluin et al., 2016). Thus, this remains inconclusive and needs replication. A final example of research supporting the idea of more connected symptoms in more severe illness is the study by Pe et al. (2015), who, using diary data, reported that patients with major depressive disorder had a denser network of negative emotions (but not positive emotions) compared to healthy controls.

The hypothesis that symptom networks get more strongly connected with increasing illness severity has some implications. One of these implications is that, if correct, the action of one symptom will have a larger impact on other symptoms in more severe stages of illness compared to earlier, milder stages of illness. The reason for this is that activation will spread more quickly throughout the network, precisely because it is more connected. Activation spreads more quickly through a network that is denser and thus, change in one symptom will have more impact on other symptoms than in earlier stages. However, at the same time, a denser network also suggests that symptoms become more 'self-predictive' (Pe et al., 2015). This means that the relative contribution of external factors decreases (i.e. the strongest predictors of the symptoms at time point t are the symptoms at time point $t - 1$). This makes it less likely that other factors can impact on the system and makes the system of experienced symptoms more rigid, less adaptive and more resistant to change (Kuppens et al., 2010; Pe et al., 2015).

Both the clinical staging framework and the network approach allow for a transdiagnostic approach. Network studies provide support for such an approach in the form of consistent findings of many interconnections between symptoms of different domains (e.g. between depressive symptoms and negative symptoms). This underlines the interpretation that these dimensions do not exist independently. The transdiagnostic character is in itself one of the core aspects of the clinical staging model and is one of the most important additions to current diagnostic systems (Fusar-Poli et al., 2014; McGorry & van Os, 2013). This transdiagnostic perspective is especially important when addressing the development of psychopathology (i.e. from a clinical staging perspective), as the level of boundary-crossing may change with phase of illness (McGorry & van Os, 2013). Multiple psychopathological dimensions may emerge sequentially and/or concurrently, in an interactive and dynamic way, especially in adolescence (McGorry, 2011). A combination of the clinical staging framework and a network analytical approach may enable us to take important steps in developing our transdiagnostic views.

Also, the network approach may help us to develop alternative ways of grouping symptoms and understanding clinical pictures, based on empirical co-occurrence. The identification of communities, for example, may offer new insights in this area. For example, Wigman et al. (2017) showed that certain psychotic experiences (e.g. 'the feeling that a double has taken the place of a significant other') were more likely to co-occur with certain experiences of anxiety (e.g. 'being scared without reason' and 'overreacting to situations'). These nuances would not have been detected with regular approaches, such as correlating sum scores of both domains. The particular patterns of co-presence could alert clinicians to the need to assess other symptom domains and, in a next phase, guide intervention strategies. Identifying communities also helps us to identify bridge symptoms that may play an important role in understanding the spreading of activation through a network. This helps us to understand comorbidity better. As bridge symptoms can relatively easily connect to other nodes in a network, they are relatively influential on the global structure of the network. This means that when a patient reports only *non*-bridge symptoms that are all clustered within one community, the chances of activation of other symptom communities is relatively small. However, when a patient *does* report a bridge symptom of this symptom community, the presence of this symptom also increases the chances of activation of the other symptom clusters (i.e. the other communities that the bridge symptom is connected to), thereby increasing the risk of comorbidity. Identifying bridge symptoms, like identifying hubs, could be an important goal for clinicians to guide treatment. Targeting a bridge symptom could prevent spreading of activation throughout the symptom network and could potentially limit or prevent the presence of comorbidity. Importantly, these typical patterns of co-occurrence and identity of bridge symptoms may change with clinical stage. Examining these aspects of the phenomenology of psychopathology across the full developmental spectrum may help us to better understand the nature of and mechanisms underlying mental illness.

Also, the clinical staging framework offers an excellent context to examine the hypothesis that mental illness is reflected in loss of complexity. Dynamic patterns between symptoms can be assessed in different stages of clinical severity and compared on network structure and characteristics. Change in the relative position (importance) of individual symptoms may illustrate how the nature of mental illness changes along the illness course, even though the same symptoms may be present at all time points.

Critical Thoughts

Applying the network approach to psychopathology is an exciting new avenue for psychiatric research, as it offers us a new array of tools to examine experiences and symptoms. Thinking from a network perspective offers us an intuitively attractive way of conceptualising psychopathology. It allows a focus on the role of individual symptoms and on the dynamics between symptoms. Also, it is very well suited to modelling psychopathology transdiagnostically. When working with time-series data, it allows us to map individual patterns of psychopathological development, facilitating more personalised diagnosis and treatment.

However, some critical thoughts are worth discussing. First, it is important to keep in mind that network analysis is a *tool* for understanding psychopathology. As with all theoretical paradigms, the network approach is a(nother) model that we use to attempt to better understand psychopathology, and it cannot provide 'the' answer to existing questions. Although the network approach is conceptually intuitive and attractive in various areas of science, its applicability in psychopathology, as well as its ability to generate replicable results, is still in its infancy. The wide applicability of network analysis is both its strength and its weakness: networks can be made out of almost anything (Newman, 2010). Thus, constructing them will not always provide useful information and should always happen from a theoretical context. In line with this is the fact that edges can represent many types of association (correlation, partial correlation, more complex associations); which choice is the best one is not always clear (yet). A variety of statistical models exist that attempt to uncover network structures between variables, and it is currently not clear which model is appropriate for a given set of research questions. Moreover, a wide variety of mathematical tools exist, and it is not certain which specific characteristics of a network are relevant to analyse.

An important limitation of network studies so far is that most work to date is cross-sectional in nature, often pertaining to (partial) correlations. This leaves questions concerning causality and dynamic associations between symptoms over time unanswered. Also, it is not known to what degree network models are suitable to describe group tendencies, given the highly individual nature of symptom dynamics that may require a within-person design rather than a between-person design. In other words, the relative contribution and merits of group-level cross-sectional networks versus individual networks over time should be further examined.

The estimation of individual dynamic networks over time comes with other problems, requiring complex analytic techniques of which the best approach to model this are yet unclear (e.g. Bos & De Jonge, 2014; Bos & Wanders, 2016; Terluin et al., 2016). Many empirical studies on diary data of symptoms, for example, assume linear developmental patterns. However, it is quite likely that the development of mental phenomena happens in a non-linear fashion (Tschacher et al., 1997). One example hereof is the phenomenon of sensitisation, which refers to an increasingly stronger response on repeated exposure to a stimulus of constant intensity (Collip et al., 2008). Sensitisation, often investigated in the context of psychopathology, may be an excellent example of non-linear dynamic development and challenges us to keep looking for the best analytical methods. At the same time, the increasing focus on complex analyses also has a down side: the risk of the analyses per se taking the lead and becoming more and more complex, just because they can. Science is a process of developing a model of reality, a simplified version of the real world, and should always aim for a good balance between the topic it investigates and the (complexity of the) methods used to the end. Clearly, much more empirical research is needed in this area.

The inclusion and interpretation of covariates in a network, while mathematically trivial, is also an open matter of research. Currently, most networks in the field of psychopathology include only symptoms. Recently other steps have been taken, for example by Isvoranu and colleagues who mapped a network of psychopathological symptoms and experiences of trauma (Isvoranu et al., 2016). Another example is the work of Galderisi et al. (2018), who modelled a network of psychopathological symptoms, contextual factors, personal factors and real-life functioning. The assumption of equivalence of these different types of nodes deserves further attention, as well as the exciting question of whether it is possible to somehow connect networks at different levels of human functioning, e.g. connecting networks of symptoms with networks of brain activity, neurotransmitter activity or physiological activity.

In the application of network theory to the phenomenology of mental illness, the nodes in the networks represent symptoms. This makes intuitive sense. However, the very nature of psychopathological symptoms poses some questions on this assumption. First, these symptoms are collected through self-report or by interviews. Compared to other fields that utilise dynamical systems analyses (e.g. physics), the signal-to-noise ratio is relatively low in psychiatry (Paulus & Braff, 2003). When assessing mental health problems via self-report, there are always issues of participants understanding the questions, giving socially desirable answers and having personal response tendencies. All these issues could lead to an increased level of noise in the information. Another problem with the use of symptoms as nodes in a network is that, if we want to investigate psychopathology in individuals with lower levels of severity (earlier stages of illness), these symptoms are often not present. How can we say something meaningful about things (i.e. symptoms) that are not there (Pickles & Angold, 2003)? However, as McGorry and van Os (2013) point out, 'mental illness has to start somewhere'. Eaton and colleagues describe a mechanism of symptom development in which subjective behaviours or experiences that have already been present for a while can intensify or develop into new experiences (Eaton et al., 1995). This, combined with the crucial dimensions of persistence and severity, can give rise to the development of need for care (McGorry & van Os, 2013). Thus, the study of the emergence and early development of mental illness (where symptoms per definition are not very severe) is possible, but we have to aim for the right construct to measure and accept that this construct can change with illness stage.

Conclusions and Future Directions

Our view on psychopathology is becoming much more complex, dynamic and increasingly focused on the development of psychiatric symptoms over time and the dynamics between symptoms. The analytic tools to disentangle these difficult issues similarly become more and more complex. The network approach offers us one exciting new avenue for examining the complex relations between symptoms and how individuals can differ herein. Finding optimal ways of mapping the dynamics between symptoms in a meaningful way, both across individuals (between-persons) and within individuals (within-person) is the first challenge to the field. As said above, most research so far has focused on mapping the network structure of a given set of psychopathological symptoms. However, the true challenge lies in the exploration of the question of whether certain network characteristics are able to predict outcome measures of interest, such as developmental course, treatment response and clinical and functional outcome (Paulus & Braff, 2003). For example, the identification of hubs in a symptom network could give rise to the development of screening tools for certain psychopathological domains or for assessing risk of further pathological development: if certain hub symptoms are present, the risk of spreading of activation is higher and the need for intervention may be more urgent compared to the presence of non-hub symptoms (Goekoop & Goekoop, 2014).

Further investigation of within-person time-series symptom dynamics could offer opportunities to explore the possibilities for personalised interventions. Also, when individual developmental pathways are known, simulation studies could be utilised to predict future pathways of symptoms and give risk profiles for transition to disorder or transition between subsequent clinical stages, including relapse or recovery (Goekoop & Goekoop, 2014; van de Leemput et al., 2014). The integration of networks across multiple levels will be an enormous challenge, but may give a new impetus to the existing biopsychosocial model. Thorough validation of network models, especially in terms of predictive validity of course and outcome of network parameters, is necessary to gain more insight into the value of this exciting approach.

References

Altman, H., Collins, M., & Mundy, P. (1997). Subclinical hallucinations and delusions in nonpsychotic adolescents. *Journal of Child Psychology and Psychiatry and Allied Disciplines, 38*(4), 413–420.

American Psychiatric Association. (2013). *Diagnostic and statistical manual of mental disorders (DSM-5)*. Arlington, VA: American Psychiatric Association.

Angst, J., Gamma, A., Benazzi, F., Ajdacic, V., Eich, D., & Rössler, W. (2003). Toward a re-definition of subthreshold bipolarity: epidemiology and proposed criteria for bipolar-II, minor bipolar disorders and hypomania. *Journal of Affective Disorders, 73*(1–2), 133–146.

Barabási, A.-L. (2010). *Bursts: the hidden patterns behind everything we do, from your e-mail to bloody crusades*. New York: Dutton.

Barabási, A. L. (2012). The network takeover. *Nature Physics, 8*(1), 14–16.

Barabási, A. L., Albert, R., & Jeong, H. (1999). Mean-field theory for scale-free random networks. *Physica A: Statistical Mechanics and Its Applications, 272*(1), 173–187.

Barabási, A. L., Gulbahce, N., & Loscalzo, J. (2011). Network medicine: a network-based approach to human disease. *Nature Reviews Genetics, 12*(1), 56–68.

Bentall, R. P., De Sousa, P., Varese, F., Wickham, S., Sitko, K., Haarmans, M., & Read, J. (2014). From adversity to psychosis: pathways and mechanisms from specific adversities to specific symptoms. *Social Psychiatry and Psychiatric Epidemiology, 49*(7), 1011–1022.

Bentall, R. P., Wickham, S., Shevlin, M., & Varese, F. (2012). Do specific early-life adversities lead to specific symptoms of psychosis? A study from the 2007 The Adult Psychiatric Morbidity Survey. *Schizophrenia Bulletin, 38*(4), 734–740.

Borsboom, D. (2017). A network theory of mental disorders. *World Psychiatry, 16*(1), 5–13.

Borsboom, D., & Cramer, A. O. J. (2013). Network analysis: an integrative approach to the structure of psychopathology. *Annual Review of Clinical Psychology, 9*, 91–121.

Borsboom, D., Cramer, A. O. J., Schmittmann, V. D., Epskamp, S., & Waldorp, L. J. (2011). The small world of psychopathology. *PLoS One, 6*(11), e27407.

Bos, E. H., & De Jonge, P. (2014). 'Critical slowing down in depression' is a great idea that still needs empirical proof. *Proceedings of the National Academy of Sciences of the United States of America, 111*(10), E878.

Bos, E. H., & Wanders, R. B. K. (2016). Group-level symptom networks in depression. *JAMA Psychiatry, 73*(4), 411.

Boschloo, L., Schoevers, R. A., van Borkulo, C. D., Borsboom, D., & Oldehinkel, A. J. (2016). The network structure of psychopathology in a community sample of preadolescents. *Journal of Abnormal Psychology, 125*(4), 599–606.

Boschloo, L., van Borkulo, C. D., Rhemtulla, M., Keyes, K. M., Borsboom, D., & Schoevers, R. A. (2015). The network structure of symptoms of the Diagnostic and Statistical Manual of Mental Disorders. *PLoS One, 10*(9), e0137621.

Breakspear, M. (2006). The nonlinear theory of schizophrenia. *Australian and New Zealand Journal of Psychiatry, 40*(1), 20–35.

Breetvelt, E. J., Boks, M. P. M., Numans, M. E., Selten, J. P., Sommer, I. E. C., Grobbee, D. E., ... Geerlings, M. I. (2010). Schizophrenia risk factors constitute general risk factors for psychiatric symptoms in the population. *Schizophrenia Research, 120*(1–3), 184–190.

Bringmann, L. F., Vissers, N., Wichers, M., Geschwind, N., Kuppens, P., Peeters, F., ... Tuerlinckx, F. (2013). A network approach to psychopathology: new insights into clinical longitudinal data. *PLoS One, 8*(4), e60188.

Buckholtz, J. W., & Meyer-Lindenberg, A. (2012). Psychopathology and the human connectome: toward a transdiagnostic model of risk for mental illness. *Neuron, 74*(6), 990–1004.

Buckley, P. F., Miller, B. J., Lehrer, D. S., & Castle, D. J. (2009). Psychiatric comorbidities and schizophrenia. *Schizophrenia Bulletin, 35*(2), 383–402.

Bystritsky, A., Nierenberg, A. A., Feusner, J. D., & Rabinovich, M. (2012). Computational non-linear dynamical psychiatry: a new methodological paradigm for diagnosis and course of illness. *Journal of Psychiatric Research,* **46**(4), 428–435.

Chapman, L. J., Chapman, J. P., Kwapil, T. R., Eckblad, M., & Zinser, M. C. (1994). Putatively psychosis-prone subjects 10 years later. *Journal of Abnormal Psychology,* **103**(2), 171–183.

Collip, D., Myin-Germeys, I., & van Os, J. (2008). Does the concept of 'sensitization' provide a plausible mechanism for the putative link between the environment and schizophrenia? *Schizophrenia Bulletin,* **34**(2), 220–225.

Costantini, G., Epskamp, S., Borsboom, D., Perugini, M., Mõttus, R., Waldorp, L. J., & Cramer, A. O. J. (2015). State of the aRt personality research: a tutorial on network analysis of personality data in R. *Journal of Research in Personality,* **54**, 13–29.

Cramer, A. O. J., Waldorp, L. J., Van Der Maas, H. L. J., & Borsboom, D. (2010). Comorbidity: a network perspective. *Behavioral and Brain Sciences,* **33**(2–3), 137–150.

de Vos, S., Wardenaar, K. J., Bos, E. H., Wit, E. C., & De Jonge, P. (2015). Decomposing the heterogeneity of depression at the person-, symptom-, and time-level: latent variable models versus multimode principal component analysis. *BMC Medical Research Methodology,* **15**(1), 88.

Dominguez, M. D. G., Saka, M. C., Lieb, R., Wittchen, H. U., & van Os, J. (2010). Early expression of negative/disorganized symptoms predicting psychotic experiences and subsequent clinical psychosis: a 10-year study. *American Journal of Psychiatry,* **167**(9), 1075–1082.

Eaton, W. W., Badawi, M., & Melton, B. (1995). Prodromes and precursors: epidemiologic data for primary prevention of disorders with slow onset. *American Journal of Psychiatry,* **152**(7), 967–972.

Epskamp, S., Cramer, A. O., Waldorp, L. J., Schmittmann, V. D., & Borsboom, D. (2011). Qgraph: network representations of relationships in data. R Package Version 0.4 10.

Eyre, H. A., Singh, A. B., & Reynolds, C. (2016). Tech giants enter mental health. *World Psychiatry,* **15**(1), 21–22.

Fleming, S., Shevlin, M., Murphy, J., & Joseph, S. (2014). Psychosis within dimensional and categorical models of mental illness. *Psychosis,* **6**(1), 4–15.

Frances, A. J., & Widiger, T. (2012). Psychiatric diagnosis: lessons from the DSM-IV past and cautions for the DSM-5 future. *Annual Review of Clinical Psychology,* **8**, 109–130.

Freeman, W. (1992). Chaos in psychiatry. *Biological Psychiatry,* **31**(11), 1079–1081.

Fried, E. I. (2015). Problematic assumptions have slowed down depression research: why symptoms, not syndromes are the way forward. *Frontiers in Psychology,* **6**, 309.

Fried, E. I., & Nesse, R. M. (2014). The impact of individual depressive symptoms on impairment of psychosocial functioning. *PLoS One,* **9**(2), e90311.

Fried, E. I., & Nesse, R. M. (2015). Depression sum-scores don't add up: why analyzing specific depression symptoms is essential. *BMC Medicine,* **13**(1), 72.

Fried, E. I., Nesse, R. M., Guille, C., & Sen, S. (2015). The differential influence of life stress on individual symptoms of depression. *Acta Psychiatrica Scandinavica,* **131**(6), 465–471.

Fusar-Poli, P., Bonoldi, I., Yung, A. R., Borgwardt, S., Kempton, M. J., Valmaggia, L., . . . McGuire, P. (2012). Predicting psychosis: meta-analysis of transition outcomes in individuals at high clinical risk. *Archives of General Psychiatry,* **69**(3), 220–229.

Fusar-Poli, P., Yung, A. R., McGorry, P., & van Os, J. (2014). Lessons learned from the psychosis high-risk state: towards a general staging model of prodromal intervention. *Psychological Medicine,* **44**(1), 17–24.

Galderisi, S., Rucci, P., Kirkpatrick, B., Mucci, A., Gibertoni, D., Rocca, P., . . . Maj, M. (2018). Interplay among psychopathologic variables, personal resources, context-related factors, and real-life functioning in individuals with schizophrenia: a network analysis. *JAMA Psychiatry,* **75**(4), 396–404.

Girvan, M., & Newman, M. E. J. (2002). Community structure in social and biological networks. *Proceedings of the National Academy of Sciences of the United States of America,* **99**(12), 7821–7826.

Goekoop, R., & Goekoop, J. G. (2014). A network view on psychiatric disorders: network clusters of symptoms as elementary syndromes of psychopathology. *PLoS One, 9*(11), e112734.

Hamaker, E. L. (2012). Why researchers should think 'within-person': a paradigmatic rationale. In M. R. Mehl and T. S. Conner (Eds), *Handbook of research methods for studying daily life* (pp. 43–61). New York: Guilford Press.

Hanssen, M., Bak, M., Bijl, R., Vollebergh, W., & van Os, J. (2005). The incidence and outcome of subclinical psychotic experiences in the general population. *British Journal of Clinical Psychology, 44*(2), 181–191.

Haslam, N., Holland, E., & Kuppens, P. (2012). Categories versus dimensions in personality and psychopathology: a quantitative review of taxometric research. *Psychological Medicine, 42*(5), 903–920.

Hetrick, S. E., Parker, A. G., Hickie, I. B., Purcell, R., Yung, A. R., & McGorry, P. D. (2008). Early identification and intervention in depressive disorders: towards a clinical staging model. *Psychotherapy and Psychosomatics, 77*(5), 263–270.

Hill, S. K., Reilly, J. L., Harris, M. S. H., Rosen, C., Marvin, R. W., DeLeon, O., & Sweeney, J. A. (2009). A comparison of neuropsychological dysfunction in first-episode psychosis patients with unipolar depression, bipolar disorder, and schizophrenia. *Schizophrenia Research, 113*(2–3), 167–175.

Hosenfeld, B., Bos, E. H., Wardenaar, K. J., Conradi, H. J., van der Maas, H. L. J., Visser, I., & De Jonge, P. (2015). Major depressive disorder as a nonlinear dynamic system: bimodality in the frequency distribution of depressive symptoms over time. *BMC Psychiatry, 15*(1), 222.

Huber, M. T., Braun, H. A., & Krieg, J. C. (2004). Recurrent affective disorders: nonlinear and stochastic models of disease dynamics. *International Journal of Bifurcation and Chaos in Applied Sciences and Engineering, 14*(2), 635–652.

Hyman, S. E. (2010). The diagnosis of mental disorders: the problem of reification. *Annual Review of Clinical Psychology, 6*, 155–179.

Insel, T. R. (2014). The NIMH Research Domain Criteria (RDoC) project: precision medicine for psychiatry. *American Journal of Psychiatry, 171*(4), 395–397.

Insel, T., Cuthbert, B., Garvey, M., Heinssen, R., Pine, D. S., Quinn, K., . . . Wang, P. (2010). Research domain criteria (RDoC): toward a new classification framework for research on mental disorders. *American Journal of Psychiatry, 167*(7), 748–751.

Isvoranu, A. M., Borsboom, D., van Os, J., & Guloksuz, S. (2016). A network approach to environmental impact in psychotic disorder: brief theoretical framework. *Schizophrenia Bulletin, 42*(4), 870–873.

Johns, L. C., & van Os, J. (2001). The continuity of psychotic experiences in the general population. *Clinical Psychology Review, 21*(8), 1125–1141.

Kapur, S., Phillips, A. G., & Insel, T. R. (2012). Why has it taken so long for biological psychiatry to develop clinical tests and what to do about it. *Molecular Psychiatry, 17*(12), 1174–1179.

Kelleher, I., Connor, D., Clarke, M. C., Devlin, N., Harley, M., & Cannon, M. (2012a). Prevalence of psychotic symptoms in childhood and adolescence: a systematic review and meta-analysis of population-based studies. *Psychological Medicine, 42*(9), 1857–1863.

Kelleher, I., Devlin, N., Wigman, J. T. W., Kehoe, A., Murtagh, A., Fitzpatrick, C., & Cannon, M. (2014). Psychotic experiences in a mental health clinic sample: implications for suicidality, multimorbidity and functioning. *Psychological Medicine, 44*(8), 1615–1624.

Kelleher, I., Keeley, H., Corcoran, P., Lynch, F., Fitzpatrick, C., Devlin, N., . . . Cannon, M. (2012b). Clinicopathological significance of psychotic experiences in non-psychotic young people: evidence from four population-based studies. *British Journal of Psychiatry, 201*(1), 26–32.

Kelleher, I., Lynch, F., Harley, M., Molloy, C., Roddy, S., Fitzpatrick, C., & Cannon, M. (2012c). Psychotic symptoms in adolescence index risk for suicidal behavior: findings from 2 population-based case-control clinical interview studies. *Archives of General Psychiatry, 69*(12), 1277–1283.

Kendell, R., & Jablensky, A. (2003). Distinguishing between the validity and utility of psychiatric diagnoses. *American Journal of Psychiatry,* **160**(1), 4–12.

Kendler, K. S. (2005a). 'A gene for...': the nature of gene action in psychiatric disorders. *American Journal of Psychiatry,* **162**(7), 1243–1252.

Kendler, K. S. (2005b). Toward a philosophical structure for psychiatry. *American Journal of Psychiatry,* **162**(3), 433–440.

Kendler, K. S., & Gardner Jr, C. O. (1998). Boundaries of major depression: an evaluation of DSM-IV criteria. *American Journal of Psychiatry,* **155**(2), 172–177.

Kendler, K. S., Zachar, P., & Craver, C. (2011). What kinds of things are psychiatric disorders? *Psychological Medicine,* **41**(6), 1143–1150.

Keshavan, M. S., Cashmere, J. D., Miewald, J., & Yeragani, V. K. (2004). Decreased nonlinear complexity and chaos during sleep in first episode schizophrenia: a preliminary report. *Schizophrenia Research,* **71**(2–3), 263–272.

Keshavan, M. S., DeLisi, L. E., & Seidman, L. J. (2011). Early and broadly defined psychosis risk mental states. *Schizophrenia Research,* **126**(1–3), 1–10.

Kessler, R. C., Berglund, P., Demler, O., Jin, R., Merikangas, K. R., & Walters, E. E. (2005a). Lifetime prevalence and age-of-onset distributions of DSM-IV disorders in the national comorbidity survey replication. *Archives of General Psychiatry,* **62**(6), 593–602.

Kessler, R. C., Birnbaum, H., Demler, O., Falloon, I. R., Gagnon, E., Guyer, M., ... Wu, E. Q. (2005b). The prevalence and correlates of nonaffective psychosis in the National Comorbidity Survey Replication (NCS-R). *Biological Psychiatry,* **58**(8), 668–676.

Kessler, R. C., McLaughlin, K. A., Green, J. G., Gruber, M. J., Sampson, N. A., Zaslavsky, A. M., ... Williams, D. R. (2010). Childhood adversities and adult psychopathology in the WHO World Mental Health Surveys. *British Journal of Psychiatry,* **197**(5), 378–385.

Kessler, R. C., Ormel, J., Petukhova, M., McLaughlin, K. A., Green, J. G., Russo, L. J., ... Üstün, T. B. (2011). Development of lifetime comorbidity in the World Health Organization World Mental Health Surveys. *Archives of General Psychiatry,* **68**(1), 90–100.

Kessler, R. C., Price, R. H., & Wortman, C. B. (1985). Social factors in psychopathology: stress, social support, and coping processes. *Annual Review of Psychology,* **36**, 531–572.

Koller, D., Friedman, N., & Getoor, L. B. T. (2007). Graphical models in a nutshell. In L. Getoor & B. Taskar (Eds), *Statistical relational learning.* Cambridge, MA: MIT Press.

Krabbendam, L., Myin-Germeys, I., De Graaf, R., Vollebergh, W., Nolen, W. A., Eidema, J., & van Os, J. (2004). Dimensions of depression, mania and psychosis in the general population. *Psychological Medicine,* **34**(7), 1177–1186.

Kramer, I., Simons, C. J. P., Wigman, J. T. W., Collip, D., Jacobs, N., Derom, C., ... Wichers, M. (2014). Time-lagged moment-to-moment interplay between negative affect and paranoia: new insights in the affective pathway to psychosis. *Schizophrenia Bulletin,* **40**(2), 278–286.

Krueger, R. F., & Markon, K. E. (2006). Reinterpreting comorbidity: a model-based approach to understanding and classifying psychopathology. *Annual Review of Clinical Psychology,* **2**, 111–133.

Krueger, R. F., & Markon, K. E. (2011). A dimensional-spectrum model of psychopathology: progress and opportunities. *Archives of General Psychiatry,* **68**(1), 10–11.

Krueger, R. F., & Piasecki, T. M. (2002). Toward a dimensional and psychometrically-informed approach to conceptualizing psychopathology. *Behaviour Research and Therapy,* **40**(5), 485–499.

Kupfer, D. J., First, M. B., & Regier, D. A. (2008). *A research agenda for DSM-V.* Washington, DC: American Psychiatric Association.

Kuppens, P., Allen, N. B., & Sheeber, L. B. (2010). Emotional inertia and psychological maladjustment. *Psychological Science,* **21**(7), 984–991.

Lauritzen, S. L. (1996). *Graphical models.* Oxford: Oxford University Press.

Lazer, D., Pentland, A., Adamic, L., Aral, S., Barabasi, A. L., Brewer, D., . . . Van Alstyne, M. (2009). Social science: computational social science. *Science, 323*(5915), 721–723.

Lin, A., Nelson, B., & Yung, A. R. (2012). 'At-risk' for psychosis research: where are we heading? *Epidemiology and Psychiatric Sciences, 21*(4), 329–334.

Linscott, R. J., & van Os, J. (2013). An updated and conservative systematic review and meta-analysis of epidemiological evidence on psychotic experiences in children and adults: on the pathway from proneness to persistence to dimensional expression across mental disorders. *Psychological Medicine, 43*(6), 1133–1149.

Loh, M., Rolls, E. T., & Deco, G. (2007). A dynamical systems hypothesis of schizophrenia. *PLoS Computational Biology, 3*(11), 2255–2265.

Maj, M. (2016). The need for a conceptual framework in psychiatry acknowledging complexity while avoiding defeatism. *World Psychiatry, 15*(1), 1–2.

Maric, N., Krabbendam, L., Vollebergh, W., De Graaf, R., & van Os, J. (2003). Sex differences in symptoms of psychosis in a non-selected, general population sample. *Schizophrenia Research, 63*(1–2), 89–95.

McGorry, P. (2011). Transition to adulthood: the critical period for pre-emptive, disease-modifying care for schizophrenia and related disorders. *Schizophrenia Bulletin, 37*(3), 524–530.

McGorry, P. D. (2013). Early clinical phenotypes, clinical staging, and strategic biomarker research: building blocks for personalized psychiatry. *Biological Psychiatry, 74*(6), 394–395.

McGorry, P. D., Hickie, I. B., Yung, A. R., Pantelis, C., & Jackson, H. J. (2006). Clinical staging of psychiatric disorders: a heuristic framework for choosing earlier, safer and more effective interventions. *Australian and New Zealand Journal of Psychiatry, 40*(8), 616–622.

McGorry, P. D., Killackey, E., & Yung, A. R. (2007). Early intervention in psychotic disorders: detection and treatment of the first episode and the critical early stages. *Medical Journal of Australia, 187*(7 Suppl.), S8–S10.

McGorry, P., & Nelson, B. (2016). Why we need a transdiagnostic staging approach to emerging psychopathology, early diagnosis, and treatment. *JAMA Psychiatry, 73*(3), 191–192.

McGorry, P., & van Os, J. (2013). Redeeming diagnosis in psychiatry: timing versus specificity. *Lancet, 381*(9863), 343–345.

McGrath, J. J., Saha, S., Al-Hamzawi, A., Alonso, J., Bromet, E. J., Bruffaerts, R., . . . Kessler, R. C. (2015). Psychotic experiences in the general population: a cross-national analysis based on 31 261 respondents from 18 countries. *JAMA Psychiatry, 72*(7), 697–705.

McGrath, J. J., Saha, S., Al-Hamzawi, A., Andrade, L., Benjet, C., Bromet, E. J., . . . Kessler, R. C. (2016). The bidirectional associations between psychotic experiences and DSM-IV mental disorders. *American Journal of Psychiatry, 173*(10), 997–1006.

McNally, R. J. (2016). Can network analysis transform psychopathology? *Behaviour Research and Therapy, 86*, 95–104.

McNally, R. J., Robinaugh, D. J., Wu, G. W. Y., Wang, L., Deserno, M. K., & Borsboom, D. (2015). Mental disorders as causal systems: a network approach to posttraumatic stress disorder. *Clinical Psychological Science, 3*(6), 836–849.

Milgram, S. (1967). The small world problem. *Psychology Today, 2*(1), 60–67.

Milton, J., & Black, D. (1995). Dynamic diseases in neurology and psychiatry. *Chaos, 5*(1), 8–13.

Mineka, S., Watson, D., & Clark, L. A. (1998). Comorbidity of anxiety and unipolar mood disorders. *Annual Review of Psychology, 49*, 377–412.

Myin-Germeys, I., Krabbendam, L., & van Os, J. (2003). Continuity of psychotic symptoms in the community. *Current Opinion in Psychiatry, 16*(4), 443–449.

Newman, M. (2010). *Networks: an introduction.* Oxford: Oxford University Press.

Nilsson, B. M., Holm, G., Hultman, C. M., & Ekselius, L. (2015). Cognition and autonomic function in schizophrenia: inferior cognitive test performance in electrodermal and niacin skin flush non-responders. *European Psychiatry, 30*(1), 8–13.

Nuevo, R., Chatterji, S., Verdes, E., Naidoo, N., Arango, C., & Ayuso-Mateos, J. L. (2012). The continuum of psychotic symptoms in the general population: a cross-national study. *Schizophrenia Bulletin, 38*(3), 475–485.

Odgers, C. L., Mulvey, E. P., Skeem, J. L., Gardner, W., Lidz, C. W., & Schubert, C. (2009). Capturing the ebb and flow of psychiatric symptoms with dynamical systems models. *American Journal of Psychiatry, 166*(5), 575–582.

Opsahl, T., Agneessens, F., & Skvoretz, J. (2010). Node centrality in weighted networks: generalizing degree and shortest paths. *Social Networks, 32*(3), 245–251.

Ozomaro, U., Wahlestedt, C., & Nemeroff, C. B. (2013). Personalized medicine in psychiatry: problems and promises. *BMC Medicine, 11*(1), 132.

Parnas, J. (2014). The RDoC program: psychiatry without psyche? *World Psychiatry, 13*(1), 46–47.

Paulus, M. P., & Braff, D. L. (2003). Chaos and schizophrenia: does the method fit the madness? *Biological Psychiatry, 53*(1), 3–11.

Paulus, M. P., Geyer, M. A., & Braff, D. L. (1996). Use of methods from chaos theory to quantify a fundamental dysfunction in the behavioral organization of schizophrenic patients. *American Journal of Psychiatry, 153*(5), 714–717.

Pe, M. L., Kircanski, K., Thompson, R. J., Bringmann, L. F., Tuerlinckx, F., Mestdagh, M., . . . Gotlib, I. H. (2015). Emotion-network density in major depressive disorder. *Clinical Psychological Science, 3*(2), 292–300.

Perlis, R. H., Uher, R., Ostacher, M., Goldberg, J. F., Trivedi, M. H., Rush, A. J., & Fava, M. (2011). Association between bipolar spectrum features and treatment outcomes in outpatients with major depressive disorder. *Archives of General Psychiatry, 68*(4), 351–360.

Phillips, M. R. (2016). Would the use of dimensional measures improve the utility of psychiatric diagnoses? *World Psychiatry, 15*(1), 38–39.

Pickles, A., & Angold, A. (2003). Natural categories or fundamental dimensions: on carving nature at the joints and the rearticulation of psychopathology. *Development and Psychopathology, 15*(3), 529–551.

Poulton, R., Caspi, A., Moffitt, T. E., Cannon, M., Murray, R., & Harrington, H. (2000). Children's self-reported psychotic symptoms and adult schizophreniform disorder: a 15-year longitudinal study. *Archives of General Psychiatry, 57*(11), 1053–1058.

Rosenman, S., Korten, A., Medway, J., & Evans, M. (2003). Dimensional vs categorical diagnosis in psychosis. *Acta Psychiatrica Scandinavica, 107*(5), 378–384.

Rosmalen, J. G. M., Wenting, A. M. G., Roest, A. M., De Jonge, P., & Bos, E. H. (2012). Revealing causal heterogeneity using time series analysis of ambulatory assessments: application to the association between depression and physical activity after myocardial infarction. *Psychosomatic Medicine, 74*(4), 377–386.

Rossi, A., & Daneluzzo, E. (2002). Schizotypal dimensions in normals and schizophrenic patients: a comparison with other clinical samples. *Schizophrenia Research, 54*(1–2), 67–75.

Rössler, W., Hengartner, M. P., Ajdacic-Gross, V., Haker, H., Gamma, A., & Angst, J. (2011). Sub-clinical psychosis symptoms in young adults are risk factors for subsequent common mental disorders. *Schizophrenia Research, 131*(1–3), 18–23.

Rössler, W., Riecher-Rössler, A., Angst, J., Murray, R., Gamma, A., Eich, D., . . . Gross, V. A. (2007). Psychotic experiences in the general population: a twenty-year prospective community study. *Schizophrenia Research, 92*(1–3), 1–14.

Rutigliano, G., Valmaggia, L., Landi, P., Frascarelli, M., Cappucciati, M., Sear, V., . . . Fusar-Poli, P. (2016). Persistence or recurrence of non-psychotic comorbid mental disorders associated with 6-year poor functional outcomes in patients at ultra high risk for psychosis. *Journal of Affective Disorders, 203*, 101–110.

Schmittmann, V. D., Cramer, A. O. J., Waldorp, L. J., Epskamp, S., Kievit, R. A., & Borsboom, D. (2013). Deconstructing the construct: a network perspective on psychological phenomena. *New Ideas in Psychology*, **31**(1), 43–53.

Scott, J., Leboyer, M., Hickie, I., Berk, M., Kapczinski, F., Frank, E., . . . McGorry, P. (2013). Clinical staging in psychiatry: a cross-cutting model of diagnosis with heuristic and practical value. *British Journal of Psychiatry*, **202**(4), 243–245.

Shaffer, F., McCraty, R., & Zerr, C. L. (2014). A healthy heart is not a metronome: an integrative review of the heart's anatomy and heart rate variability. *Frontiers in Psychology*, **5**, 1040.

Shevlin, M., Murphy, J., Dorahy, M. J., & Adamson, G. (2007). The distribution of positive psychosis-like symptoms in the population: a latent class analysis of the National Comorbidity Survey. *Schizophrenia Research*, **89**(1–3), 101–109.

Smith, K. P., & Christakis, N. A. (2008). Social networks and health. *Annual Review of Sociology*, **34**, 405–429.

Stefanis, N. C., Hanssen, M., Smirnis, N. K., Avramopoulos, D. A., Evdokimidis, I. K., Stefanis, C. N., . . . van Os, J. (2002). Evidence that three dimensions of psychosis have a distribution in the general population. *Psychological Medicine*, **32**(2), 347–358.

Terluin, B., de Boer, M. R., & de Vet, H. C. (2016). Differences in connection strength between mental symptoms might be explained by differences in variance: reanalysis of network data did not confirm staging. *PLoS One*, **11**(11), e0155205.

Tien, A. Y., & Eaton, W. W. (1992). Psychopathologic precursors and sociodemographic risk factors for the schizophrenia syndrome. *Archives of General Psychiatry*, **49**(1), 37–46.

Torous, J., & Baker, J. T. (2016). Why psychiatry needs data science and data science needs psychiatry connecting with technology. *JAMA Psychiatry*, **73**(1), 3–4.

Tschacher, W., Scheier, C., & Hashimoto, Y. (1997). Dynamical analysis of schizophrenia courses. *Biological Psychiatry*, **41**(4), 428–437.

van Borkulo, C. D., Borsboom, D., Epskamp, S., Blanken, T. F., Boschloo, L., Schoevers, R. A., & Waldorp, L. J. (2014). A new method for constructing networks from binary data. *Scientific Reports*, **4**, 5918.

van Borkulo, C., Boschloo, L., Borsboom, D., Penninx, B. W. J. H., Lourens, J. W., & Schoevers, R. A. (2015). Association of symptom network structure with the course of longitudinal depression. *JAMA Psychiatry*, **72**(12), 1219–1226.

van de Leemput, I. A., Wichers, M., Cramer, A. O. J., Borsboom, D., Tuerlinckx, F., Kuppens, P., . . . Scheffer, M. (2014). Critical slowing down as early warning for the onset and termination of depression. *Proceedings of the National Academy of Sciences of the United States of America*, **111**(1), 87–92.

van Os, J., Gilvarry, C., Bale, R., Van Horn, E., Tattan, T., White, I., & Murray, R. (1999). A comparison of the utility of dimensional and categorical representations of psychosis. *Psychological Medicine*, **29**(3), 595–606.

van Os, J., Krabbendam, L., Myin-Germeys, I., & Delespaul, P. (2005). The schizophrenia envirome. *Current Opinion in Psychiatry*, **18**(2), 141–145.

van Os, J., Linscott, R. J., Myin-Germeys, I., Delespaul, P., & Krabbendam, L. (2009). A systematic review and meta-analysis of the psychosis continuum: evidence for a psychosis proneness–persistence–impairment model of psychotic disorder. *Psychological Medicine*, **39**(2), 179–195.

van Os, J., & Reininghaus, U. (2016). Psychosis as a transdiagnostic and extended phenotype in the general population. *World Psychiatry*, **15**(2), 118–124.

Verdoux, H., & van Os, J. (2002). Psychotic symptoms in non-clinical populations and the continuum of psychosis. *Schizophrenia Research*, **54**(1–2), 59–65.

Verdoux, H., van Os, J., Maurice-Tison, S., Gay, B., Salamon, R., & Bourgeois, M. (1998). Is early adulthood a critical developmental stage for psychosis proneness? A survey of delusional ideation in normal subjects. *Schizophrenia Research*, **29**(3), 247–254.

Vieta, E., Reinares, M., & Rosa, A. R. (2011). Staging bipolar disorder. *Neurotoxicity Research*, **19**(2), 279–285.

Vinogradov, S., King, R. J., & Huberman, B. A. (1992). An associationist model of the paranoid process: application of phase transitions in spreading activation networks. *Psychiatry (New York)*, **55**(1), 79–94.

Vollema, M. G., & Hoijtink, H. (2000). The multidimensionality of self-report schizotypy in a psychiatric population: an analysis using multidimensional Rasch models. *Schizophrenia Bulletin*, **26**(3), 565–575.

Wanders, R. B. K., Wardenaar, K. J., Kessler, R. C., Penninx, B. W. J. H., Meijer, R. R., & De Jonge, P. (2015). Differential reporting of depressive symptoms across distinct clinical subpopulations: what DIFference does it make? *Journal of Psychosomatic Research*, **78**(2), 130–136.

Wardenaar, K. J., & De Jonge, P. (2013). Diagnostic heterogeneity in psychiatry: towards an empirical solution. *BMC Medicine*, **11**(1), 201.

Wardenaar, K. J., Van Veen, T., Giltay, E. J., Den Hollander-Gijsman, M., Penninx, B. W. J. H., & Zitman, F. G. (2010). The structure and dimensionality of the Inventory of Depressive Symptomatology Self Report (IDS-SR) in patients with depressive disorders and healthy controls. *Journal of Affective Disorders*, **125**(1–3), 146–154.

Watts, D. J., & Strogatz, S. H. (1998). Collective dynamics of 'small-world' networks. *Nature*, **393**, 440.

Weiser, M., van Os, J., & Davidson, M. (2005). Time for a shift in focus in schizophrenia: from narrow phenotypes to broad endophenotypes. *British Journal of Psychiatry*, **187**, 203–205.

Werbeloff, N., Drukker, M., Dohrenwend, B. P., Levav, I., Yoffe, R., van Os, J., . . . Weiser, M. (2012). Self-reported attenuated psychotic symptoms as forerunners of severe mental disorders later in life. *Archives of General Psychiatry*, **69**(5), 467–475.

Wichers, M. (2014). The dynamic nature of depression: a new micro-level perspective of mental disorder that meets current challenges. *Psychological Medicine*, **44**(7), 1349–1360.

Wichers, M., & Groot, P. C. (2016). Critical slowing down as a personalized early warning signal for depression. *Psychotherapy and Psychosomatics*, **85**(2), 114–116.

Wichers, M., Wigman, J. T. W., & Myin-Germeys, I. (2015). Micro-level affect dynamics in psychopathology viewed from complex dynamical system theory. *Emotion Review*, **7**(4), 362–367.

Widiger, T. A., & Clark, L. A. (2000). Toward DSM-V and the classification of psychopathology. *Psychological Bulletin*, **126**(6), 946–963.

Widiger, T. A., & Samuel, D. B. (2005). Diagnostic categories or dimensions? A question for the Diagnostic and Statistical Manual of Mental Disorders – Fifth Edition. *Journal of Abnormal Psychology*, **114**(4), 494–504.

Wigman, J. T. W., De Vos, S., Wichers, M., van Os, J., & Bartels-Velthuis, A. A. (2017). A transdiagnostic network approach to psychosis. *Schizophrenia Bulletin*, **43**(1), 122–132.

Wigman, J. T. W., Van Nierop, M., Vollebergh, W. A. M., Lieb, R., Beesdo-Baum, K., Wittchen, H. U., & van Os, J. (2012). Evidence that psychotic symptoms are prevalent in disorders of anxiety and depression, impacting on illness onset, risk, and severity: implications for diagnosis and ultra-high risk research. *Schizophrenia Bulletin*, **38**(2), 247–257.

Wigman, J. T. W., van Os, J., Borsboom, D., Wardenaar, K. J., Epskamp, S., Klippel, A., . . . Wichers, M. (2015). Exploring the underlying structure of mental disorders: cross-diagnostic differences and similarities from a network perspective using both a top-down and a bottom-up approach. *Psychological Medicine*, **45**(11), 2375–2387.

Wigman, J. T. W., van Os, J., Thiery, E., Derom, C., Collip, D., Jacobs, N., & Wichers, M. (2013). Psychiatric diagnosis revisited: towards a system of staging and profiling combining nomothetic and idiographic parameters of momentary mental states. *PLoS One*, **8**(3), e59559.

World Health Organization. (1993). *The ICD-10 classification of mental and behavioural disorders: diagnostic criteria for research.* Geneva: World Health Organization.

Yang, A. C., & Tsai, S. J. (2013). Is mental illness complex? From behavior to brain. *Progress in Neuro-Psychopharmacology and Biological Psychiatry,* **45**, 253–257.

Yung, A. R., Buckby, J. A., Cotton, S. M., Cosgrave, E. M., Killackey, E. J., Stanford, C., . . . McGorry, P. D. (2006). Psychotic-like experiences in nonpsychotic help-seekers: associations with distress, depression, and disability. *Schizophrenia Bulletin,* **32**(2), 352–359.

Yung, A. R., Phillips, L. J., Yuen, H. P., & McGorry, P. D. (2004). Risk factors for psychosis in an ultra high-risk group: psychopathology and clinical features. *Schizophrenia Research,* **67**(2–3), 131–142.

A Moving Target

How Risk for Mental Disorder Can Be Modelled in Dynamic Rather than Static Terms

Barnaby Nelson, Patrick D. McGorry and
Jessica A. Hartmann

Introduction

Recent decades have witnessed an increased focus on subthreshold stages of mental disorders, with attempts to predict which individuals will progress to full-threshold (i.e. DSM or ICD diagnosable) disorder (McGorry, 2010; 2013). A prototype for this line of research has been prediction of onset of psychotic disorder in high-risk cohorts defined through a combination of risk factors (Fusar-Poli et al., 2013), although this prediction work has extended to other disorders (Hartmann et al., 2019) and transdiagnostic risk criteria are currently being trialled (Hartmann et al., in press; McGorry & Nelson, 2016). The standard research approach in these prediction studies consists of assessing a range of variables (clinical, neurocognitive, neurobiological, etc.) at clinical service entry and investigating whether these variables predict the emergence of more severe psychopathology (i.e. onset of psychotic disorder) over time. In the case of psychosis prediction research, this point of disorder onset has traditionally been defined as 'transition' to first-episode psychosis (Yung et al., 2010). Comparable outcome points have been operationalised in other disorders (Hartmann et al., 2019). The assumption here is that a single baseline assessment of clinical variables (e.g. intensity of paranoid ideation or frequency of perceptual disturbances) may index level of risk for emergence of diagnosable mental disorder (schizophrenia, major depression, etc.) over time (Fusar-Poli & Schultze-Lutter, 2016). In other words, the approach assumes that a one-off sampling of cross-sectional data (i.e. a 'snapshot' of clinical state and other risk markers) can reliably predict future emergence of a particular mental disorder or progression to more advanced stages of disorder (McGorry, 2007; McGorry & Nelson, 2016).

However, there is increasing recognition of psychopathology as being highly dynamic and changeable in nature (van Os, 2013). Symptoms can vary substantially over time both on a 'macro' (months, years) level and a 'micro' (momentary, day-to-day) level and also defy diagnostic boundaries, changing from one clinical picture to another, particularly in the early phases of disorder (McGorry & van Os, 2013). In addition, these patterns of symptom development can differ substantially *between* individuals, adding to the heterogeneous nature of emerging psychopathology. These characteristics of psychopathology suggest that the 'static' model of prediction described above (i.e. predictions based on single baseline assessments) may not be fit for purpose (Nelson et al., 2017). This is also reflected in the modest accuracy and replicability of static prediction models in the psychosis prediction field (Fusar-Poli et al., 2013; Strobl et al., 2012; Yuen et al., 2018). Rather, theoretical models and associated analytic techniques built on the dynamic nature of psychopathology may be more powerful for predicting which individuals (and *when* such individuals) may change from one clinical state to another (subthreshold to threshold states and vice versa) (McGorry & van Os, 2013; Nelson et al., 2017; van Os, 2013; Vinogradov et al., 1992; Yuen et al., 2018).

Clinical Staging

The clinical staging model in psychiatry is consistent with this picture of dynamic change in psychopathology (Hickie et al., 2013; McGorry, 2007; McGorry et al., 2006). This model, which parallels staging models in general medicine (e.g. cancer or renal disease), moves beyond the traditional cross-sectional categorical approach to psychiatric diagnosis by defining the extent of disease progression based on severity, duration and course of symptoms. The model attempts to determine the position of an individual along a *continuum* of illness, defined according to stages. The differentiation of early and milder clinical phenomena from more severe and chronic phenomena lies at the heart of the concept, and allows the clinician to select appropriate treatments according to stage. While highly congruent with notions of an extended phenotype for individual disorders (van Os & Linscott, 2012), involving continuity with the healthy population, it places strong diagnostic emphasis on where a person sits in the evolution of the clinical phenotype transdiagnostically. The model, which does impose an empirically defined categorical structure on a fluid reality to aid treatment decisions, acknowledges that a person may (repeatedly) move between stages of disorder and cross traditional diagnostic boundaries. In terms of prediction research, there may be factors that can aid identification of patients most likely to progress to another stage of disorder (or indeed to remit and return to earlier stages of disorder), and there may also be dynamic change in mental state and other parameters *within* a stage of disorder that can aid these identification and prediction efforts.

A number of other models of dynamic change have emerged from other disciplines. Expanding on Chapter 3, we briefly present a number of cross-disciplinary models of system change (dynamical systems theory, network theory, instability mechanisms, chaos theory and catastrophe theory) and suggest how these may be conceptually and empirically applied to psychopathology prediction research, whether this is in the context of the clinical staging model of disorder or more broadly in psychiatric research.

Dynamical Systems Theory

Dynamical systems theory (Scheffer, 2009), originating in the fields of mathematics and physics, aims to explain the behaviour of complex systems such as the climate, ecosystems and financial markets. It proposes that complex systems can have different types of constitutive architecture. While some systems are made up of parts that are diverse and only marginally connected, other systems consist of similar, highly interconnected components (Scheffer, 2010; Scheffer et al., 2012). In the first type of system, change tends to occur gradually, while the second type of system may initially resist change and then reach a 'tipping point' that involves a relatively sudden and dramatic shift to an alternative state (Figures 4.1c and 4.2). Particular system changes have been described that identify how *close* a system is to such transitions. While some system transitions occur gradually in response to changing conditions (Figure 4.1a), others may be triggered by a massive external shock (Figure 4.1b). Other system transitions are foreshadowed by an increase in random variance

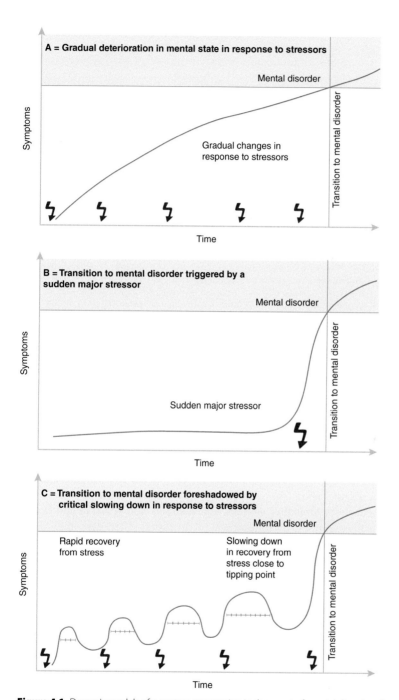

Figure 4.1 Dynamic models of symptom progression in the onset of mental disorders. Stressors are indicated by a lightning bolt. Reproduced with permission (Nelson et al., 2017).

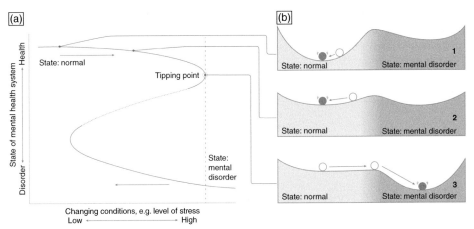

Figure 4.2 Critical slowing down as an early warning sign for transition in mental state. (a) The figure shows a system with two alternative states, a normal state and a mental disorder state. With changing conditions (e.g. increased stress), the system is pushed towards a critical threshold (tipping point). The closer it gets to the tipping point, the less resilient it becomes. (b) This principle of resilience can be represented using a ball-in-a-valley diagram. In 1, the valley is deep, and the system is resilient; after a perturbation, the ball will quickly return to its original position. In 2, the valley becomes shallower, demonstrating that the ball requires less perturbation to move to the alternative valley (to the right). The increased shallowness also means that the ball will take more time to return to its original position after a perturbation (critical slowing down). In 3, the valley is even shallower, so a small perturbation (e.g. an argument) was sufficient to push the ball beyond the threshold to the valley to the right and trigger a system change: the whole system transitioned to a different state (in this case, mental disorder). Panel (a) is adapted with permission from Scheffer et al. (2012); panel (b) is adapted with permission from Lenton (2011).

and volatility or, alternatively, a 'critical slowing down' of activity (Figure 4.1c). *Critical slowing down* refers to a system slowing down in returning to a state of equilibrium in response to disturbances ('perturbations') when it is close to a tipping point (Figure 4.2). This phenomenon has been demonstrated in mathematical models (e.g. in paleoclimatic transitions such as the Earth's shift from icehouse to greenhouse states) and has been demonstrated experimentally in biological systems (e.g. the food web of a lake and cyano-bacterial population changes in response to increasing light stress) (Carpenter et al., 2011; Dai et al., 2012; Veraart et al., 2012). The concept has also been used in general medicine. Olde Rikkert and colleagues (2016), for example, argue that system slow-down can predict acute transitions in chronic diseases such as asthma, cardiac arrhythmias, migraine and epilepsy.

Several studies have applied dynamical systems theory to mood disorders using eco-logical momentary assessment (i.e. frequently assessing individuals' mood states in the flow of their everyday lives). In a large sample of healthy individuals and depressed patients, van de Leemput and colleagues (2014) found that shifts between depressed and normal states were preceded by increased connectivity of an emotional state *with itself* over time (increased temporal autocorrelation), increased variance in recorded emotions, and stronger positive correlation between emotions with the same valence (e.g. cheerful and content) and stronger negative correlation between emotions with different valences (e.g. cheerful and anxious). A very similar pattern of early warning signals was reported in a single-person case study prior to a clinically and statistically significant transition to depression after discontinuation of antidepressant medication (Wichers et al., 2016). These findings are consistent with the notion of a critical slowing down in a person's response to perturbations (e.g. slower recovery from depressed affect after a life stressor, such as the end of an intimate relationship) as an early warning sign for a tipping point in mood state (from normal to depressed state and possibly vice versa; Figure 4.2) (van de Leemput et al., 2014; Wichers, 2014; Wichers et al., 2015; 2016; Wigman et al., 2013b). However, while related ideas have been applied to psychotic symptomatology (Arzouan et al., 2014; Gharibzadeh et al., 2011; Loh et al., 2007), this approach to modelling critical transitions in complex systems has not been applied to predicting transitions in people at clinical high risk of psychosis. It would be of interest to investigate whether transitions in psychotic and other psychiatric disorders (e.g. transition from prodrome to first-episode disorder or from remission/recovery to relapse) are foreshadowed by a critical slowing down in the system's (i.e. the person's) various domains of subjective experience and functioning (cognition, affect, corporeality, interpersonal functioning, etc.) in response to perturbations (e.g. life stressors, trauma, etc.). For example, a person at high risk of psychosis may describe becoming 'stuck' in paranoid thoughts and may take longer to return to non-paranoid thinking in response to situational stressors as a signal of an imminent 'tipping point' into first-episode psychosis (Figures 4.1c and 4.2). Critical slowing down may also apply to domains such as neurocognitive functioning and EEG patterns. It is also possible, of course, that the critical slowing down model is less applicable to some disorders, with gradual changes in a system (Figure 4.1a) or sudden shifts in response to a sudden strong external impact (Figure 4.1b), or possibly also increased variability and volatility in mental state, being more accurate models of disorder onset and relapse (Early Warning Signals Toolbox). There may also be individual differences: critical slowing down may foreshadow some patients' transitions, while there may be alternative courses for other patients.

Network Theory

A related area of research that has already gained some traction in psychiatric research is that of network models (Borsboom, 2017). In network models, correlations between symptoms are not explained by a common cause (the underlying mental disorder), as in the traditional latent disease model (e.g. lung cancer being a common cause of symptoms such as shortness of breath, chest pain, and coughing up blood). Rather, mental disorders are seen as complex dynamic systems in which symptoms and psychological, biological and sociological components have autonomous causal power to influence each other (Borsboom & Cramer, 2013; Isvoranu et al., 2016; van Borkulo et al., 2015). By this account, symptoms are not passive expressions of an underlying disturbance but may *actively trigger* other symptoms (e.g. psychosocial circumstances may produce anxiety, which in turn may activate paranoid ideation) (Hofmann et al., 2016). If symptoms engage in patterns of mutual reinforcement and feedback loops, the system as a whole may become trapped or 'locked' in a state of extended symptom activation, a point at which a mental disorder may be diagnosed. Using a network approach, Isvoranu and colleagues (2017), for example, recently showed that general psychopathological symptoms (anxiety, poor impulse control, motor retardation) connect different types of childhood trauma with positive and negative psychotic symptoms. This finding suggests that these general psychopathological symptoms may activate and reinforce psychotic symptoms in patients with a history of childhood trauma, which points towards mechanisms of onset of psychotic disorder and variables that may be incorporated into dynamic predictive models in those at high risk. Accordingly, the network perspective may be useful in predicting transition to frank disorder in those with emerging signs and symptoms (e.g. from clinical high-risk state to psychotic disorder) (Wigman et al., 2013a). The network approach would benefit from further fine-grained longitudinal data to test its theoretical robustness and clinical applicability (see the following) (Guloksuz et al., 2017).

Stable versus Unstable Systems

Another relevant area of research is that of *instability mechanisms* identified in environmental geography (Dunlop et al., 2008; Fowler, 2010a; 2010b). In 'unstable' systems, small natural variations or disturbances are amplified through the operation of positive feedback loops, eventually disrupting consistency in a pattern. Mathematical analysis and computer modelling have established that instability mechanisms are responsible for many natural formations and patterns. For example, on an initially flat sand surface on a beach, a small variation in the sand thickness encourages the accumulation of local sediment and the sand thickness consequently grows. With regards to psychopathology, it is possible that analogous mechanisms drive the intensification of symptoms over time. For example, in the area of psychosis risk, such instability mechanisms may exacerbate minor anomalous subjective experiences (e.g. mild dissociative phenomena) into frank psychotic symptoms over time. Interestingly, many writers in the phenomenological tradition have posited an underlying instability in basic processes of conscious awareness (awareness of time, space, body, self, intersubjectivity, etc.) as being *le trouble générateur* (Minkowski, 1926) (generative disorder or underlying causal mechanism) in schizophrenia-spectrum disorders (Conrad, 1958; Jaspers, 1963), reflected in the 'basic symptoms' (Schultze-Lutter, 2009) and most recently formulated in the minimal self or 'ipseity' disturbance model (Parnas & Henriksen, 2014). Conrad's (1958) classic account of the psychosis prodrome, including such key concepts as trema, apophany, anastrophy, hyperreflexivity and transparence, captures the emergence and stages of such instability, as well as Jasper's (1963) concept of primary delusion ('a new world has come into being', which arguably represents instability reaching a new stable plateau). Although some work has applied the concept of instability to brain functioning in schizophrenia (Levit-Binnun et al., 2010; Loh et al., 2007), the predictive value of such models has not yet been tested.

Non-linear and Chaotic Systems

Finally, non-linear and chaos-based theories have been used to examine a wide array of phenomena ranging from biological population models to the functioning of modern work organisations. These theories posit that, although a series of observations over time or space may *appear* complex, relatively simple underlying 'generators' may in fact be responsible for these seemingly complex observations or behaviours. Chaotic dynamical systems are characterised by a lawful but extreme sensitivity to initial conditions, which can lead to a striking divergence of behavioural patterns over time, popularly referred to as the 'butterfly effect'. In such systems, small differences in initial conditions yield widely diverging outcomes. 'Initial conditions' in terms of psychosocial development, such as adverse childhood experiences, or effectiveness of treatment in early stages of illness may influence the ultimate trajectory of psychiatric symptoms and syndromes, or may set the basic parameters within which a system can develop. A similar approach is that of catastrophe theory, a mathematical theory that models how sudden changes may occur even though the underlying causal variables are essentially continuous (Poston & Steward, 1978). The approach shows that phenomena or systems that show sudden quantitative shifts from one state to another may be under the influence of two or more independent mechanisms which themselves do *not* show any sudden shifts or jumps in magnitude. In the emergence of psychopathology it may be that the steady accumulation of a range of risk factors (e.g. obstetric complications, trauma, social adversity) forces the person to reach a rather sudden change ('catastrophe' or 'tipping point') in mental state. Again, although there has been some discussion of non-linear, chaos-based (Bystritsky et al., 2012; Paulus & Braff, 2003; Tschacher et al., 1997) or catastrophe-based (Scott, 1985) models of mental disorder, it has not yet been applied to prediction of transition from subthreshold to full-threshold psycho-pathology. For example, Scott (1985) applied the mathematical principles of catastrophe theory to bipolar disorder, modelling how the variables of anxiety, self-esteem and aberrant salience of environmental stimuli may interact over time to produce depressive and manic episodes. Such dynamic models could be tested for their predictive utility in high-risk samples.

Applications to Psychopathology Research

These overlapping models each attempt to capture the dynamic and shifting nature of complex systems and may be fruitfully applied to psychopathological research, i.e. model-ling and predicting the movement from less severe to more severe stages of disorder formulated in terms of the clinical staging model. Psychosis and mood disorder prediction research, in particular, are at junctures where they could move beyond static or baseline 'snapshot' prediction to modelling a complex system with resilience and fragilities built into its structure that can reach 'tipping points' (transitions) in response to internal and/or external stressors. These dynamic models of emerging psychopathology require different methodological designs and analytical techniques from those to which we are accustomed and also indicate the value of cross-disciplinary collaboration, for example with mathemat-icians and physicists. Although machine learning methods (Bedi et al., 2015; Koutsouleris et al., 2009) and a 'high-risk calculator' (Cannon et al., 2016) have gained much attention in recent years, these methods are still built on prediction from 'single snapshot' baseline data, albeit applied on an individual patient level, and tend not to take into account the time-to-event nature of prediction research. In order to examine the value of dynamic models, methodology that uses repeated longitudinal assessments of relevant features (time-series methods) are required. This may be either, or a combination of, moment-to-moment ecological assessment (micro-level assessment of psychopathology) or repeated assessments over more extended periods of time (macro-level assessment; Figure 4.3) (Wichers, 2014). The most widely used method for the former is ecological momentary assessments tech-niques (Myin-Germeys et al., 2009). Techniques for the latter, such as joint modelling of time-to-event outcome with time-dependent predictors, which can take into account the time-to-event nature of predicting onset of disorder, are also currently being developed (Yuen & Mackinnon, 2016) and have in fact already been found to outperform standard statistical prediction based solely on baseline data (Yuen et al., 2018). Other applicable time-series metric-based and model-based methods are also available. Of course, one of the challenges of these time-series methods of detecting imminent transitions is the large amount of repeat data required per research participant (Wichers et al., 2016). However, with an increased use of technology aiding data collection (e.g. mobile applications for

Measurement for static prediction

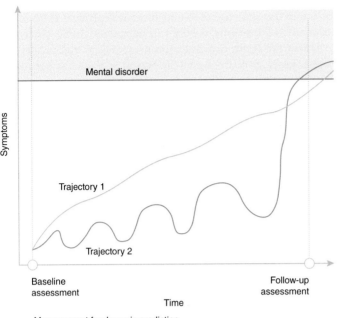

Measurement for dynamic prediction

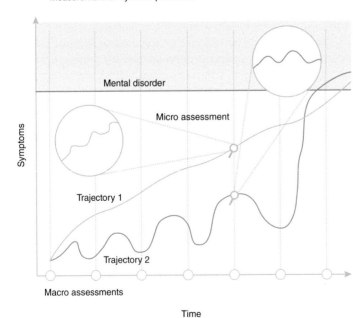

Figure 4.3 Measurement required in static and dynamic predictive models. Two different trajectories to threshold-level mental disorder are presented. The circles on the *x*-axis represent measurement time points. Macro-level assessments involve repeated assessment time points, e.g. at monthly intervals. Micro-level assessments are represented by the magnifying-glass symbol. These assessments involve high-resolution, granular-level assessments (e.g. repeated assessments over the course of a day). Reproduced with permission (Nelson et al., 2017).

ambulatory assessments, online surveys) and more than two decades of experience with engaging clinical high risk for psychosis populations, we are better equipped than ever to gather the required high-resolution, longitudinal data. In-depth qualitative methods with smaller samples (e.g. retrospective first-person accounts of subjectively experienced changes associated with the onset of disorder) should also be considered.

There are a number of important questions raised by these models that can push the field of prediction research in psychiatry forward. All of these models emphasise *systems* rather than *categories*. While the concept of psychopathology/mental disorders as being disordered systems is not a new one (Globus & Arpaia, 1994; Mandell & Selz, 1992; Odgers et al., 2009), it has not yet been directly applied to prediction of outcome in clinical high-risk populations (Hartmann et al., 2019). What sort of system exactly is psychopathology, with what sort of constitutive architecture, and what factors are this architecture most sensitive to? Which of the overlapping but distinct concepts of dynamical systems theory, network models, instability mechanisms or non-linear/chaos- or catastrophe-based theories are most appropriate for modelling change in psychopathological states? As mentioned above, it may be that mental disorder cannot be characterised as a single type of system, but may consist of *different types* of systems (e.g. some disorders with high heterogeneity, others more homogeneous in structure, which will influence response to stressors) and may vary between individuals (Scheffer et al., 2012). Certainly, common psychiatric language (e.g. 'flight into health', 'psychotic break') suggests that system change can be quite abrupt for some individuals. It would be valuable to characterise and quantify the abrupt-onset psychoses versus the gradual-onset cases in clinical high-risk samples (i.e. the 'psychotic break', Figures 4.1b and 4.1c vs 'psychotic slide', Figure 4.1a) in order to improve our understanding of these issues, rather than simply categorise patients according to 'transitioned' or 'non-transitioned' cases. The nature of the early warning signals of system change will vary depending on the type of system: for some individuals or for some disorders the critical slowing down phenomenon (slowed reattainment of equilibrium in response to stressors; Figures 4.1c and 4.2) may be predictive, whereas for others variability and volatility in the system (rapid cycling mood episodes, wildly fluctuating affective or mental states, etc.) or sensitivity to particular conditions (low thresholds for particular affective or cognitive responses, dissociation, etc.) may be predictive. A challenge for the next wave of research in this field is to determine which of these concepts is clinically useful, and to translate these models from group-level to individual-level prediction, akin to the concept of an individual's 'relapse signature' (Birchwood, 1995), which Wichers and colleagues have already shown is possible (Wichers et al., 2016). The theoretical richness of these dynamic models needs to be balanced with clinical applicability (Bak et al., 2016).

In a sense, these dynamic models are more sophisticated versions of diathesis–stress models, incorporating architectural features of a system, feedback loops and interactive effects between symptoms, which raises a number of issues: what factors determine why transitions occur at particular points in time? What is it about *particular* stressors and not others that trigger system change? Why does a system manifest particular clusters of symptoms (e.g. psychotic or mood symptoms) rather than other symptom clusters? There may be architectural features of the system and biopsychosocial interactions within the system (e.g. hypothalamic-pituitary-adrenal (HPA) axis dysregulation interacting with cognitive biases) that prime it for reacting to stressors in a particular way (resulting in emergence of a certain type or intensity of symptoms over others). Metacognition (i.e. the individual's *reaction* to symptoms) is also of relevance and may introduce cascading or self-reinforcing cycles, although possibly also present opportunities for recovery and resilience (Lysaker et al., 2011).

From a practical point of view, baseline prediction (the snapshot model) is appealing because it would provide an opportunity based on an initial assessment to inform a patient of their level of risk for a particular disorder. However, there may be a limit to the utility and accuracy of this approach as it may not do justice to the dynamic and complex nature of psychopathology and the progression or regression of the illness. It may ultimately be most effective to supplement baseline prediction with repeated assessment (a time-series) of the person's psychopathology and other factors. From a treatment point of view, such longitudinal modelling would facilitate being able to identify 'danger times' or activate 'alerts' for possible mental state deterioration (analogous to a 'relapse signature'), either in the context of in-person therapy or via tools such as mobile phone applications. It also more closely mimics what actually happens in clinical practice: an initial impression of level of risk, which is updated and adjusted based on subsequent clinical contact (Yuen et al., 2018).

Conclusion

The models reviewed in this chapter show the benefits of engaging with cross-disciplinary approaches to modelling complex systems and present challenges to the current theoretical and analytical templates used in psychopathology prediction research. The ability to predict change from subthreshold- to threshold-level disorder (i.e. progression through stages of disorder), both on the group and individual level, may benefit from incorporating dynamic change into predictive modelling rather than relying on static data from a baseline assessment point. This requires enhanced understanding of the structural features of mental disorder and indicators of imminent system change. Future studies require study designs with repeat longitudinal assessment of relevant variables, achieved through either, or a combination of, micro- and macro-level assessments of psychopathology and other variables (e.g. neurocognition and neuroimaging). Ecological momentary assessment is a data collection technique appropriate for micro-level assessment. Relevant statistical approaches include joint modelling and time-series analysis, including metric- and model-based methods that draw on the mathematical principles of dynamical systems.

References

Arzouan, Y., Moses, E., Peled, A., & Levit-Binnun, N. (2014). Impaired network stability in schizophrenia revealed by TMS perturbations. *Schizophrenia Research*, **152** (1), 322–324.

Bak, M., Drukker, M., Hasmi, L., & van Os, J. (2016). An n=1 clinical network analysis of symptoms and treatment in psychosis. *PLoS One*, **11**(9), e0162811.

Bedi, G., Carrillo, F., Cecchi, G. A., Slezak, D. F., Sigman, M., Mota, N. B., . . . Corcoran, C. M. (2015). Automated analysis of free speech predicts psychosis onset in high-risk youths. *NPJ Schizophrenia*, **1**, 15030.

Birchwood, M. (1995). Early intervention in psychotic relapse: cognitive approaches to detection and management. *Behaviour Change*, **12**, 2–9.

Borsboom, D. (2017). A network theory of mental disorders. *World Psychiatry*, **16**(1), 5–13.

Borsboom, D., & Cramer, A. O. (2013). Network analysis: an integrative approach to the structure of psychopathology. *Annual Review of Clinical Psychology*, **9**, 91–121.

Bystritsky, A., Nierenberg, A. A., Feusner, J. D., & Rabinovich, M. (2012). Computational non-linear dynamical psychiatry: a new methodological paradigm for diagnosis and course of illness. *Journal of Psychiatric Research, 46*(4), 428–435.

Cannon, T. D., Yu, C., Addington, J., Bearden, C. E., Cadenhead, K. S., Cornblatt, B. A., ... Kattan, M. W. (2016). An individualized risk calculator for research in prodromal psychosis. *American Journal of Psychiatry, 173*(10), 980–988.

Carpenter, S. R., Cole, J. J., Pace, M. L., Batt, R., Brock, W. A., Cline, T., ... Weidel, B. (2011). Early warnings of regime shifts: a whole-ecosystem experiment. *Science, 332*(6033), 1079–1082.

Conrad, K. (1958). *Die beginnende Schizophrenie. Versuch einer Gestaltanalyse des Wahns.* Stuttgart: Thieme.

Dai, L., Vorselen, D., Korolev, K. S., & Gore, J. (2012). Generic indicators for loss of resilience before a tipping point leading to population collapse. *Science, 336*(6085), 1175–1177.

Dunlop, P., Clark, C. D., & Hindmarsh, R. C. A. (2008). Bed ribbing instability explanation: testing a numerical model of ribbed moraine formation arising from coupled flow of ice and subglacial sediment. *Journal of Geophysical Research: Earth Surface, 113*(F3), F03005.

Early Warning Signals Toolbox. What is a critical transition? Retrieved from www.early-warning-signals.org/theory/what-is-a-critical-transition.

Fowler, A. C. (2010a). The formation of subglacial streams and mega-scale glacial lineations. *Proceedings of the Royal Society A: Mathematical Physical and Engineering Sciences, 466*(2123), 3181–3201.

Fowler, A. C. (2010b). The instability theory of drumlin formation applied to Newtonian viscous ice of finite depth. *Proceedings of the Royal Society A: Mathematical Physical and Engineering Sciences, 466*(2121), 2673–2694.

Fusar-Poli, P., Borgwardt, S., Bechdolf, A., Addington, J., Riecher-Rossler, A., Schultze-Lutter, F., ... Yung, A. (2013). The psychosis high-risk state: a comprehensive state-of-the-art review. *JAMA Psychiatry, 70*(1), 107–120.

Fusar-Poli, P., & Schultze-Lutter, F. (2016). Predicting the onset of psychosis in patients at clinical high risk: practical guide to probabilistic prognostic reasoning. *Evidence Based Mental Health, 19*(1), 10–15.

Gharibzadeh, S., Zendehrouh, S., Vafadoost, M., & Bakouie, F. (2011). Is the functional state of schizophrenic patients located in the vicinity of a bifurcation point? *Journal of Neuropsychiatry and Clinical Neurosciences, 23*(2), E11.

Globus, G. G., & Arpaia, J. P. (1994). Psychiatry and the new dynamics. *Biological Psychiatry, 35*(5), 352–364.

Guloksuz, S., Pries, L. K., & van Os, J. (2017). Application of network methods for understanding mental disorders: pitfalls and promise. *Psychological Medicine, 47*(16), 2743–2752.

Hartmann, J., Nelson, B., Ratheesh, A., Treen, D., & McGorry, P. D. (2019). At-risk studies and clinical antecedents of psychosis, bipolar disorder and depression: a scoping review in the context of clinical staging. *Psychological Medicine, 49*(2), 177–189.

Hartmann, J., Nelson, B., Spooner, R., Amminger, G. P., Chanen, A., Davey, C. G., ... McGorry, P. D. (in press). Broad clinical high-risk mental state (CHARMS): methodology of a cohort study validating criteria for pluripotent risk. *Early Intervention in Psychiatry*, in press.

Hickie, I. B., Scott, E. M., Hermens, D. F., Naismith, S. L., Guastella, A. J., Kaur, M., ... McGorry, P. D. (2013). Applying clinical staging to young people who present for mental health care. *Early Intervention in Psychiatry, 7*(1), 31–43.

Hofmann, S. G., Curtiss, J., & McNally, R. J. (2016). A complex network perspective on clinical science. *Perspectives on Psychological Science, 11*(5), 597–605.

Isvoranu, A. M., Borsboom, D., van Os, J., & Guloksuz, S. (2016). A network approach to environmental impact in psychotic disorder: brief theoretical framework. *Schizophrenia Bulletin, 42*(4), 870–873.

Isvoranu, A. M., van Borkulo, C. D., Boyette, L. L., Wigman, J. T., Vinkers, C. H., Borsboom, D.; Group Investigators. (2017). A network approach to psychosis: pathways between childhood trauma and psychotic symptoms. *Schizophrenia Bulletin, 43*(1), 187–196.

Jaspers, K. (1963). *General psychopathology.* Trans. J. H. a. M. W. Hamilton. Chicago, IL: University of Chicago Press.

Koutsouleris, N., Meisenzahl, E. M., Davatzikos, C., Bottlender, R., Frodl, T., Scheuerecker, J., . . . Gaser, C. (2009). Use of neuroanatomical pattern classification to identify subjects in at-risk mental states of psychosis and predict disease transition. *Archives of General Psychiatry, 66*(7), 700–712.

Lenton, T. M. (2011). Early warning of climate tipping points. *Nature Climate Change, 1,* 201–209.

Levit-Binnun, N., Litvak, V., Pratt, H., Moses, E., Zaroor, M., & Peled, A. (2010). Differences in TMS-evoked responses between schizophrenia patients and healthy controls can be observed without a dedicated EEG system. *Clinical Neurophysiology, 121*(3), 332–339.

Loh, M., Rolls, E. T., & Deco, G. (2007). A dynamical systems hypothesis of schizophrenia. *PLoS Computational Biology, 3*(11), e228.

Lysaker, P. H., Dimaggio, G., Buck, K. D., Callaway, S. S., Salvatore, G., Carcione, A., . . . Stanghellini, G. (2011). Poor insight in schizophrenia: links between different forms of metacognition with awareness of symptoms, treatment need, and consequences of illness. *Comprehensive Psychiatry, 52*(3), 253–260.

Mandell, A. J., & Selz, K. A. (1992). Dynamical systems in psychiatry: now what? *Biological Psychiatry, 32*(4), 299–301.

McGorry, P. D. (2007). Issues for DSM-V: clinical staging – a heuristic pathway to valid nosology and safer, more effective treatment in psychiatry. *American Journal of Psychiatry, 164*(6), 859–860.

McGorry, P. D. (2010). Risk syndromes, clinical staging and DSM V: new diagnostic infrastructure for early intervention in psychiatry. *Schizophrenia Research, 120*(1–3), 49–53.

McGorry, P. D. (2013). Early clinical phenotypes, clinical staging, and strategic biomarker research: building blocks for personalized psychiatry. *Biological Psychiatry, 74*(6), 394–395.

McGorry, P. D., Hickie, I. B., Yung, A. R., Pantelis, C., & Jackson, H. J. (2006). Clinical staging of psychiatric disorders: a heuristic framework for choosing earlier, safer and more effective interventions. *Australian and New Zealand Journal of Psychiatry, 40*(8), 616–622.

McGorry, P., & Nelson, B. (2016). Why we need a transdiagnostic staging approach to emerging psychopathology, early diagnosis, and treatment. *JAMA Psychiatry, 73*(3), 191–192.

McGorry, P., & van Os, J. (2013). Redeeming diagnosis in psychiatry: timing versus specificity. *Lancet, 381*(9863), 343–345.

Minkowski, E. (1926). *La Notion de Perte de Contact Vital avec la Réalité et ses Applications en Psychopathologie.* Paris: Jouve & Cie.

Myin-Germeys, I., Oorschot, M., Collip, D., Lataster, J., Delespaul, P., & van Os, J. (2009). Experience sampling research in psychopathology: opening the black box of daily life. *Psychological Medicine, 39*(9), 1533–1547.

Nelson, B., McGorry, P. D., Wichers, M., Wigman, J. T. W., & Hartmann, J. (2017). Moving from static to dynamic models of the onset of mental disorder. *JAMA Psychiatry, 74*(5), 528–534.

Odgers, C. L., Mulvey, E. P., Skeem, J. L., Gardner, W., Lidz, C. W., & Schubert, C. (2009). Capturing the ebb and flow of psychiatric symptoms with dynamical systems models. *American Journal of Psychiatry, 166*(5), 575–582.

Olde Rikkert, M. G., Dakos, V., Buchman, T. G., Boer, R., Glass, L., Cramer, A. O., . . . Scheffer, M. (2016). Slowing down of recovery as generic risk marker for acute severity transitions in chronic diseases. *Critical Care Medicine, 44*(3), 601–606.

Parnas, J., & Henriksen, M. G. (2014). Disordered self in the schizophrenia spectrum: a clinical and research perspective. *Harvard Review of Psychiatry,* **22**(5), 251–265.

Paulus, M. P., & Braff, D. L. (2003). Chaos and schizophrenia: does the method fit the madness? *Biological Psychiatry,* **53**, 3–11.

Poston, T., & Steward, I. (1978). *Catastrophe theory and its applications.* London: Pitman.

Scheffer, M. (2009). *Critical transitions in nature and society.* Princeton, NJ: Princeton University Press.

Scheffer, M. (2010). Complex systems: foreseeing tipping points. *Nature,* **467**(7314), 411–412.

Scheffer, M., Carpenter, S. R., Lenton, T. M., Bascompte, J., Brock, W., Dakos, V., . . . Vandermeer, J. (2012). Anticipating critical transitions. *Science,* **338**(6105), 344–348.

Schultze-Lutter, F. (2009). Subjective symptoms of schizophrenia in research and the clinic: the basic symptoms concept. *Schizophrenia Bulletin,* **35**(1), 5–8.

Scott, D. W. (1985). Catastrophe theory applications in clinical psychology: a review. *Current Psychological Research and Reviews,* **4**(1), 69–86.

Strobl, E. V., Eack, S. M., Swaminathan, V., & Visweswaran, S. (2012). Predicting the risk of psychosis onset: advances and prospects. *Early Intervention in Psychiatry,* **6**(4), 368–379.

Tschacher, W., Scheier, C., & Hashimoto, Y. (1997). Dynamical analysis of schizophrenia courses. *Biological Psychiatry,* **41**(4), 428–437.

van Borkulo, C., Boschloo, L., Borsboom, D., Penninx, B. W., Waldorp, L. J., & Schoevers, R. A. (2015). Association of symptom network structure with the course of longitudinal depression. *JAMA Psychiatry,* **72** (12), 1219–1226.

van de Leemput, I. A., Wichers, M., Cramer, A. O. J., Borsboom, D., Tuerlinckx, F., Kuppens, P., . . . Scheffer, M. (2014). Critical slowing down as early warning for the onset and termination of depression. *Proceedings of the National Academy of Sciences of the United States of America,* **111**(1), 87–92.

van Os, J. (2013). The dynamics of subthreshold psychopathology: implications for diagnosis and treatment. *American Journal of Psychiatry,* **170**(7), 695–698.

van Os, J., & Linscott, R. J. (2012). Introduction: the extended psychosis phenotype – relationship with schizophrenia and with ultrahigh risk status for psychosis. *Schizophrenia Bulletin,* **38**(2), 227–230.

Veraart, A. J., Faassen, E. J., Dakos, V., van Nes, E. H., Lurling, M., & Scheffer, M. (2012). Recovery rates reflect distance to a tipping point in a living system. *Nature,* **481**(7381), 357–359.

Vinogradov, S., King, R. J., & Huberman, B. A. (1992). An associationist model of the paranoid process: application of phase transitions in spreading activation networks. *Psychiatry,* **55**(1), 79–94.

Wichers, M. (2014). The dynamic nature of depression: a new micro-level perspective of mental disorder that meets current challenges. *Psychological Medicine,* **44**(7), 1349–1360.

Wichers, M., Groot, P. C., & Psychosystems, ESM Group, EWS Group. (2016). Critical slowing down as a personalized early warning signal for depression. *Psychotherapy and Psychosomatics,* **85**(2), 114–116.

Wichers, M., Wigman, J. T. W., & Myin-Germeys, I. (2015). Micro-level affect dynamics in psychopathology viewed from complex dynamical system theory. *Emotion Review,* 7(4), 362–367.

Wigman, J. T., Collip, D., Wichers, M., Delespaul, P., Derom, C., Thiery, E., . . . van Os, J. (2013a). Altered transfer of momentary mental states (ATOMS) as the basic unit of psychosis liability in interaction with environment and emotions. *PLoS One,* **8**(2), e54653.

Wigman, J. T. W., van Os, J., Thiery, E., Derom, C., Collip, D., Jacobs, N., & Wichers, M. (2013b). Psychiatric diagnosis revisited: towards a system of staging and profiling combining nomothetic and idiographic parameters of momentary mental states. *PLoS One, 8*(3), e59559.

Yuen, H. P., & Mackinnon, A. (2016). Performance of joint modelling of time-to-event data with time-dependent predictors: an assessment based on transition to psychosis data. *PeerJ, 4,* e2582.

Yuen, H. P., Mackinnon, A., & Nelson, B. (2018). A new method for analysing transition to psychosis: joint modelling of time-to-event outcome with time-dependent predictors. *International Journal of Methods in Psychiatric Research, 27*(1), e1588.

Yung, A. R., Nelson, B., Thompson, A., & Wood, S. J. (2010). The psychosis threshold in ultra high risk (prodromal) research: is it valid? *Schizophrenia Research, 120*(1–3), 1–6.

The Utility of Clinical Staging in Youth Mental Health Settings
Neurobiological and Longitudinal Data from Sydney-Based Studies of Transdiagnostic Cohorts

Ian B. Hickie, Joanne S. Carpenter, Frank Iorfino, Elizabeth Scott, Shane Cross and Daniel F. Hermens

Introduction

Internationally, there is widespread recognition of the premature death and disability attributable to major mental disorders, and most notably the anxiety, mood and psychotic disorders (Bloom et al., 2012; Erskine et al., 2015; Gustavsson et al., 2011). The burden derives from their early age of onset, population prevalence, chronicity, comorbidity with physical illness and the degree of resultant impairment (Gore et al., 2011; Gustavsson et al., 2011; Lopez et al., 2006). To reduce that burden, earlier identification and enhanced long-term care of those who are at risk of developing, or are in the early phases of life-threatening or chronic disorders has been prioritised (Hickie et al., 2013c; Insel, 2007; 2009; Lopez et al., 2006; McGorry et al., 2014; Scott et al., 2012).

For the major anxiety, mood or psychotic disorders, a progressive illness trajectory typically has its onset in late childhood or early puberty and then recurs or continues progressively into adult life (Hafner et al., 2008; Merikangas et al., 2010; Paus et al., 2008). Although 75 per cent of major mental disorders begin before the age of 25 years (Gore et al., 2011), current diagnostic and research criteria used to identify these subjects are derived largely from the experiences reported by middle-aged persons with recurring or chronic illness. These mid-life phenotypes often map poorly onto earlier and often less specific phases of the illness experience (Hickie et al., 2013c; McGorry, 2007; 2010; McGorry et al., 2008). Our current research systems also assume that multiple parallel pathways or pathophysiologies underpin each 'independent' or 'clinical' category – an assumption which is not readily supported by modern family, genetic and neurobiological risk factor studies (Buckholtz & Meyer-Lindenberg, 2012; Lichtenstein et al., 2009; Sullivan et al., 2012; Waszczuk et al., 2014).

Diagnostic symptom sets for 'single' disorders prioritise phenomena such as delusions, hallucinations, periods of elevated mood or increased energy, psychomotor slowing, emotional blunting or cognitive slowing for schizophrenia, bipolar disorder or severe depression. Data from recent community studies that assess subjects longitudinally from childhood or adolescence, however, emphasise the extent to which many of these phenomena are shared, both at onset and across the whole illness trajectory (Copeland et al., 2013; Kelleher et al., 2012; Merikangas et al., 2008; 2010; 2012; Murray & Jones, 2012; Ormel et al., 2015). Additionally, earlier risk states such as anxiety, conduct and developmental disorders that are evident in children before age 12 years predict the full spectrum of later depressive, bipolar and psychotic disorders (Kim-Cohen et al., 2003). Our great clinical challenge is to derive new dynamic diagnostic systems that are not only consistent with developmental epidemiology and neurobiology but also useful when applied in everyday clinical practice.

A major response to this challenge has been to apply the general medical concept of clinical staging in mental health practice. In other areas of medicine, it is commonly accepted that it is totally inadequate to choose treatments, or plan health care, for persons who suffer from conditions that are likely to progress or recur simply on the basis of a broad illness category (e.g. breast cancer or cardiovascular disease). We suggest that it is equally meaningless in mental health to expect to plan preventive or early intervention strategies or select specific treatments on the basis of recognition of broad categories such as schizophrenia, bipolar disorder or major depression. There is indeed a wealth of evidence indicating that subjects at different points along the illness continuum of all of these conditions show quite different patterns of response to various psychological or pharmacological interventions (McGorry et al., 2006; 2007; Scott, 2011; Scott et al., 2006). Consequently, we have proposed a general framework for clinical staging (see Chapter 2) that can be applied to the more severe mood or psychotic disorders (Hickie et al., 2013c; McGorry et al., 2006).

Utilising Clinical Staging Framework in Youth Mental Health Services

The clinical staging framework, when applied to young people (ages 12–30) presenting for health care, proposes that earlier stages are characterised by lower rates of impairment and predict lower risk of progression to later, more severe, disabling or persistent disorders. We apply this framework to young people who present for health care and clearly differentiate those in early phases (Stages 1a 'seeking help' or 1b 'attenuated syndromes') from those who have reached a higher threshold for disorder (Stage 2 and above). Within the earlier (and assumed typically non-progressive) Stage 1 disorders we differentiate the 'attenuated syndromes' (which often meet DSM-4 or -5 or ICD-10 criteria for specific anxiety or mood disorders) from the more non-specific anxiety and depressive syndromes. A simple and reliable decision-tree (Figure 5.1) for making these key distinctions is incorporated in our clinical practice systems. We have previously demonstrated the inter-rater reliability of this structured approach (Hickie et al., 2013c). Where there is uncertainty about the appropriate stage to assign, we rate down to the earlier and less severe category.

A Transdiagnostic Approach

Importantly, the approach we have undertaken (Hickie et al., 2013c; 2013d; Scott et al., 2013b; Scott et al., 2014) is consistent with that proposed by the National Institute of Mental Health (NIMH) developed 'Research Domain Criteria' (Cuthbert & Insel, 2013; Insel et al., 2010; Kozak & Cuthbert, 2016). That is, establishing new ways for classifying mental disorders based on correlations with independent neurobiological measures. These approaches also place an appropriate emphasis on recognising developmental trajectories and the active bidirectional impacts of interaction with the environment.

Further, our emphasis on non-selective recruitment from enhanced primary care and youth-focused service environments is consistent with the recommendations by NIMH's Bruce Cuthbert (Casey et al., 2013) that such research should recruit cohorts from common service settings that are likely to also demonstrate appropriate variance along relevant dimensions of interest (e.g. neuropsychological function, cortical or subcortical brain structure).

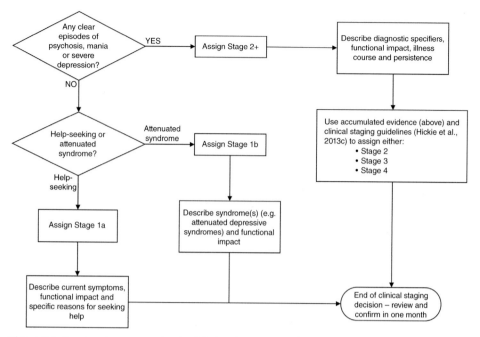

Figure 5.1 The stepwise process taken in clinical services to assign those presenting to care to the appropriate stage.

The Brain and Mind Youth Cohorts (BMYC)

Over the last decade, we have continuously recruited young people from our enhanced primary care and youth-focused mental health services to cross-sectional, longitudinal and interventional studies, with concurrent participation in relevant neuropsychological, brain imaging, circadian and metabolic assessments. This cohort has unique characteristics in terms of its: (1) size; (2) emphasis on early clinical phases of illness; (3) recruitment based on presentation for services rather than specific anxiety, mood or psychotic diagnoses; (4) patterns of comorbidity; and (5) concurrent collection of relevant neurobiological data.

Outcomes of BMYC Cases

A key aspect of our work with the BMYC has been to articulate a multidimensional outcomes framework (Figure 5.2). This framework recognises the key domains of interest in our youth-focused early intervention work. Most importantly, the domain that has dominated most research work in the early psychosis field, namely transition from 'at-risk' states to 'full-threshold' psychotic syndromes (i.e. mental illness trajectory) constitutes only one of our concerns here. In fact, within a transdiagnostic perspective, transition from earlier to later stages (rather than transition within one narrow diagnostic category) is the equivalent concept. In our work, the key 'clinical transition' is from Stage 1b to Stage 2.

Much of our work in this area has placed much greater emphasis on the other major outcome domains, notably the longitudinal course of functional impairment. As we recruit broadly, we are then able to examine the relative predictive power of specific diagnostic

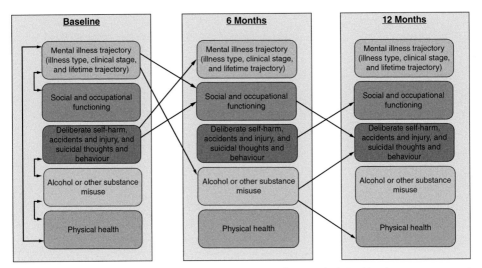

Figure 5.2 Multidimensional outcome domains and examples of potential relationships that operate across the various domains over time.

features as compared with other key aspects, such as neuropsychological function or patterns of comorbidity.

Cross-Sectional and Longitudinal Validation of the Clinical Staging Framework

We have reported extensively on the demographic, clinical (illness type and stage), disability, neuropsychological, brain imaging, and circadian characteristics of this cohort (see Table 5.1).

Our initial studies have utilised both cross-sectional data with regards to social participation, educational and employment status and longitudinal outcome data characterising clinical course to test the construct and predictive validity of the clinical staging model in this relevant population. First, with regards to levels of impairment, there is clear support across our various studies that earlier stages are associated with lower degrees of functional impairment. This is not unexpected as the clinical phenotype used for staging purposes is, to some degree, inclusive of current levels of function.

Second, it has also been relevant in our studies to determine the extent to which the clinical staging system is a better predictor of functional impairment than classical diagnostic systems in this population. Typically, those who work with clinical cohorts that are older with more persistent or recurring disorders, and are also limited to those with more distinct 'bipolar' or 'psychotic/schizophrenia' (having excluded those with other relevant comorbid patterns of developmental difficulties, personality disturbance, repeated self-harm, alcohol or other substance misuse or physical health problems) expect that specific diagnoses will be more predictive of functional impairment, longitudinal course or independent neurobiological phenomena (see below). In our view, these important differences are a consequence of the differences in sampling frameworks; we focus on early phases of disorder and *include* all relevant clinical (i.e. 'transdiagnostic') presentations.

Table 5.1 Key publications linking clinical stage with demographic, clinical (illness type), disability, neuropsychological, brain imaging, and circadian characteristics of the BMYC

Study design		Authors	Sample (stage, n)	Key results	Other relevant information
Clinical	Cross-Sectional	Hamilton et al. (2011)	1a = 110; 1b = 126; 2 = 47; 3+ = 24	Distress, disability and socio-occupational functioning all gradually worsened with higher stages of illness	Age and gender did not predict clinical stage
		Scott et al. (2012)	1a = 293; 1b = 292; 2 = 121; 3+ = 133	Clinician-rated SOFAS strongly related to stages; later stages having more impaired role function	Stage 2 had highest levels of distress and role function impairment
		Hickie et al. (2013a)	1b = 286; 2+ = 289	Impairments in functioning and general behavioural disturbance were less marked in Stages 1b cf. 2+	Interaction between stage and tripartite classification; 1b less common in developmental psychosis
		Purcell et al. (2015)	1a = 285; 1b = 412; 2+ = 96	Stage 1a better than Stages 1b and 2+ on all symptom and functioning scores	Stages 1b & 2+ comparable on all measures (except CGI, SOFAS)
	Longitudinal	Hickie et al. (2013c)	1a = 21; 1b = 112; 2+ = 53	Transition (median = 48 weeks): 11 per cent of Stage 1a; 19 per cent of Stage 1b; 33 per cent of Stage 2	Those who remained within the same stage may have had persistent symptoms/dysfunction or responded to clinical interventions
		Cross et al. (2016)	1a = 601; 1b = 257; 2+ = 31	Psychological distress (K10) and SOFAS improved over 1 to 6 to 10 sessions of care for both Stages 1b and 1a	Stage 1b remained impaired after 10 sessions; Stage 1a commenced with better SOFAS, less psychological distress
		Cross et al. (2017a)	1a = 579; 1b = 249	Stage 1b made and missed more appointments than Stage 1a	Social functioning best predictor of female attendance; age and stage best predicted male attendance

Table 5.1 (cont.)

Study design		Authors	Sample (stage, n)	Key results	Other relevant information
		Cross et al. (2017b)	1b = 243	About 17 per cent experienced transition to a major mental disorder. Independent of syndromal diagnosis, transition more likely in NEET cases, females and those with more negative psychological symptoms (e.g. social withdrawal)	NEET status and negative symptoms are modifiable predictors of illness trajectory across diagnostic categories and are not specific to transition to psychosis
		Cross et al. (2018)	1b = 243	Approx. one-quarter to one-quarter of Stage 1b showed reliable improvement and approx. 10 per cent showed reliable deterioration for both symptoms (K10 and BPRS) and functioning (SOFAS) over six months. Many individuals did not show linear improvement or deterioration	Individual patterns of symptomatic and functional change are diverse in this group over time, highlighting the importance of routine outcome monitoring in treatment
Neuropsychological	Cross-sectional	Hermens et al. (2013)	1b = 94; 2+ = 100	Stage 2+ had most impaired neuropsychological profile; Stage 1b had intermediate profile (cf. controls)	Greatest impairments in verbal memory and executive functioning
	Longitudinal	Tickell et al. (in press)	1b = 262; 2+ = 235	Baseline: Stage 2+ worse than Stage 1b in verbal learning, verbal memory, visual memory, set-shifting. Both showed stability in processing speed, sustained attention and visual memory at follow-up	Neuropsychological stability corresponded with stability in clinical and functional status, despite stage of illness

Domain	Study design	Study	Sample	Findings	
Neuroimaging	Cross-sectional	Lagopoulos et al. (2012)	1b = 23; 2+ = 24	Stage 2+ had decreased GM in frontal brain regions cf. Stage 1b	Cf. controls, Stage 1b showed similar pattern of GM loss, albeit not to the same degree as their peers in Stage 2+
		Lagopoulos et al. (2013)	1b = 73; 2+ = 69	Both Stages 1b and 2+ showed reduced WM integrity in left ACR; Stage 2+ had additional demyelination	ACR = junction point of three major long association fibres; impacts projections from thalamus to frontal lobes
Circadian	Cross-sectional	Naismith et al. (2012)	1b = 28; 2+ = 16	Stage 2+ had markedly reduced levels of melatonin secretion cf. their peers in 1b	In Stage 2+ only, reduced melatonin correlated with poorer verbal memory
		Scott et al. (2016)	1a = 18; 1b = 82; 2+ = 54	Delayed sleep phase (weekdays) increased progressively across illness stages	Older age, medication & later sleep offset strongest predictors of later stage

SOFAS, Social and Occupational Functioning Assessment Scale; CGI, Clinical Global Impression scale; K10, Kessler Psychological Distress Scale; NEET, not in education, employment or training; BPRS, Brief Psychiatric Rating Scale; GM, grey matter; WM, white matter; ACR, anterior thalamic radiation.

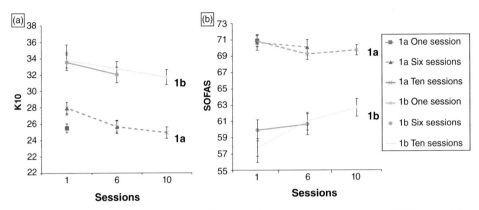

Figure 5.3 Psychological distress (K10, panel (a)) and social and occupational functioning (SOFAS, panel (b)) following one, six or ten sessions of treatment in individuals classified as Stage 1a and 1b at baseline, from Cross et al. (2016). Reproduced with permission.

Our preliminary longitudinal work using this clinical staging system, among subjects who present to our primary care services typically with severe mood or anxiety disorders, indicates that in the short term, those initially classified as Stage 1b remain significantly impaired following ten sessions of treatment despite using more services and improving modestly (Figure 5.3). Within 12 months, approximately 17 per cent of those rated as Stage 1b at initial assessment progress to a later stage (despite receiving clinical care) (Cross et al., 2017b). A significant proportion of these 'clinical transitions' occur within the first three months, indicating the need for very close clinical supervision and monitoring following initial presentation. The transition rate varies between pathophysiological pathways; 11 per cent for depression, 40 per cent for psychosis and 22 per cent for bipolar (Cross et al., 2017b). Regardless of the pathway, transition was found to be predicted by NEET (not in education, employment or training) status (Figure 5.4) and negative symptoms, and not by general psychological distress (K10) or positive symptoms, which is consistent with findings from other studies (Fusar-Poli et al., 2010; Valmaggia et al., 2013).

Beyond the risks associated with the initial clinical episode, however, the ongoing risks are significant. In our ongoing longitudinal studies, which focus on those who have an ongoing need for clinical care, such 'clinical transitions' continue to occur over the next 3–5 years in a large subpopulation of the initial cohort. Within these studies, one can map the changes in functional outcomes as a function of the initial clinical stage (Figure 5.5). These patterns of initial and ongoing functional impairment support preliminary construct and predictive validation of the clinical staging model. Of considerable interest, those initially classified as Stage 2+ demonstrated the most sustained improvement over the longer-term clinical follow-up (with 29 per cent improving at least 10 points on SOFAS from baseline to time last seen, as compared to 15 per cent of Stage 1b and 13 per cent of Stage 1a) – presumably reflecting greater engagement with long-term and more specialised care.

To advance this work and, more specifically, to plan relevant early intervention and secondary prevention trials, we need to identify more accurately those who may be at particularly high risk of illness progression. Our related work (Scott et al., 2013a; Scott et al., 2014) focusing on identifying those subjects in the early course of bipolar disorder has

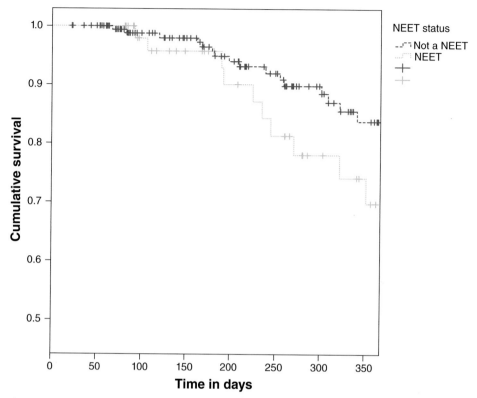

Figure 5.4 Kaplan–Meier curve representing time to transition in groups defined by NEET (not in education, employment or training) status at baseline, from Cross et al. (2017b). Reproduced with permission.

indicated how difficult this is to achieve on the basis of clinical features or neuropsychological testing. Specifically, one study has highlighted the importance of family history of bipolar disorder, psychosis or substance misuse in predicting this transition (Scott et al., 2013a).

Neurocognitive and Neuroimaging Evidence to Support Staging

We have conducted a number of studies to determine whether there are neurobiological features that distinguish key stages of illness. To date, these studies have utilised neuroimaging (Lagopoulos et al., 2012; 2013), sleep/circadian (Naismith et al., 2012; Scott et al., 2016) and neuropsychological (Hermens et al., 2013; Tickell et al., in press) measures. Across these studies, consistent with a neuroprogressive model of illness, the data show that while those with an attenuated syndrome (compared to controls) have reduced grey matter volumes (Figure 5.6a), compromised white matter integrity (Figure 5.6b), delayed sleep phase (see Figure 5.7) and reductions in neuropsychological performance, their peers at later stages of illness (i.e. with discrete disorders) have significantly greater deficits across these domains. Furthermore, these differences were generally in the absence of any differences in clinical (including diagnosis, clinical state) and functional (e.g. socio-occupational) measures, suggesting that the staging model has utility in terms of distinguishing putative phenotypes, particularly with respect to underlying neurobiology. It should be noted that

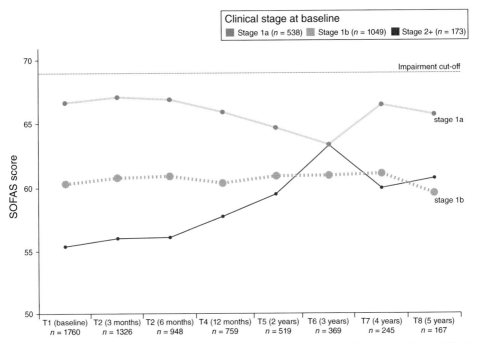

Figure 5.5 Longitudinal change in mean SOFAS scores during care in those classified as Stage 1a (n = 538), 1b (n = 1049) and 2+ (n = 173) at baseline.

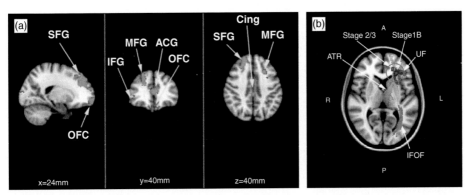

Figure 5.6 (a) Grey matter volume changes in Stage 1 versus Stage 2+ subjects (regions of grey matter loss are in green). SFG = superior frontal gyrus; OFC = orbitofrontal cortex; IFG = inferior frontal gyrus; MFG = middle frontal gyrus; ACG = anterior cingulate gyrus; Cing = cingulate, from Lagopoulos et al. (2012). (b) Graphical overlay of the fractional anisotropy results for Stage 1b (red) and Stage 2+ (blue) subjects along with the coregistered fibre tracts for anterior thalamic radiation (ATR), inferior fronto-occipital fasciculus (IFOF) and uncinate fasciculus (UF), from Lagopoulos et al. (2013). *A black and white version of this figure will appear in some formats. For the colour version, please refer to the plate section.*

these studies focused on the two major stages of illness in our cohort, that being attenuated syndrome (1b) and discrete disorder (2+). The other stages within our model, that is, help-seeking (Stage 1a) and persistent/unremitting (Stage 4), were intentionally not included in these studies because our aim was to determine the neurocognitive and neurobiological features that occur around the major demarcation point in these syndromes.

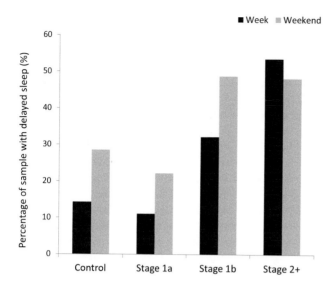

Figure 5.7 Percentages of individuals with a delayed sleep phase profile in each stage group. Results from the chi-square analyses indicated a significant difference for week (χ^2 (3 df) = 17.3, p = 0.001), but not weekend days (χ^2 (3 df) = 7.3, p = 0.063), from Scott et al. (2016). Reproduced with permission.

Hermens et al. (2013) examined the neuropsychological profiles between young people based on attenuated syndromes (n = 94) compared to those with discrete disorders (n = 100). The latter showed the most impaired neuropsychological profile, with the earlier Stage (1b) group showing an intermediate profile, compared to controls. Greatest impairments were seen in verbal memory and executive functioning. To address potential confounds created by 'diagnosis', profiles for those with a mood syndrome or disorder but not psychosis were also examined and the neuropsychological impairments for the Stage 2/3 group remained. Thus, the degree of neuropsychological impairment discriminated those with attenuated syndromes from those with a discrete disorder, independent of diagnostic status and current symptoms. Our findings support the notion that neuropsychological assessment is a key tool of clinical evaluation in early stages of major psychiatric illness in young adults. Other studies from our group have illustrated the nature of neuropsychological functioning as a strong predictor of functioning longitudinally, over and above psychiatric symptomatology (Lee et al., 2013; 2014; 2015). Additionally, more recent studies examining subjects at risk of schizophrenia identified neuropsychological dysfunction as a potential risk factor for illness onset/transition (e.g. executive function, verbal fluency, attention, visual memory, verbal memory and working memory) (Lin et al., 2013; Maziade et al., 2011; Sumiyoshi et al., 2013).

As a follow-up to our first staging by neuropsychology study, we examined a larger sample (n = 497) of help-seeking young people (aged 21.2 ± 3 years; 56 per cent female) of whom 262 were rated as 'attenuated syndrome' (Stage 1b) and 235 as 'discrete' or 'persistent' disorder (Stage 2+) at baseline (Tickell et al., in press). Of this sample, 170 individuals (54 per cent at Stage 1b) were reassessed neuropsychologically after 19.8 ± 9 months (range: 3–51 months). We found that at baseline the attenuated and discrete/persistent disorder groups significantly differed in four of the nine neuropsychological measures (verbal learning, verbal memory, visual memory and set-shifting). Despite this, both groups showed similar stability in neuropsychological functioning at follow-up, particularly in processing speed, sustained attention and visual memory. Furthermore, longitudinal stability in cognition corresponded with increases in socio-occupational functioning.

Importantly, we found again (note: there was a 38 per cent overlap in the baseline sample with our previous study; Hermens et al., 2013) that the degree of baseline neuropsychological dysfunction discriminated those with attenuated syndromes from those with a discrete/persistent disorder. Furthermore, stability in neuropsychological functioning corresponded with stability in clinical and functional status, despite stage of illness. This suggests that neuropsychological functioning remains relatively stable in young people with a mental illness and may be a critical window for intervention.

We conducted two neuroimaging studies to examine whether attenuated syndrome and discrete disorder patient groups could be distinguished in terms of grey matter (GM) and white matter (WM) integrity. Findings from a voxel-based morphometry study (Lagopoulos et al., 2012) revealed that compared to Stage 1B patients ($n = 23$) and controls ($n = 33$), the Stage 2+ patients ($n = 24$) were found to have decreased GM volumes within distributed frontal brain regions. The greatest GM loss for Stage 2+ occurred within an overlapping region bounded by the superior and middle frontal gyri on the right side. Additional loss of GM volume was also observed in the inferior aspects of the frontal gyrus as well as the anterior cingulate and the orbitofrontal cortex on the right side and the medial prefrontal cortex midline. Of note, we did not find any evidence of GM loss that extended outside the prefrontal cortex. Overall the findings of this study suggested that, in terms of frontal GM changes, a major transition point may occur in the course of affective illness between early attenuated syndromes and later discrete illness stages (see Figure 5.6a).

In a subsequent study (Lagopoulos et al., 2013) we examined WM integrity – more specifically, fractional anisotropy in $n = 74$ patients in Stage 1b as well as in $n = 69$ patients in Stage 2+, and these were contrasted with $n = 39$ healthy controls. Interestingly, we found a significant disruption in WM integrity in the left anterior corona radiata and in particular the anterior thalamic radiation for both the patients groups when separately contrasted with healthy controls (see Figure 5.6b). Our results suggested that patients with sub-syndromal symptoms exhibit discernible early WM changes when compared with healthy controls and more significant disruptions are associated with clinical evidence of illness progression.

Despite limitations (i.e. mainly cross-sectional studies, relatively small sample sizes and the potential effects of medication), collectively these studies are consistent with a progression-of-illness model. Across these studies the overall pattern was that Stages 1b and 2+ groups did not differ in their current levels of functioning (SOFAS) nor clinical symptomatology (depression ratings, psychological distress, etc.) nor the proportions being treated with antidepressants.

Sleep and Circadian Evidence to Support Staging

Abnormalities in the sleep–wake cycle and circadian rhythms are found across a range of psychiatric disorders, and have been highlighted as potentially transdiagnostic factors (Benca et al., 1992; Dolsen et al., 2014; Harvey et al., 2011; Jones & Benca, 2015; Karatsoreos, 2014). Across adolescence and young adulthood, developmental changes in sleep–wake and circadian systems typically result in delayed sleep and circadian rhythms (Carpenter et al., 2015a; Gradisar et al., 2011), which may predispose the circadian system to be particularly vulnerable to perturbations across this period. In our cohort of young people, we have found that delays in sleep timing and increases in wakefulness across the night are found across multiple diagnoses (Robillard et al., 2015), and we have also found sleep–wake delays to be particularly prominent in adolescents and young adults (Robillard et al., 2014).

To examine sleep–wake cycles in young people at different stages of psychiatric illness, we used actigraphy monitoring to measure average rest and activity timing over multiple days of recording, and compared those with attenuated syndromes ($n = 82$), and those with discrete disorders ($n = 54$), to control participants ($n = 21$) (Scott et al., 2016). We found delayed sleep timing in both patient groups compared to controls, with more severe delays in those with discrete disorders (Stage 2+) compared to those with attenuated syndromes (Stage 1b). The proportion of individuals with a delayed sleep–wake profile also increased across illness stages (see Figure 5.7). In addition to being related to more established and severe illness stages, these sleep–wake delays may also be indicative of a more bipolar type of illness, with our research finding delayed sleep phase to be more common in those with bipolar syndromes (over 60 per cent) as compared to those with unipolar mood disorders (30 per cent) and controls (10 per cent) (Robillard et al., 2013a). These findings suggest that sleep–wake delays may be an important feature to distinguish between stage of illness as well as being potentially indicative of a specific illness phenotype characterised by circadian dysregulation and bipolar-type symptoms. We have also shown sleep–wake disturbances to be predictive of longitudinal outcomes in our cohort; Robillard et al. (2016) report on 50 young people with sleep–wake assessment (actigraphy) followed up after 11–47 months (average 18.9 months). This study found that lower sleep efficiency (i.e. more time spent awake during the night) was predictive of worsening of manic symptoms at follow-up, and both shorter sleep and poorer circadian rhythmicity of 24-hour activity patterns were predictive of worsening in verbal memory, demonstrating the utility of sleep–wake assessment in prediction of outcomes.

Disturbance of biological circadian systems is likely to underlie these delays of rest and activity behaviour, and we have investigated this by measuring melatonin levels prior to habitual sleep in a subset of participants. While we found no difference in the timing of melatonin secretion across stages of illness, those at Stage 2+ ($n = 16$) had reduced levels of evening melatonin as compared to those at Stage 1b ($n = 28$), and shorter phase angles (time differences) between melatonin onset and sleep onset (Naismith et al., 2012) (see Figure 5.8). Abnormal phase angles indicate that internal circadian rhythms may not be optimally timed in relation to each other or the external environment, which may be indicative of severe disruption to the circadian system. Reduced evening melatonin secretion may also be a result of circadian misalignment, or may be reflective of reduced circadian rhythm amplitude and weaker circadian signalling. These findings suggest that such disruptions are linked to stage of illness, and the circadian system may become increasingly disrupted with progression of illness. Notably, in this study we did not find any associations between melatonin measures and depressive symptoms, further suggesting that relationships with illness stage may be independent of current symptom levels (Naismith et al., 2012).

In concordance with the actigraphy findings, we have also found reduced evening melatonin in those with bipolar disorders as compared to unipolar depressive disorders, as well as relatively delayed melatonin profiles in those with bipolar disorders (Robillard et al., 2013b). This provides further support for a distinct circadian profile with delayed rhythms and links to bipolar type symptoms. However, it is important to note that while such a profile may be linked to bipolar type symptoms, it likely exists across multiple psychiatric diagnoses, rather than being linked to the strict traditional diagnosis of bipolar disorder. In support of this, we have used a data-driven technique to identify clusters of individuals in our cohort with similar sleep–wake profiles, and found these profiles to be

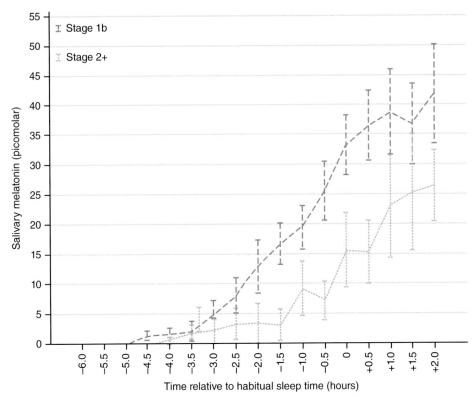

Figure 5.8 Graph demonstrating reduced salivary melatonin data (mean ± standard error) for patients with Stage 2+ affective disorders, relative to Stage 1b. According to prior actigraphy monitoring, habitual sleep onset would normally occur at sample 0. From Naismith et al. (2012).

distinct from traditional diagnostic categories (Carpenter et al., 2015b; 2017b). We found that those with a profile of delayed sleep show evidence of delayed biological circadian rhythms of melatonin and core temperature (Carpenter et al., 2017b), highlighting a biological basis of delayed sleep–wake presentations.

There is also evidence for interactions between sleep–wake and circadian abnormalities and neural structure and function in this cohort of young people with psychiatric disorders. We have observed links between sleep–wake and circadian disturbances and neuropsychological performance, with one study finding impaired visual memory in those with a profile of long sleep (Carpenter et al., 2015b), and another finding lower melatonin levels are related to poorer verbal memory functioning in those with discrete disorders (Naismith et al., 2012). An MRI investigation suggests that structural differences in the brain may underlie circadian outputs, with significant correlations between pineal volume and evening melatonin secretion (Carpenter et al., 2017a). We have also linked circadian disturbances with neurochemical changes, using proton magnetic resonance spectroscopy. These studies have found that later sleep timing is associated with higher levels of glutamine in the anterior cingulate cortex (Naismith et al., 2014), and that later melatonin onset is associated with lower myo-inositol concentrations in the anterior cingulate cortex (Robillard et al., 2017). These various relationships suggest that observed abnormalities in sleep–wake behaviour may be reflective of disturbed circadian and related neural systems, with potential transdiagnostic relevance to illness progression.

Designing Personalised Treatments Based on these Approaches

Internationally, there is an increasing move to manage actively in clinical settings adolescents and young adults who present for care in the early phases of major mood or psychotic disorders. However, the symptom complexes presented are often an admixture of anxiety, depressive, hypomanic, psychotic or substance misuse-related symptoms (Hickie et al., 2013c), and typically do not meet the diagnostic thresholds employed for more specific disorders. The evidence-base for providing specific treatments for many of these subthreshold or first-episode-type disorders is sparse and there is also an increasing desire to link interventions more closely to underlying developmental or specific pathophysiological pathways (Hickie et al., 2013c; 2013d; 2013e). While we have proposed the potential utility of adapting a clinical staging strategy to guide assessment and treatment selection for such early or less-differentiated cases of major mood or psychotic disorders, our view is that essentially this approach is adjunctive to more conventional diagnostic practice.

Consequently, we have developed preliminary approaches to plotting both clinical stage and major pathophysiological pathways, while also proposing likely objective neurobiological markers that can be tracked concurrently (Figure 5.9). We have proposed three major developmental trajectories, putatively linked with more specific (but not mutually exclusive) pathophysiologies (ANXIETY – depression; CIRCADIAN – mania/fatigue; NEURODEVELOPMENTAL – psychotic) (Hickie et al., 2013a). These approaches also recognise likely preceding childhood risk phenotypes and differential patterns of comorbidity (notably

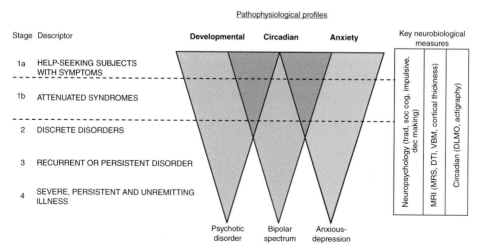

Figure 5.9 Clinical staging model for post-pubertal onset and course of major mental disorders: developmental, circadian or anxiety pathophysiological pathways progress from non-specific to discrete syndromes. Trad, traditional; soc cog, social cognition; dec, decision; MRI, magnetic resonance imaging; MRS, magnetic resonance spectroscopy; DTI, diffusion tensor imaging; VBM, voxel-based morphometry; DLMO, dim light melatonin onset. *A black and white version of this figure will appear in some formats. For the colour version, please refer to the plate section.*

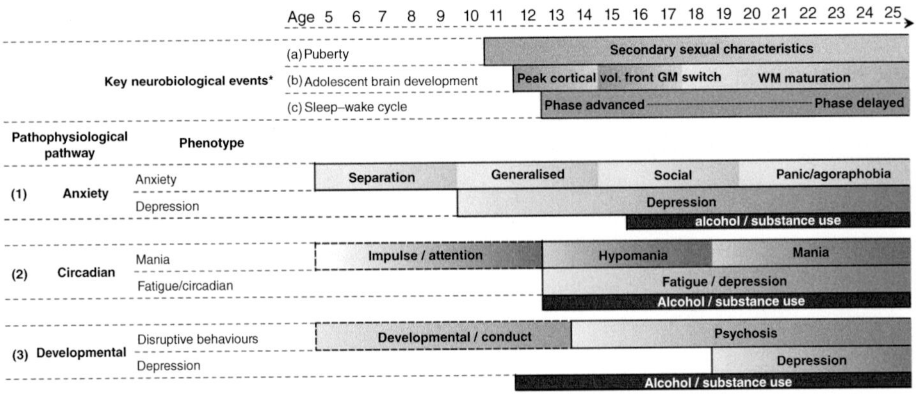

Figure 5.10 Pathophysiological pathways to early-onset depressive disorders. There are at least three common trajectories that lead to depression in the teenage and early-adult years. These are characterised by (1) 'anxiety–central nervous system reactivity'; (2) 'circadian and 24-hour sleep–wake cycle dysfunction'; and (3) 'developmental brain abnormalities'. The six corresponding phenotypic patterns have distinct ages of onset and characteristics. From age 8–10 years onwards these processes are transformed by key neurobiological phenomena: (a) puberty, (b) adolescent brain development and (c) sleep–wake cycle. From Hickie et al. (2013b). *A black and white version of this figure will appear in some formats. For the colour version, please refer to the plate section.*

differential ages of onset of alcohol or other substance misuse; Figure 5.10). Within such a model the majority of our work is located currently at the threshold between Stages 1b and 2, and draws extensively from young people recruited uniquely through our enhanced headspace services and affiliated research clinics.

Complementary to this pathway model, we have commenced the development of a treatment-selection model (Table 5.2), demonstrating the capacity to, first, prioritise psychological, social and behavioural approaches and, second, only later to choose pharmacological approaches that may be most relevant to the underlying pathophysiological pathway (inferred from the observed phenotype or concurrent neurobiological testing). For example, 24-hour sleep–wake cycle behavioural interventions or melatonin-based antidepressants may be preferred for some depressive disorders in those who have phenotypic, actigraphic or laboratory-based evidence of underlying circadian disturbance. This approach is the subject of ongoing clinical testing and refinement.

Conclusion

In these Sydney-based studies over the last decade, we have been able to test the clinical utility and predictive validity of clinical staging when applied to young people presenting with anxiety, mood or psychotic syndromes. The range of studies summarised here provides a firm evidence-base for further elaboration of this model. Of greatest importance now are: (1) longitudinal studies evaluating the ongoing relationships between independent neurobiological correlates of clinical stage and illness progression; (2) the design and implementation of stage-specific secondary prevention trials; and (3) the testing of the clinical utility of stage-specific and pathophysiologically oriented treatment options. Compared with practice based on traditional diagnostic systems, however, it now appears that we can use clinical staging to underpin the development of much more personalised, and youth-relevant, models of care.

Table 5.2 Putative stepped care therapies for relevant depressive subtypes

Depression type	First-line therapy: psychological/behavioural	Second-line therapy: pharmacological	Experimental therapies
1. Anxious-depression	CBT, IPT, problem-solving, e-health-based anxiety management, exposure therapy, CBCM, MCT	SSRIs, SNRIs	Fish oils, DCS, oxytocin, ketamine
2. Circadian-fatigue/depression	Behavioural regulation, physical activity, sleep–wake cycle/circadian CBT, rumination-focused CBT, DBT, CBCM, MCT	Melatonin, melatonin analogues, lithium, pregabalin, lamotrigine	Sleep deprivation suvorexant, stimulants, modafinil, TMS, tDCS, ketamine, fish oils
3. Developmental/psychosis	Problem-solving, social skills training, cognitive training, social recovery therapy, CBCM, MCT, IPS	Atypical antipsychotics	Ketamine, cannabidiol, oxytocin, novel neuropeptides, hormonal therapies, fish oils

CBT, cognitive behavioural therapy; IPT, interpersonal therapy; CBCM, cognitive behavioural case management; MCT, meta-cognitive therapy; SSRI, selective serotonin reuptake inhibitor; SNRI, selective serotonin and norepinephrine reuptake inhibitor; DCS, d-cycloserine; DBT, dialectic behaviour therapy; TMS, transcranial magnetic stimulation; tDCS, transcranial direct current stimulation; IPS, individual placement and support.

References

Benca, R. M., Obermeyer, W. H., Thisted, R. A., & Gillin, J. C. (1992). Sleep and psychiatric disorders: a meta-analysis. *Archives of General Psychiatry*, **49**(8), 651–668.

Bloom, D., Cafiero, E., Jane-Llopis, E., Abrahams-Gessel, S., Bloom, L., Fathima, S., ... Weiss, J. (2012). *The global economic burden of non-communicable diseases*. Geneva: World Economic Forum.

Buckholtz, J. W., & Meyer-Lindenberg, A. (2012). Psychopathology and the human connectome: toward a transdiagnostic model of risk for mental illness. *Neuron*, **74**(6), 990–1004.

Carpenter, J. S., Abelmann, A. C., Hatton, S. N., Robillard, R., Hermens, D. F., Bennett, M. R., ... Hickie, I. B. (2017a). Pineal volume and evening melatonin in young people with affective disorders. *Brain Imaging and Behavior*, **11**(6), 1741–1750.

Carpenter, J. S., Robillard, R., Hermens, D. F., Naismith, S. L., Gordon, C., Scott, E. M., & Hickie, I. B. (2017b). Sleep–wake profiles and circadian rhythms of core temperature and melatonin in young people with affective disorders. *Journal of Psychiatric Research*, **94**, 131–138.

Carpenter, J. S., Robillard, R., & Hickie, I. B. (2015a). Variations in the sleep–wake cycle from childhood to adulthood: chronobiological perspectives. *ChronoPhysiology and Therapy*, **5**, 37–49.

Carpenter, J. S., Robillard, R., Lee, R. S., Hermens, D. F., Naismith, S. L., White, D., ... Hickie, I. B. (2015b). The relationship between sleep–wake cycle and cognitive functioning in young people with affective disorders. *PLoS One*, **10**(4), e0124710.

Casey, B. J., Craddock, N., Cuthbert, B. N., Hyman, S. E., Lee, F. S., & Ressler, K. J. (2013). DSM-5 and RDoC: progress in psychiatry research? *Nature Reviews Neuroscience,* **14**(11), 810–814.

Copeland, W. E., Adair, C. E., Smetanin, P., Stiff, D., Briante, C., Colman, I., ... Angold, A. (2013). Diagnostic transitions from childhood to adolescence to early adulthood. *Journal of Child Psychology and Psychiatry,* **54**(7), 791–799.

Cross, S. P., Hermens, D. F., & Hickie, I. B. (2016). Treatment patterns and short-term outcomes in an early intervention youth mental health service. *Early Intervention in Psychiatry,* **10**(1), 88–97.

Cross, S. P. M., Hermens, D. F., Scott, J., Salvador-Carulla, L., & Hickie, I. B. (2017a). Differential impact of current diagnosis and clinical stage on attendance at a youth mental health service. *Early Intervention in Psychiatry,* **11**(3), 255–262.

Cross, S. P., Scott, J. L., Hermens, D. F., & Hickie, I. B. (2018). Variability in clinical outcomes for youths treated for subthreshold severe mental disorders at an early intervention service. *Psychiatric Services,* **69**(5), 555–561.

Cross, S. P. M., Scott, J., & Hickie, I. B. (2017b). Predicting early transition from sub-syndromal presentations to major mental disorders. *British Journal of Psychiatry Open,* **3**(5), 223–227.

Cuthbert, B. N., & Insel, T. R. (2013). Toward the future of psychiatric diagnosis: the seven pillars of RDoC. *BMC Medicine,* **11**, 126.

Dolsen, M. R., Asarnow, L. D., & Harvey, A. G. (2014). Insomnia as a transdiagnostic process in psychiatric disorders. *Current Psychiatry Reports,* **16**(9), 471.

Erskine, H. E., Moffitt, T. E., Copeland, W. E., Costello, E. J., Ferrari, A. J., Patton, G., ... Scott, J. G. (2015). A heavy burden on young minds: the global burden of mental and substance use disorders in children and youth. *Psychological Medicine,* **45**(7), 1511–1563.

Fusar-Poli, P., Byrne, M., Valmaggia, L., Day, F., Tabraham, P., Johns, L., ... Team, O. (2010). Social dysfunction predicts two years clinical outcome in people at ultra high risk for psychosis. *Journal of Psychiatric Research,* **44**(5), 294–301.

Gore, F. M., Bloem, P. J. N., Patton, G. C., Ferguson, J., Joseph, V., Coffey, C., ... Mathers, C. D. (2011). Global burden of disease in young people aged 10–24 years: a systematic analysis. *Lancet,* **377**(9783), 2093–2102.

Gradisar, M., Gardner, G., & Dohnt, H. (2011). Recent worldwide sleep patterns and problems during adolescence: a review and meta-analysis of age, region, and sleep. *Sleep Medicine,* **12**(2), 110–118.

Gustavsson, A., Svensson, M., Jacobi, F., Allgulander, C., Alonso, J., & Beghi, E.; CDBE 2010 Study Group (2011). Cost of disorders of the brain in Europe 2010. *European Neuropsychopharmacology,* **21**(10), 718–779.

Hafner, H., an der Heiden, W., & Maurer, K. (2008). Evidence for separate diseases? Stages of one disease or different combinations of symptom dimensions? *European Archives of Psychiatry and Clinical Neuroscience,* **258** (Suppl. 2), 85–96.

Hamilton, B. A., Naismith, S. L., Scott, E. M., Purcell, S., & Hickie, I. B. (2011). Disability is already pronounced in young people with early stages of affective disorders: data from an early intervention service. *Journal of Affective Disorders,* **131**(1–3), 84–91.

Harvey, A. G., Murray, G., Chandler, R. A., & Soehner, A. (2011). Sleep disturbance as transdiagnostic: consideration of neurobiological mechanisms. *Clinical Psychology Review,* **31**(2), 225–235.

Hermens, D. F., Naismith, S. L., Lagopoulos, J., Lee, R. S. C., Guastella, A. J., Scott, E. M., & Hickie, I. B. (2013). Neuropsychological profile according to the clinical stage of young persons presenting for mental health care. *BMC Psychology,* **1**, 8.

Hickie, I. B., Hermens, D. F., Naismith, S. L., Guastella, A. J., Glozier, N., Scott, J., & Scott, E. M. (2013a). Evaluating differential developmental trajectories to adolescent-onset mood and psychotic disorders. *BMC Psychiatry,* **13**, 303.

Hickie, I. B., Naismith, S. L., Robillard, R., Scott, E. M., & Hermens, D. F. (2013b). Manipulating the sleep–wake cycle and circadian rhythms to improve clinical management of major depression. *BMC Medicine,* **11,** 79.

Hickie, I. B., Scott, E. M., Hermens, D. F., Naismith, S. L., Guastella, A. J., Kaur, M., ... McGorry, P. D. (2013c). Applying clinical staging to young people who present for mental health care. *Early Intervention in Psychiatry,* **7**(1), 31–43.

Hickie, I. B., Scott, J., Hermens, D. F., Scott, E. M., Naismith, S. L., Guastella, A. J., ... McGorry, P. D. (2013d). Clinical classification in mental health at the crossroads: which direction next? *BMC Medicine,* **11,** 125.

Hickie, I. B., Scott, J., & McGorry, P. D. (2013e). Clinical staging for mental disorders: a new development in diagnostic practice in mental health. *Medical Journal of Australia,* **198**(9), 461–462.

Insel, T. R. (2007). The arrival of preemptive psychiatry. *Early Intervention in Psychiatry,* **1**(1), 5–6.

Insel, T. R. (2009). Translating scientific opportunity into public health impact: a strategic plan for research on mental illness. *Archives of General Psychiatry,* **66**(2), 128–133.

Insel, T., Cuthbert, B., Garvey, M., Heinssen, R., Pine, D. S., Quinn, K., ... Wang, P. (2010). Research Domain Criteria (RDoC): toward a new classification framework for research on mental disorders. *American Journal of Psychiatry,* **167**(7), 748–751.

Jones, S. G., & Benca, R. M. (2015). Circadian disruption in psychiatric disorders. *Sleep Medicine Clinics,* **10**(4), 481–493.

Karatsoreos, I. N. (2014). Links between circadian rhythms and psychiatric disease. *Frontiers in Behavioral Neuroscience,* **8,** 162.

Kelleher, I., Keeley, H., Corcoran, P., Lynch, F., Fitzpatrick, C., Devlin, N., ... Cannon, M. (2012). Clinicopathological significance of psychotic experiences in non-psychotic young people: evidence from four population-based studies. *British Journal of Psychiatry,* **201**(1), 26–32.

Kim-Cohen, J., Caspi, A., Moffitt, T. E., Harrington, H., Milne, B. J., & Poulton, R. (2003). Prior juvenile diagnoses in adults with mental disorder: developmental followback of a prospective-longitudinal cohort. *Archives of General Psychiatry,* **60**(7), 709–717.

Kozak, M. J., & Cuthbert, B. N. (2016). The NIMH Research Domain Criteria Initiative: background, issues, and pragmatics. *Psychophysiology,* **53**(3), 286–297.

Lagopoulos, J., Hermens, D. F., Hatton, S. N., Battisti, R. A., Tobias-Webb, J., White, D., ... Hickie, I. B. (2013). Microstructural white matter changes are correlated with the stage of psychiatric illness. *Translational Psychiatry,* **3,** e248.

Lagopoulos, J., Hermens, D. F., Naismith, S. L., Scott, E. M., & Hickie, I. B. (2012). Frontal lobe changes occur early in the course of affective disorders in young people. *BMC Psychiatry,* **12,** 4.

Lee, R. S., Hermens, D. F., Naismith, S. L., Lagopoulos, J., Jones, A., Scott, J., ... Hickie, I. B. (2015). Neuropsychological and functional outcomes in recent-onset major depression, bipolar disorder and schizophrenia-spectrum disorders: a longitudinal cohort study. *Translational Psychiatry,* **5,** e555.

Lee, R. S., Hermens, D. F., Redoblado-Hodge, M. A., Naismith, S. L., Porter, M. A., Kaur, M., ... Hickie, I. B. (2013). Neuropsychological and socio-occupational functioning in young psychiatric outpatients: a longitudinal investigation. *PLoS One,* **8**(3), e58176.

Lee, R. S., Hermens, D. F., Scott, J., Redoblado-Hodge, M. A., Naismith, S. L., Lagopoulos, J., ... Hickie, I. B. (2014). A meta-analysis of neuropsychological functioning in first-episode bipolar disorders. *Journal of Psychiatric Research,* **57C,** 1–11.

Lichtenstein, P., Yip, B. H., Björk, C., Pawitan, Y., Cannon, T. D., Sullivan, P. F., & Hultman, C. M. (2009). Common genetic determinants of schizophrenia and bipolar disorder in Swedish families: a population-based study. *Lancet,* **373,** 234–239.

Lin, A., Yung, A. R., Nelson, B., Brewer, W. J., Riley, R., Simmons, M., ... Wood, S. J. (2013). Neurocognitive predictors of transition to psychosis: medium- to long-term findings from a sample at ultra-high risk for psychosis. *Psychological Medicine,* **43**(11), 2349–2360.

Lopez, A. D., Mathers, C. D., Ezzati, M., Jamison, D. T., & Murray, C. J. L. (2006). Global and regional burden of disease and risk factors, 2001: systematic analysis of population health data. *Lancet,* **367**(9524), 1747–1757.

Maziade, M., Rouleau, N., Merette, C., Cellard, C., Battaglia, M., Marino, C., . . . Roy, M. A. (2011). Verbal and visual memory impairments among young offspring and healthy adult relatives of patients with schizophrenia and bipolar disorder: selective generational patterns indicate different developmental trajectories. *Schizophrenia Bulletin,* **37**(6), 1218–1228.

McGorry, P. (2007). Issues for DSM-V: clinical staging – a heuristic pathway to valid nosology and safer, more effective treatment in psychiatry. *American Journal of Psychiatry,* **164**(6), 859–860.

McGorry, P. D. (2010). Risk syndromes, clinical staging and DSM V: new diagnostic infrastructure for early intervention in psychiatry. *Schizophrenia Research,* **120**(1–3), 49–53.

McGorry, P. D., Goldstone, S. D., Parker, A. G., Rickwood, D. J., & Hickie, I. B. (2014). Cultures for mental health care of young people: an Australian blueprint for reform. *Lancet Psychiatry,* **1**(7), 559–568.

McGorry, P. D., Hickie, I. B., Yung, A. R., Pantelis, C., & Jackson, H. J. (2006). Clinical staging of psychiatric disorders: a heuristic framework for choosing earlier, safer and more effective interventions. *Australian and New Zealand Journal of Psychiatry,* **40**, 616–622.

McGorry, P. D., Purcell, R., Hickie, I. B., Yung, A. R., Pantelis, C., & Jackson, H. J. (2007). Clinical staging: a heuristic model for psychiatry and youth mental health. *Medical Journal of Australia,* **187**, S40–S42.

McGorry, P. D., Yung, A. R., Bechdolf, A., & Amminger, P. (2008). Back to the future: predicting and reshaping the course of psychotic disorder. *Archives of General Psychiatry,* **65**(1), 25–26.

Merikangas, K. R., Cui, L., Kattan, G., Carlson, G. A., Youngstrom, E. A., & Angst, J. (2012). Mania with and without depression in a community sample of US adolescents. *Archives of General Psychiatry,* **69**(9), 943–951.

Merikangas, K. R., He, J.-P., Burstein, M., Swanson, S. A., Avenevoli, S., Cui, L., . . . Swendsen, J. (2010). Lifetime prevalence of mental disorders in U.S. adolescents: results from the National Comorbidity Survey Replication – Adolescent Supplement (NCS-A). *Journal of the American Academy of Child and Adolescent Psychiatry,* **49**(10), 980–989.

Merikangas, K. R., Herrell, R., Swendsen, J., Rossler, W., Ajdacic-Gross, V., & Angst, J. (2008). Specificity of bipolar spectrum conditions in the comorbidity of mood and substance use disorders: results from the Zurich Cohort Study. *Archives of General Psychiatry,* **65**(1), 47–52.

Murray, G. K., & Jones, P. B. (2012). Psychotic symptoms in young people without psychotic illness: mechanisms and meaning. *British Journal of Psychiatry,* **201**(1), 4–6.

Naismith, S. L., Hermens, D. F., Ip, T. K., Bolitho, S., Scott, E., Rogers, N. L., & Hickie, I. B. (2012). Circadian profiles in young people during the early stages of affective disorder. *Translational Psychiatry,* **2**(5), e123.

Naismith, S. L., Lagopoulos, J., Hermens, D. F., White, D., Duffy, S. L., Robillard, R., . . . Hickie, I. B. (2014). Delayed circadian phase is linked to glutamatergic functions in young people with affective disorders: a proton magnetic resonance spectroscopy study. *BMC Psychiatry,* **14**, 345.

Ormel, J., Raven, D., van Oort, F., Hartman, C. A., Reijneveld, S. A., Veenstra, R., . . . Oldehinkel, A. J. (2015). Mental health in Dutch adolescents: a TRAILS report on prevalence, severity, age of onset, continuity and co-morbidity of DSM disorders. *Psychological Medicine,* **45**(2), 345–360.

Paus, T., Keshavan, M., & Giedd, J. N. (2008). Why do many psychiatric disorders emerge during adolescence? *Nature Reviews Neuroscience,* **9**(12), 947–957.

Purcell, R., Jorm, A. F., Hickie, I. B., Yung, A. R., Pantelis, C., Amminger, G. P., . . . McGorry,

P. D. (2015). Demographic and clinical characteristics of young people seeking help at youth mental health services: baseline findings of the Transitions Study. *Early Intervention in Psychiatry,* 9(6), 487–497.

Robillard, R., Hermens, D. F., Lee, R. S., Jones, A., Carpenter, J. S., White, D., . . . Hickie, I. B. (2016). Sleep–wake profiles predict longitudinal changes in manic symptoms and memory in young people with mood disorders. *Journal of Sleep Research,* 25(5), 549–555.

Robillard, R., Hermens, D. F., Naismith, S. L., White, D., Rogers, N. L., Ip, T. K., . . . Hickie, I. B. (2015). Ambulatory sleep–wake patterns and variability in young people with emerging mental disorders. *Journal of Psychiatry and Neuroscience,* 40(1), 28–37.

Robillard, R., Lagopoulos, J., Hermens, D. F., Naismith, S. L., Rogers, N. L., White, D., . . . Hickie, I. B. (2017). Lower in vivo myo-inositol in the anterior cingulate cortex correlates with delayed melatonin rhythms in young persons with depression. *Frontiers in Neuroscience,* 11, 336.

Robillard, R., Naismith, S. L., Rogers, N. L., Ip, T. K., Hermens, D. F., Scott, E. M., & Hickie, I. B. (2013a). Delayed sleep phase in young people with unipolar or bipolar affective disorders. *Journal of Affective Disorders,* 145(2), 260–263.

Robillard, R., Naismith, S. L., Rogers, N. L., Scott, E. M., Ip, T. K., Hermens, D. F., & Hickie, I. B. (2013b). Sleep-wake cycle and melatonin rhythms in adolescents and young adults with mood disorders: comparison of unipolar and bipolar phenotypes. *European Psychiatry,* 28(7), 412–416.

Robillard, R., Naismith, S. L., Smith, K. L., Rogers, N. L., White, D., Terpening, Z., . . . Hickie, I. B. (2014). Sleep–wake cycle in young and older persons with a lifetime history of mood disorders. *PLoS One,* 9(2), e87763.

Scott, E. M., Hermens, D. F., Glozier, N., Naismith, S. L., Guastella, A. J., & Hickie, I. B. (2012). Targeted primary care-based mental health services for young Australians. *Medical Journal of Australia,* 196(2), 136–140.

Scott, E. M., Hermens, D. F., Naismith, S. L., Guastella, A. J., De Regt, T., White, D., . . . Hickie, I. B. (2013a). Distinguishing young people with emerging bipolar disorders from those with unipolar depression. *Journal of Affective Disorders,* 144(3), 208–215.

Scott, E. M., Hermens, D. F., Naismith, S. L., Guastella, A. J., White, D., Whitwell, B. G., . . . Hickie, I. B. (2013b). Distress and disability in young adults presenting to clinical services with mood disorders. *International Journal of Bipolar Disorders,* 1, 23.

Scott, E. M., Robillard, R., Hermens, D. F., Naismith, S. L., Rogers, N. L., Ip, T. K., . . . Hickie, I. B. (2016). Dysregulated sleep–wake cycles in young people are associated with emerging stages of major mental disorders. *Early Intervention in Psychiatry,* 10(1), 63–70.

Scott, J. (2011). Bipolar disorder: from early identification to personalized treatment. *Early Intervention in Psychiatry,* 5(2), 89–90.

Scott, J., Paykel, E., Morriss, R., Bentall, R., Kinderman, P., Johnson, T., . . . Hayhurst, H. (2006). Cognitive-behavioural therapy for severe and recurrent bipolar disorders: randomised controlled trial. *British Journal of Psychiatry,* 188, 313–320.

Scott, J., Scott, E. M., Hermens, D. F., Naismith, S. L., Guastella, A. J., White, D., . . . Hickie, I. B. (2014). Functional impairment in adolescents and young adults with emerging mood disorders. *British Journal of Psychiatry,* 205(5), 362–368.

Sullivan, P. F., Daly, M. J., & O'Donovan, M. (2012). Genetic architectures of psychiatric disorders: the emerging picture and its implications. *Nature Reviews Genetics,* 13(8), 537–551.

Sumiyoshi, T., Miyanishi, T., Seo, T., & Higuchi, Y. (2013). Electrophysiological and neuropsychological predictors of conversion to schizophrenia in at-risk subjects. *Frontiers in Behavioral Neuroscience,* 7, 148.

Tickell, A. M., Lee, R. S. C., Hickie, I. B., & Hermens, D. F. (in press). The course of neuropsychological functioning in young people with attenuated vs discrete mental disorders. *Early Intervention in Psychiatry.* DOI: 10.1111/eip.12499.

Valmaggia, L. R., Stahl, D., Yung, A. R., Nelson, B., Fusar-Poli, P., McGorry, P. D., & McGuire, P. K. (2013). Negative psychotic symptoms and impaired role functioning predict transition outcomes in the at-risk mental state: a latent class cluster analysis study. *Psychological Medicine, 43*(11), 2311–2325.

Waszczuk, M. A., Zavos, H. M., Gregory, A. M., & Eley, T. C. (2014). The phenotypic and genetic structure of depression and anxiety disorder symptoms in childhood, adolescence, and young adulthood. *JAMA Psychiatry, 71*(8), 905–916.

Chapter

Neuroimaging and Staging
Do Disparate Mental Illnesses Have Distinct Neurobiological Trajectories?

6

Cali F. Bartholomeusz and Christos Pantelis

Introduction

Integration of brain structural information into prognostic and treatment formulation is key for achieving an all-encompassing biopsychosocial approach in psychiatry and to enabling personalised medicine in the future. Uncovering biological markers of specific mental illnesses, specific illness stages and of remission, may help to: (1) further our understanding of the aetiology and precipitators of certain types of psychopathologies; (2) identify central neurobiological processes as distinct from epiphenomena; (3) validate boundaries of clinical groups (diagnostic or otherwise); and (4) potentially aid in predicting response to treatment.

Currently, no biological markers have been identified for any mental illness, and being able to discover neurobiological distinctions between illness stages will depend on the slope of the trajectory of change across time (Figure 6.1). Hypothetically, if neurobiological changes occur rapidly and in parallel to when an individual's *phenotypic presentation* moves them from one stage to the next within a distinct time window (the light grey line in Figure 6.1), this steep slope would suggest the discovery of biological markers of illness progression is attainable. However, if neurobiological changes take place gradually over a longer time period (the dark grey line in Figure 6.1) and do not map onto phenotypic changes, distinctions may be more difficult to detect, particularly if research is cross-sectional, if longitudinal studies have short follow-up periods or if illness stage is defined by behavioural indices (as it is currently).

This chapter will review the current structural neuroimaging evidence in three prominent mental illness domains and discuss the degree to which the literature supports a psychiatric clinical staging model. We address three key questions: (1) Do biological distinctions, in this case brain structural indices, that are deemed abnormal relative to the healthy population exist between broad illness groups? (2) Are there more subtle yet detectable neurobiological distinctions between the clinical stages within a given illness? (3) Are changes within the longitudinal trajectory of each disorder apparent in the same or in different brain regions across illness stages? We first summarise the well-established structural magnetic resonance imaging (MRI) abnormalities in cohorts with schizophrenia-spectrum, bipolar and depressive disorders, focusing on chronic illness stages, as this is where differences are expected to be most prominent. Given the sheer abundance of literature in this area, we will draw heavily on findings from meta-analyses. We will outline the findings supporting abnormalities in brain morphology that appear to depend on stage of a given illness (McGorry et al., 2007), that is, the evidence for differences between the prodromal (Stages 1a and 1b), first-episode (Stage 2) and established illness stages (Stages 3 and 4). The bulk of these studies have been conducted in the schizophrenia-spectrum

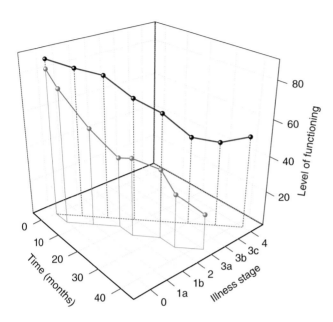

Figure 6.1 Model of differing illness stage trajectories over time. Two examples are displayed which show different rates of change in level of functioning and associated amount of time spent within certain illness stages.

psychoses, but we will also touch on the limited literature in this area that involved the other mental illness domains mentioned above. This latter section will highlight the differences between early illness stages, given the clinical implications this has for prevention and early intervention. Lastly, we will discuss the concept of a clinical staging model in relation to remission and relapse signatures, before outlining the limitations and caveats of this chapter.

Neural Structural Abnormalities Associated with Schizophrenia-Spectrum, Bipolar and Depressive Disorders in the Established Illness Stages

Neuroimaging studies in psychiatry have primarily focused on characterising grey matter (GM) volumetric abnormalities in the context of searching for neurobiological illness markers, which by way of practicality and feasibility took place in a silo fashion rather than across the mental illness domains.[1] Of the broad mental illness groups, psychotic disorders have been the most widely studied.

Schizophrenia-Spectrum Disorders

In meta-analyses of primarily cross-sectional research, individuals with a diagnosed schizophrenia-spectrum disorder have been consistently shown to have bilateral reductions in hippocampal volumes (Adriano et al., 2012; Davidson & Heinrichs, 2003; Ellison-Wright

---

[1] The studies that will be described in this section are presumed to have involved primarily individuals who are in the established illness Stages 3 and 4, as the majority of these past studies did not adopt a staging model and typically included individuals if they met the criteria for having a clinical diagnosis, based on the DSM or ICD.

et al., 2008; Fornito et al., 2009; Haijma et al., 2013; Nelson et al., 1998; Wright et al., 2000; Zakzanis et al., 2000), a subcortical GM structure of the medial temporal lobes that forms part of the limbic system. (The hippocampus is primarily responsible for declarative (long-term) and associative memory, specifically encoding and retrieving information (Eichenbaum, 2004), but is also thought to play a role in learning and cognitive-emotional control, given its connections with other limbic and frontal regions (Wall & Messier, 2001).) These meta-analyses each comprised between 18 and 155 studies and between 522 and 4043 patients, and despite overlap in the individual studies analysed, reduced hippocampal volume is a consistent finding in established schizophrenia. A meta-review suggests this evidence is of a relatively high standard and that the deficit is of moderate magnitude (effect size $d = -0.38$ to -0.58) (Shepherd et al., 2012). Recently, a worldwide initiative known as the Enhancing NeuroImaging Genetics through Meta-Analysis (ENIGMA) consortium meta-analysed subcortical brain volumes of 2028 participants with schizophrenia and 2540 healthy control (HC) participants (from 15 research centres) (van Erp et al., 2016). Findings confirmed that reduced hippocampal volumes (of moderate magnitude, $d = -0.64$) are a significant characteristic of schizophrenia (van Erp et al., 2016). Van Erp and colleagues (van Erp et al., 2016) additionally found schizophrenia patients displayed volume reduction of the amygdala ($d = -0.31$), thalamus ($d = -0.31$) and the accumbens ($d = -0.25$), along with enlargement of the pallidum ($d = 0.21$), relative to controls. GM regions that other meta-analyses have identified as significantly abnormal and specifically reduced in schizophrenia include the amygdala, uncus, insula, thalamus, nucleus accumbens, cerebellum, cingulate cortices, prefrontal cortices, dorsomedial frontal cortex, orbitofrontal cortices, fusiform gyrus, inferior, medial and superior temporal regions, parahippocampus, inferior parietal lobe and frontal, occipital, parietal and temporal lobes (Chan et al., 2011; Davidson & Heinrichs, 2003; Ellison-Wright & Bullmore, 2010; Ellison-Wright et al., 2008; Fornito et al., 2009; Haijma et al., 2013; Wright et al., 2000; Zakzanis et al., 2000). A mega-analysis of data collected from 784 schizophrenia patients via 23 scanning sites across Europe similarly found widespread reductions in cortical GM concentration, with the largest differences being in the superior temporal gyrus, inferior frontal gyrus and insula, relative to controls ($n = 936$) (Gupta et al., 2015). In contrast, there was some evidence for increased GM concentration in regions of the cerebellum and brainstem of patients (Gupta et al., 2015). Meta-analysis of nine studies that focused on pituitary gland volume failed to find any significant difference between schizophrenia-spectrum patients (although this group also comprised first-episode psychosis (FEP) samples) and HCs (Nordholm et al., 2013). White matter (WM) deficits have been observed in the corpus callosum (Walterfang et al., 2006; Zhuo et al., 2016), prefrontal and frontal regions, temporal regions and the internal capsule (Di et al., 2009; Ellison-Wright & Bullmore, 2009; Haijma et al., 2013). While not all meta-analyses identified exactly the same regions, the general findings of GM reductions in temporal, frontal, limbic and striatal regions are relatively consistent, despite the variation in methodology used (i.e. automated or manually parcellated volumetry (mm^3) or voxel-based morphometry (VBM)). Moreover, these findings indicate that GM loss is widespread in people who have an established schizophrenia-spectrum disorder and are (most likely) in the latter illness phases (see Figure 6.2 for an example of the distribution of cortical and subcortical GM loss relative to HCs (Fornito et al., 2009)). Meta-analyses of longitudinal studies support the association between established illness and reductions in grey (and white) matter volume (Fusar-Poli et al., 2013; Olabi et al., 2011). Moreover, these meta-analyses further suggest that volume loss is *progressive* in nature, where the rate of

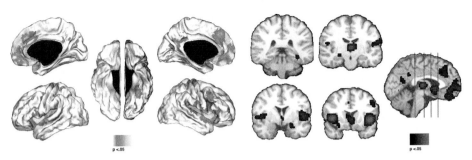

Figure 6.2 Extent of cortical and subcortical GM loss in schizophrenia-spectrum disorders. Regions showing significant GM reductions in patients with schizophrenia across all 37 studies included in the anatomical likelihood estimation analysis (Fornito et al., 2009). The left hemisphere is on the right side of the brain images; statistics are displayed on brain templates. (Image reproduced with permission). *A black and white version of this figure will appear in some formats. For the colour version, please refer to the plate section.*

volume change over the course of the illness is significantly greater than that of the general population. However, whether the cause of this volume loss is directly related to the pathophysiology of the illness has recently been brought into question (Zipursky et al., 2013). This is supported by evidence showing cumulative antipsychotic exposure over time (median = 74.2 weeks) is significantly associated with GM reductions in schizophrenia (Fusar-Poli et al., 2013). However, Haijma et al. (2013) found that antipsychotic-naïve patients (n = 771) still presented with significant volume reductions, suggesting that to some degree, volumetric brain changes are indeed driven by the illness itself.

In addition to GM abnormalities, and what is often considered to be the most reproducible brain structural finding in schizophrenia-spectrum disorders, is enlargement of the ventricles (Shenton et al., 2001). The ventricular system consists of four interconnecting cavities: the left and right hemisphere lateral ventricles, the third ventricle (located in the diencephalon of the forebrain) and the fourth ventricle (located in the hindbrain) (Kandel et al., 2000). The ventricles are involved in the production and circulation of cerebrospinal fluid, and enlargement of these structures implicates loss of epithelial cells that line these cavities or possibly a 'receding' of the brain tissue boundaries (which may be related to GM or WM loss in close or farther proximity). Enlargement of the ventricles in mental illness was discovered before the advent of antipsychotic medication, using pneumoencephalography (Moore et al., 1935). Johnstone et al. (1976) were the first to identify lateral ventricular enlargement (VE) in schizophrenia using computer tomography, and since then VE has been the most consistently reported brain abnormality in schizophrenia (Kempton et al., 2010; Shenton et al., 2001). Cross-sectional meta-analyses, which included substantial numbers of drug-naïve patients (Haijma et al., 2013; Wright et al., 2000), show significant VE (e.g. global VE = 126 per cent) of moderate magnitude (e.g. Cohen's d = 0.45 to 0.60) in schizophrenia patients relative to HCs. Of the subdivisions of the ventricular system, the greatest differences tend to be in lateral and third ventricles (Haijma et al., 2013; van Erp et al., 2016; Wright et al., 2000). Recently, three systematic reviews of longitudinal neuroimaging studies in schizophrenia confirmed significant progressive VE of small to moderate effect size (Cohen's d = 0.45–0.53; Hedges' g = 0.21–0.45) in established schizophrenia, where follow-up ranged from one to approximately ten years (Fusar-Poli et al., 2013; Kempton et al., 2010; Olabi et al., 2011). Interestingly, lateral VE was not linked with exposure to antipsychotic medications, as was the case with GM volume loss mentioned earlier (Fusar-Poli et al., 2013).

Collectively, in light of the multitude of abnormalities in this illness domain, some of which are consistent, it has been suggested that structural pathophysiological changes may not necessarily occur via a common singular process (Fornito et al., 2009). This begs the question of whether these structural abnormalities are specific to schizophrenia-spectrum disorders, which is crucial for clarifying whether integration of neuroimaging data into a clinical staging model is viable, at least in the near term.

Bipolar Disorders

As with schizophrenia-spectrum disorders, an abundance of neuroimaging research has been conducted in people with established bipolar disorders (BDs). In comparison to the schizophrenia literature, overall there are less consistent and less extensive structural neural abnormalities in BD. The amygdala has been a key region of interest (ROI) in many BD studies, given that this subcortical GM structure, part of the limbic system, plays a prominent role in emotion and social behaviour (Adolphs, 2001). Despite this, meta-analyses have failed to find a significant difference in amygdala volume of BD patients when compared to HCs (Arnone et al., 2009; Bora et al., 2010; Hajek et al., 2009; Hibar et al., 2016; Houenou et al., 2011; Kempton et al., 2008; McDonald et al., 2004; Selvaraj et al., 2012). This is possibly related to the difficulty associated with delineating amygdalae GM boundaries on T1-weighted images. Potential explanations for heterogeneity of this region in meta-analyses have been inconsistent, with some suggesting volume is dependent on age where reductions were specific to children and adolescents with BD (Hajek et al., 2009), while others have reported no effects of age (Kempton et al., 2008) or age of illness onset (Hibar et al., 2016). Interestingly, although Arnone et al. (2009) found no difference between BD patients and HCs, they did find BD patients had significantly enlarged right amygdala volume when compared to schizophrenia patients. Mixed findings may be partly due to illness severity or type of bipolar illness, as Hibar and colleagues (2016) found that amygdala volume reductions only reached significance after dividing the patient groups into BD-I ($n = 1349$) and BD-II ($n = 361$), where BD-I patients had smaller volumes in comparison to HCs.

Meta-analyses (of primarily whole-brain VBM studies) have also reported GM reductions of the hippocampus, thalamus, precentral gyrus, anterior cingulate, insula, prefrontal cortex, inferior frontal cortex, temporal cortex and claustrum, and WM reduction of the corpus callosum, in people with BD (Bora et al., 2010; Ellison-Wright & Bullmore, 2010; Hajek et al., 2012; Hibar et al., 2016; Houenou et al., 2011; Kempton et al., 2008; Selvaraj et al., 2012). Fractional anisotropy (FA) abnormalities have also been observed in the superior longitudinal fasciculus, forceps minor, inferior fronto-occipital fasciculus, cingulum and cerebellum of BD patients (Jenkins et al., 2016). These meta-analyses involved 14–141 studies and 215–3509 BD patients and found effects ranging from $d = -0.15$ to -0.45 (see Figure 6.3 for an example of GM reductions in BD and regional overlap with schizophrenia (Ellison-Wright & Bullmore, 2010)). Similar to schizophrenia-spectrum disorders, significant VE has also been found in BD, albeit of slightly smaller magnitude (effect size = 0.26–0.39) (Arnone et al., 2009; Hibar et al., 2016; Kempton et al., 2008; McDonald et al., 2004). Review of 20 longitudinal structural MRI studies suggested GM loss of the prefrontal cortex, anterior cingulate cortex and subgenual regions is progressive in nature in BD (Lim et al., 2013).

Medication effects on the brain also need to be considered in BD. Many of the BD meta-analyses found use of mood stabilisers impacted significantly on total GM volume

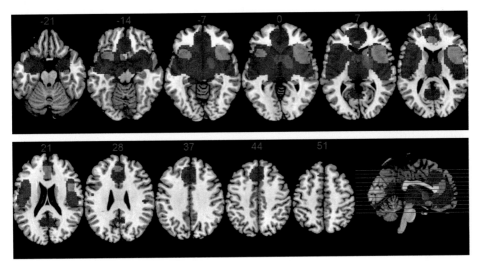

Figure 6.3 Regions of GM change in people with BD and people with schizophrenia. Regions of GM decreases in bipolar subjects compared with controls (yellow), regions of GM decreases in schizophrenia subjects compared with controls (red) and regions of GM increases in schizophrenia subjects compared with controls (purple), displayed on a brain template (Ellison-Wright & Bullmore, 2010). The left side of the image represents the left side of the brain. (Image reproduced with permission). *A black and white version of this figure will appear in some formats. For the colour version, please refer to the plate section.*

(Kempton et al., 2008), and specifically the globus pallidus (Arnone et al., 2009), hippocampus (Hajek et al., 2012) and anterior cingulate (Bora et al., 2010). However, the direction of this effect is in contrast with the schizophrenia-spectrum literature, as mood stabilisers (in particular lithium) are associated with GM *increases*, which is suggested to be linked to neurotrophic and other neuroprotective effects (Moore et al., 2000).

Despite the inconsistencies in this illness domain, particularly with regard to regional GM volumes, there is some evidence to show that WM hyperintensities are consistently found in BD (Beyer et al., 2009), a neuropathological anomaly suggested to be particularly prevalent in a range of affective disorders (Lyoo et al., 2002). Although WM volumetric abnormalities have often been reported in schizophrenia as mentioned above, report of hyperintensities tends to be relatively rare. Deep WM and periventricular hyperintensities are suggested to be reflective of microangiopathy (Hahn et al., 2014) and, as might be expected, are associated with ageing (Sachdev et al., 2007). Thus, it has been proposed that WM hyperintensities may be specific characteristics of 'late-onset' mental illnesses, namely schizophrenia and BD (Hahn et al., 2014). However, Hahn et al.'s (2014) review comprised only six studies that specifically investigated WM hyperintensities in late-onset patients. Further, such anomalies have been observed in early-onset illness, which will be discussed later in this chapter. It is worth noting that WM hyperintensities have been shown to be independent of the use of mood stabilisers (Kempton et al., 2008).

In recent years, BD has been suggested to sit on a continuum with schizophrenia-spectrum psychoses, given that there is significant overlap in symptom characteristics, neurophysiological anomalies and genetic factors that are linked to these mental illness groups (Ivleva et al., 2010). Despite this, a review of 11 spectrum criteria (set out by the DSM-5 Study Group), ranging from shared neural substrates to shared endophenotypes, concluded that evidence for grouping BD in the psychosis domain was relatively weak

(Carpenter et al., 2009). Ellison-Wright and Bullmore's (2010) meta-analysis found that, while GM deficits were common in the cingulate and insula for both illness groups, a region of the anterior pregenual cingulate (Brodmann area 24) was reduced in GM for BD patients only. Similarly, while there appears to be a high degree of overlap in regions of reduced FA for BD cohorts when qualitatively compared to other emotion-type disorders (e.g. major depressive disorder (MDD)), some unique features emerge, specifically the BD group was the only illness cohort to display increased FA in any region, and to have a more bilateral pattern of WM abnormalities (Jenkins et al., 2016).

Schnack and colleagues (2014) used a machine learning technique to directly test the utility of structural GM MRI information in differentiating between BD, schizophrenia and HC individuals. An astounding 88 per cent of schizophrenia patients were, on average, accurately distinguished from BD patients, and an average of 90 per cent were correctly distinguished from controls (Schnack et al., 2014). However, mean accuracy of classifying BD when grouped with controls was only 53 per cent. Nonetheless, this evidence suggests it is possible for an algorithm to be effective in discriminating between different mental illnesses based on GM density. Future research should endeavour to explore machine learning approaches further by integrating data from across multiple modalities, such as physiological, genetic and neurocognitive information (Orru et al., 2012).

Depressive Disorders

Depressive disorders are the most common of the mental illnesses worldwide, with lifetime prevalence ranging between 3 and 17 per cent (World Federation for Mental Health, 2012). The hippocampus and amygdala, along with other frontostriatal and thalamic circuitry involved in mood regulation, are regions that have received much attention in the study of MDD, the most widely studied of the depressive disorders. However, as with BD, the evidence for these regions being structurally abnormal is somewhat inconsistent. Meta-analyses involving 11 to 143 studies and 176 to 6063 patients have shown that individuals with MDD, when compared to HCs, display GM reductions in the hippocampus, parahippocampus, thalamus, basal ganglia, putamen, caudate, globus pallidus, superior, middle and inferior frontal gyri, gyrus rectus, and prefrontal, orbitofrontal, frontomedial, paracingulate and anterior cingulate cortices (Bora et al., 2012; Du et al., 2012; Kempton et al., 2011; Koolschijn et al., 2009; Lai, 2013; Sacher et al., 2012; Schmaal et al., 2016; Zhao et al., 2014), with effect sizes ranging from $d = -0.14$ to -1.11 (Bora et al., 2012; Koolschijn et al., 2009; Schmaal et al., 2016). The largest effect was observed in the left anterior cingulate cortex (Koolschijn et al., 2009). GM thinning of the medial orbitofrontal cortex was recently discovered in the ENGIMA recurrent MDD adult cohort ($n = 1302$) (Schmaal et al., 2017). Conversely, adolescents with recurrent MDD ($n = 104$) did not have any cortical thinning but were found to display widespread bilateral surface area reductions, including within parietal, frontal, orbitofrontal, occipital, motor, somatosensory and temporal areas (Schmaal et al., 2017). White matter reductions have been found in the frontal lobes, fusiform gyrus and occipital lobe (Liao et al., 2013). Meta-analyses of 8–11 diffusion tensor imaging studies found reduced FA in regions of the anterior thalamic radiation, superior longitudinal fasciculus, cerebellum, corpus callosum, arcuate network and the fronto-occipital and uncinate fasciculi in MDD (Jenkins et al., 2016; Jiang et al., 2017). Significant VE has also been observed in MDD, albeit less frequently than that observed for schizophrenia-spectrum psychoses, but of comparable magnitude ($d = 0.41–0.47$) (Kempton et al., 2011).

Deep WM hyperintensities are considered to be one of the more consistent neuropathological findings in MDD (Desmyter et al., 2011; Kempton et al., 2011). Meta-analysis of nine studies comprising 324 patients shows periventricular hyperintensities are significantly increased in MDD compared to HCs (effect size = 0.29) (Kempton et al., 2011). Interestingly, direct comparison between depressed and BD cohorts suggests that WM hyperintensities are significantly more common in BD (Cardoso de Almeida & Phillips, 2013; Kempton et al., 2011), with as much as a twofold increased incidence rate than that of MDD patients (Kempton et al., 2011). A small review of neuroimaging studies that directly compared MDD to BD further suggested that reduction of the habenula (a set of nuclei that is connected to the limbic system and is thought to be involved in a range of processes, including value-based decision-making (Hikosaka, 2010)), may be specific to BD (Cardoso de Almeida & Phillips, 2013).

In line with the putative protective effects of mood stabilisers in general, antidepressants specifically have been suggested to normalise brain volumetric changes in MDD (Duman et al., 2001). Campbell and MacQueen (2004) suggested that antidepressant medications prevent hippocampal volume loss by way of protecting against the harmful effects of elevated glucocorticoids (e.g. excitotoxicity) associated with the neuropathophysiology of MDD. The meta-analysis by Bora and colleagues (2012) found that non-medicated compared to medicated MDD patients had smaller orbitofrontal, anterior cingulate and subgenual anterior cingulate cortices. This suggests that (1) certain brain regions may benefit preferentially from antidepressant exposure over others, and (2) regional volume loss of the prefrontal cortex, caudate, putamen and thalamus, which were no different between non-medicated and medicated patient groups, may be due to trait-like pathological changes associated with MDD.

Given the overlap in phenotypic presentation particularly between MDD and BD, identification of neurobiological risk markers that uniquely predict whether a person will develop one illness over the other would be of great clinical importance. Indeed, initial misdiagnosis is common in BD (Hirschfeld et al., 2003), as individuals with BD experience depression symptoms more often than hypomanic or manic states, which typically occurs between 1 and 9 per cent of the time (Judd et al., 2002; 2003). Thus, future research into structural brain abnormalities should move away from diagnostic silos and begin by implementing designs that encompass cohorts from across the spectrum of affective disorders, as well as other mental illness domains.

Summary and Implication of Evidence Across the Three Mental Illness Domains

Overall, the number of brain regions implicated in what is presumed the latter stages (i.e. Stages 3 and 4) of these mental illness domains is large. While some regions, such as the hippocampus and ventricles, are consistently abnormal in schizophrenia psychoses, and WM hyperintensities are commonly found in BD and MDD, *specificity* continues to be an issue. In addition, many demographic factors, as well as age of illness onset and use of psychiatric medications, need to be considered when interpreting the evidence. There is clearly a substantial degree of overlap in the brain regions implicated across these disorders (for an example see Figure 6.3), with no specific neural anomaly that presents as a definitive biological 'marker' of a given illness. Thus, evidence points towards machine learning approaches and the search for patterns of widespread deficits across multiple neural networks as a means of differentiating between illness groups in the future.

Thus far we have focused largely on cross-sectional research of individuals in the typically chronic illness stages, and touched on the *progressive* nature of volume loss over time, particularly in regards to schizophrenia-spectrum disorders. We now turn to the early illness stages, where brain changes appear to be more dynamic, and hence the *trajectory of change* more telling in the context of a clinical staging heuristic.

Neural Structural Abnormalities Associated with Schizophrenia-Spectrum Psychoses, Bipolar Disorder and Depression in the Early Illness Stages

It is now known that during adolescence and through to early adulthood (around age 25) the brain undergoes substantial GM and WM changes as part of normal neurodevelopment (Shaw et al., 2008). Specifically, much of the frontal, temporal, parietal and occipital cortices develop along a cubic trajectory, where during childhood there is an initial increase in the thickness of the cortex, but this then declines during adolescence and stabilises in adulthood (Shaw et al., 2008). However, the insula and anterior cingulate mostly develop along a quadratic trajectory, while regions of the orbitofrontal, piriform, medial temporal and occipitotemporal cortices, as well as the hippocampus, frontal operculum and subgenual areas, develop along a gradual downward linear trajectory (Shaw et al., 2008). These trajectories need to be taken into consideration when evaluating neuroimaging data in the context of clinical stages (Cropley & Pantelis, 2014). Several recent papers have outlined the potential applicability of neuroimaging evidence to a clinical staging model in psychiatry, with particular emphasis on the early illness stages which typically occur during adolescence, within this critical neurodevelopmental window (Frank et al., 2015; Lin et al., 2013; McGorry et al., 2014; Wood et al., 2011). As with the latter illness stages, the majority of the research in this area has been in schizophrenia-spectrum psychoses. We will focus primarily on Stages 2 (first episode (FE) of illness) and 1b (ultra-high risk (UHR)).

Schizophrenia-Spectrum Psychoses
First-Episode Psychosis

As with established schizophrenia disorders, meta-analyses of cross-sectional studies in FEP (excluding psychoses associated with a primary affective disorder) demonstrate that reductions in hippocampal volumes, relative to HCs, are consistent (Adriano et al., 2012; Steen et al., 2006; Vita & de Peri, 2007; Vita et al., 2006). Interestingly, this deficit is comparable in magnitude to that of individuals in the chronic illness stages, with Cohen's *d* ranging from −0.47 to −0.66 (Adriano et al., 2012; Vita et al., 2006). Taking into account the linear developmental trajectory of this subcortical structure, these findings suggest that reduced hippocampal volume may be a biological trait marker of psychotic illness. VE is also a consistent finding in FEP (effect size range = 0.47–0.61) (De Peri et al., 2012; Steen et al., 2006; Vita et al., 2006). These ROI-based meta-analyses involved between 13 and 52 studies and 114 and 1424 FEP patients, indicating that findings are robust.

Other meta-analyses (*n* patient range = 271–965) that employed voxel-based methods have found reduced GM volume of the cerebellum, insula, caudate, operculum, superior temporal, medial frontal, prefrontal and anterior cingulate cortices (Chan et al., 2011; Fusar-Poli et al., 2012b; 2014; Radua et al., 2012), and WM deficits (reduced FA) in the corpus callosum (Zhuo et al., 2016), and deep in the frontal and temporal lobes (Yao et al.,

2013). One region that appears to be of normal volume in FEP is the amygdala (Velakoulis et al., 2006; Vita & de Peri, 2007; Vita et al., 2006). As mentioned previously, amygdala volume reductions are observed in established schizophrenia, suggesting that volume loss occurs post illness onset, which may be pathologically driven or a secondary consequence related to other factors (e.g. medication; see discussion below). Nonetheless, if amygdala volume is intact at the first episode, this has implications for early interventions that may protect this region from later decline and possibly improve certain phenomenology associated with amygdala function (e.g. emotion regulation).

Interestingly, Radua and colleagues (2012) additionally found that the lingual and precentral gyri were significantly *enlarged* in comparison to age-matched HCs (mean age = 24 and 26, respectively; range = 15–35 years). Possible explanations for this may be related to the second (or third)-hit neurodevelopmental hypothesis, which posits that underlying pathophysiological mechanisms may lead to 'arrest' or potentially 'delay' of normal brain development during adolescence (Pantelis et al., 2005). Given that these gyri would normally develop along a cubic trajectory and generally are not found to be abnormal in established schizophrenia-spectrum illnesses, arrest or delay in the maturation of this region (i.e. a halt or delay in the natural reduction in thickness and subsequent stabilisation) is possible. However, the evidence presented here is cross-sectional in nature. Identifying neurobiological markers during the early stages of illness onset, which coincides with dynamic neurodevelopmental changes, is in essence like 'searching for a moving target' (Pantelis et al., 2009). Thus, longitudinal designs are far more informative.

A recent meta-analysis of nine longitudinal studies in FEP ($n = 500$) generally supports the findings from cross-sectional research (Vita et al., 2012). Specifically, in addition to whole-brain GM volume reductions, FEP patients displayed significant GM reductions in the frontal, temporal (including transverse gyri) and parietal lobes over time in comparison to controls (mean years inter-MRI interval = 2.5). One prominent study conducted by Sun and colleagues (2009b; see Figure 6.4) demonstrated that from the first psychotic episode cortical surface contraction, particularly the dorsal regions of the frontal lobes, occurs at twice the rate as that observed in HCs over a period of 1–4 years, implying that the normal pattern of development is altered in FEP by way of excessive cortical thinning. Work from

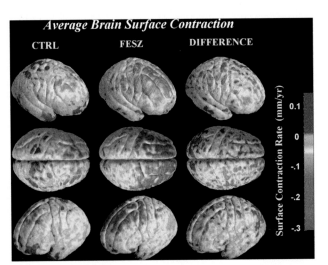

Figure 6.4 Average brain surface contraction in FE psychosis. Displayed are the average rates of brain surface contraction (mm per year) in control individuals (CTRL), first-episode schizophrenia patients (FESZ) and the absolute difference between the two groups. Negative values (warm colours) denote surface contraction (Sun et al., 2009b; image reproduced with permission). *A black and white version of this figure will appear in some formats. For the colour version, please refer to the plate section.*

this same research group has further demonstrated progressive GM reductions of the insula and several superior temporal subregions in FEP (Takahashi et al., 2009a; 2009c).

The Iowa Longitudinal Study is one of the largest and longest follow-up studies of FEP patients, with a subsample of 202 patients having on average two follow-up MRI scans, occurring up to 15 years after intake (mean time between first and last scan = 7.2 years) (Andreasen et al., 2011). Andreasen et al. (2011) found that total GM volume/yr (specifically GM of the frontal, temporal and parietal lobes) and total WM volume/yr (specifically WM of the frontal and temporal lobes) decreased and that sulcal cerebrospinal fluid (CSF) increased significantly for FEP patients over time when compared to HCs. Interestingly, when they examined *pattern of change* it was only at the first inter-scan interval (approximately two years post-baseline) that FEP volume changes were statistically different to control participants, highlighting that the most severe brain changes occur during the critical early illness stages. Surprisingly, there were no significant group differences in volume change for parietal WM or for the lateral ventricles. However, as time progressed higher doses of antipsychotic medications corresponded to greater reductions in total cerebral and lobar WM, caudate and cerebellar volumes, and greater enlargements in sulcal CSF, lateral ventricular and putamen volumes (Ho et al., 2011). Irrespective of illness duration and illness severity, higher antipsychotic dose was associated with smaller GM and larger putamen volumes (Ho et al., 2011). Despite this, cross-sectional research has shown that medication-naïve FEP patients present with reduced superior temporal, insula and cerebellum volumes (Fusar-Poli et al., 2012b), indicating that although brain changes across the illness stages may be partially due to the effects of antipsychotic medications, alterations in brain structure also appear to be intrinsic to the illness. Overall, findings are in line with cross-sectional research into medication effects on the brain in FEP (Ansell et al., 2014; Lesh et al., 2015; Radua et al., 2012). (For further discussion on the effects of antipsychotic class on brain structure, see Ansell et al. (2014) and Ho et al. (2011).) One reason for researchers turning their focus to the at-risk mental state was indeed to escape the confounding effects of antipsychotic medication use.

Ultra-High Risk of Psychosis

Study of individuals at 'clinical' or 'ultra-high risk' of psychosis (i.e. Stage 1b) is essential for uncovering the potential predictors of both illness progression and response to treatment (be it either pharmacological or psychosocial). However, readers should be mindful that interpretation of cross-sectional research in this area is challenging, given that a large proportion (approximately 65–73 per cent) will *not* transition to a full-threshold psychotic disorder in the short term (e.g. two years; Simon et al., 2013) or long term (e.g. ten years; Nelson et al., 2013). Additionally, there is a distinction between individuals at UHR (i.e. clinically help-seeking and functioning suboptimally) and individuals at genetic high risk (GHR; i.e. Stages 0–1a), who may be functioning normally and tend to have a lower risk of transition (one in ten lifetime risk when one first-degree relative is affected by psychotic illness (Mueser & McGurk, 2004)). (For a review of genetic high risk populations, see Bois et al. (2015), Boos et al. (2007), Cooper et al. (2014), Fusar-Poli et al. (2014) and McIntosh et al., (2011).)

Meta-analysis of 14 VBM studies has shown that UHR individuals ($n = 198$) present with significant GM reductions in the middle frontal gyrus, middle and superior temporal gyri, hippocampus, parahippocampus and anterior cingulate in comparison to matched HCs (Fusar-Poli et al., 2012b). However, in relation to FEP patients, GM volumes of the superior temporal gyrus, anterior cingulate, cerebellum and insula were significantly larger in UHR (Fusar-Poli et al., 2012b). Although these studies were cross-sectional, findings imply that *additional* volume loss may occur in specific structures (i.e. superior temporal and anterior cingulate gyri) during the transition phase from Stage 1b to Stage 2. Similarly, findings suggest certain regions, namely the insula and cerebellum, may be preserved prior to the first psychotic episode and deteriorate thereafter (Fusar-Poli et al., 2012b). However, this is challenged by research showing these regions to be reduced in UHR relative to HCs (Borgwardt et al., 2007). Some studies have also failed to find any between-group differences in whole-brain or regional GM, WM or cortical thickness (Klauser et al., 2015). Mixed findings may in part be the result of a dilution effect, which comes from averaging the volumes across a broad UHR population comprising both people who will and will not end up developing a psychotic disorder. Thus, numerous studies have followed up UHR individuals over several years to assess UHR status.

It has been shown that UHR individuals who later transition to psychosis (UHR-P) in comparison to UHR individuals who do not transition to psychosis (UHR-NP) have reduced insula volumes, thinning in regions of the anterior cingulate and anterior genu of the corpus callosum, but normal cerebellar volumes at baseline (Fornito et al., 2008; Pantelis et al., 2003; Takahashi et al., 2009b; Walterfang et al., 2008b). Larger baseline pituitary volume (thought to be indicative of a heightened hypothalamic-pituitary-adrenal (HPA) axis response to stress) has been found in UHR-P compared to UHR-NP and HCs (Buschlen et al., 2011; Garner et al., 2005). Evidence for WM is somewhat mixed (when comparing UHR-P to UHR-NP) where WM volume was reported as increased in regions of the frontal lobes (Fusar-Poli et al., 2011; Walterfang et al., 2008a) and decreased in medial temporal and superior parietal regions (Fusar-Poli et al., 2011), while FA has been found both decreased and increased in disparate temporal lobe regions (Bloemen et al., 2010). FA in a subregion of the corpus callosum has been found to be significantly reduced in UHR-NP individuals (but not UHR-P) relative to HCs, although UHR-P did show a trend in the same direction (Katagiri et al., 2015). A recent study that used a whole-brain structural covariance approach (which examines GM correlations between *a priori* ROIs) found aberrant structural interconnectedness between nodes within several well-defined networks (salience, executive control, auditory and motor) in UHR-P relative to UHR-NP (Heinze et al., 2015).

Contrary to evidence that distinguishes transitioned individuals from non-transitioned individuals, volume of the superior temporal gyrus was equally reduced in UHR-P and UHR-NP relative to HCs, suggestive of a more generalised deficit for persons with an at-risk mental state (Takahashi et al., 2010; Wood et al., 2010). Findings regarding the amygdala have been fairly consistent thus far, with UHR individuals presenting with normal baseline volumes, irrespective of later transition (Dazzan et al., 2012; Velakoulis et al., 2006; Witthaus et al., 2010).

Despite the somewhat reduced heterogeneity within the broad UHR group by prospective classification of transition status, numerous other underlying factors appear unaccounted for, as findings continue to be inconsistent. For example, studies have found hippocampal volumes of both UHR-P and UHR-NP to be: no different to HCs (Velakoulis et al., 2006); equally reduced compared to HCs (Wood et al., 2010); or have found UHR-NP (but not UHR-P) to be reduced compared to HCs (Phillips et al., 2002). In addition, dividing the UHR sample into subgroups is proving increasingly difficult, given the low (and declining) transition rate, which impacts on statistical power. It has been postulated that the inconsistencies in this cross-sectional literature (for review, see Smieskova et al.,

2010) are due to, in part, abnormalities being dependent on the interactions between illness stage, developmental trajectory of the given brain structure and age/life stage (Gogtay et al., 2011; Pantelis et al., 2005; 2008) and/or illness/symptom acuity (Cropley & Pantelis, 2014), which further highlights the importance of longitudinal designs.

Longitudinal UHR studies (most of which used an ROI approach) with follow-up between 1 and 2.5 years have found the UHR-P individuals (but not UHR-NP) to have significant volume reductions in the insula, cingulate cortex, orbitofrontal cortex, superior temporal gyrus, fusiform gyrus and parahippocampus (Pantelis et al., 2003; Takahashi et al., 2009b), as well as reduced FA in frontal (Carletti et al., 2012) and reduced WM in cerebellar-thalamic (Mittal et al., 2014) regions, during the transition to psychosis. Similarly, cortical thinning of the anterior cingulate, precuneus and subregions of superior temporal and temporo-parieto-occipital cortices has been found to be more pronounced in UHR-P relative to HCs, although no differences were found when compared to UHR-NP (Ziermans et al., 2012). However, Sun and colleagues (2009a), using a cortical pattern-matching technique, did find that the rate of surface contraction was significantly exaggerated in the prefrontal lobe of UHR-P compared to UHR-NP individuals, consistent with their study in FEP (described earlier) (Sun et al., 2009b). While there are various morphological brain abnormalities that appear to be more common in UHR-P, cerebellar (Pantelis et al., 2003) and hippocampal (Walter et al., 2012) volumes have been found to decrease over time (1–4 years) in UHR individuals irrespective of transition status.

One of the largest longitudinal UHR studies to date (North American Prodromal Longitudinal Study; NAPLS) has recently confirmed that cortical thinning of the superior and middle frontal, as well as orbitofrontal, cortices occurs at a significantly faster rate in UHR-P ($n = 35$) compared to UHR-NP ($n = 239$) and HCs ($n = 135$), which was of moderate to large magnitude ($d = -0.30$ to -1.0) (Cannon et al., 2015). This was demonstrated with an average inter-scan interval of only 141 days in individuals who transitioned, suggesting that structural brain changes can occur in a short time period. Several other regions, including the parahippocampus and regions of the parietal and superior temporal cortices, also demonstrated abnormal rates of change (however, these did not survive correction). Interestingly, Cannon et al. (2015) further examined the impact of duration of prodrome on brain changes; that is, whether a shorter time in Stage 1b corresponds to more severe neural abnormalities. Indeed, they found that UHR-P individuals with a shorter duration (<26 months) had a steeper reduction in prefrontal cortical thickness compared to those with a long duration of prodromal symptoms (>26 months). In addition, UHR-P participants had greater enlargement of the third ventricle in comparison to UHR-NP and HC participants, but there were no longitudinal group differences in other ventricular regions, subcortical GM structures or various other cortical regions not mentioned above. It is noteworthy that no baseline differences existed between any of the groups, and changes occurred irrespective of antipsychotic exposure. Taken together with the heterogeneity in findings from cross-sectional studies across different stages of the illness, we propose that mapping trajectories of pathophysiological brain changes is needed, particularly if neuroimaging is to have a place within a clinical staging framework.

Summary

Some abnormalities that are consistently observed in the chronic illness stages, namely hippocampal volume reductions and VEs, appear to also be present in FEP (Stage 2), suggesting that these are potential biological risk markers of schizophrenia-spectrum disorders. In addition, GM (and to a lesser extent WM) reductions are widespread across multiple regions of the frontal, temporal (especially superior regions), insular and parietal cortices in FEP. Moreover, GM in particular continues to develop abnormally (e.g. greater volume reductions, cortical thinning) for at least several years following the initial onset of illness, which includes regions that develop along differing trajectories (i.e. cubic, quadratic and linear). The UHR literature is considerably more mixed but, importantly, the severity and degree of neural abnormalities in Stage 1b is significantly less than that observed in later, more established illness stages. Initial evidence suggests that VE and reduced hippocampal volumes are not typical characteristic features of the 1b illness stage. However, certain neural abnormalities, particularly volume reductions of the insula, cingulate and superior temporal cortices as well as a faster rate of frontal cortical thinning, may act as predisposing risk factors that could aid in predicting transition to psychosis. Many studies have examined predictive ability of specific neural abnormalities. For example, Garner et al.'s (2005) cross-sectional study showed that for every 10 per cent increase in baseline pituitary volume, risk of transition increased by 20 per cent. Similarly, Walterfang et al. (2008b) showed that for every 1 mm reduction in mean thickness of the anterior genu, UHR participants had a 52 per cent increase in risk for transition. However, a whole-brain approach appears to be more advantageous, as multivariate neuroanatomical pattern classification has been found to accurately identify UHR individuals who later transition for 88 per cent of cases, when grouped with UHR-NP and HCs (Koutsouleris et al., 2009). Thus, machine learning, as mentioned earlier, as well as multimodal stepwise prediction models (Clark et al., 2015), may prove most useful for applying a clinical staging model to schizophrenia-spectrum and more broadly psychiatric illness in the future.

Bipolar Disorders
First-Episode Bipolar Disorder

Unlike schizophrenia-spectrum psychoses, research into early illness stages of BDs is somewhat scarce and complicated by issues of diagnostic uncertainty. Two small meta-analyses have been conducted in first-episode (i.e. Stage 2) BD (FEBD; note that this is typically defined as presentation of first *manic* episode, which is usually preceded by a history of one or several depressive episodes). These comprised 5–11 studies (n = 64–221 patients) and found that total WM, but not GM, was significantly reduced (Hedges' g = –0.35) compared to HCs (De Peri et al., 2012; Vita et al., 2009). There were no group differences for ventricular volume (De Peri et al., 2012). While these studies report on volumes of gross neuroanatomical structures, a number of region-specific investigations have been conducted.

As mentioned earlier, meta-analyses suggest that amygdala volume abnormalities are specific to children and adolescents with BD (Hajek et al., 2009; Pfeifer et al., 2008). However, because these meta-analyses did not focus on first-episode cases (i.e. those with a short duration of illness), it is unknown whether the amygdala reductions are related to early illness stage (irrespective of age of onset), to length of illness, or are a marker relevant to onset in childhood (i.e. a putative marker of a paediatric form of the illness). The latter is unlikely, as Rosso et al. (2007) found significant reductions in amygdala volumes of FEBD individuals (mean age = 23 years) who had been ill for <1 year, suggesting it may be early illness stage-related.

White matter hyperintensities have been found in children with BD compared with age-equivalent controls, and compared to children with schizophrenia (Lyoo et al., 2002), which is consistent with established forms of these disorders in adulthood (see above). Lyoo et al. (2002), however, did not report on duration of illness, thus it is possible that patients had already passed from Stage 2 into Stage 3. To our knowledge, only one study examined WM hyperintensities in individuals with FEBD; investigators failed to find any group differences in the degree of WM hyperintensities between FEBD, FEP and controls, where prevalence in controls was approximately 29 per cent (Zanetti et al., 2008). Further research is needed in this area, including studies to identify whether WM hyperintensity load, or the regions affected, might be relevant.

A number of other studies have investigated specific ROIs in FEBD. Koo et al. (2008) focused on the anterior cingulate and found the subgenual subregion was significantly smaller in FEBD in comparison to HCs, and this was more pronounced if patients had a family history of mood disorder. Mills et al. (2005) examined the vermal subregion of the cerebellum, a region suggested to be involved in mood regulation, given its neuronal projections to limbic brain regions. While they found that FEBD patients did not differ from HCs, multiple-episode BD patients had volume reductions in two vermal subregions relative to HCs, and one subregion relative to FEBD patients. However, the authors concluded that this was likely confounded by exposure to antidepressant medication, which was a significant predictor of vermal subregion V3 volume. Atmaca et al. (2007) examined the corpus callosum in a unique medication-naïve FEBD sample (mean illness duration = 3.6 months; mean age = 28 years), and found that total corpus callosum area was significantly smaller compared to HCs. Kozicky et al. (2013) measured dorsolateral prefrontal cortex (DLPFC) and caudate volumes and found that only the latter structure was abnormal (enlarged) in FEBD patients who were up to three months in remission from their first manic episode.

Studies that adopted a whole-brain approach have produced mixed findings. There is evidence of significant GM enlargements of the thalamus, basal ganglia, fusiform gyrus, paracentral lobule, regions of the cingulate and temporal cortices, and of the cerebellum in FEBD (Adler et al., 2007; Chen et al., 2012). Additionally, FA has been found reduced in parietal WM of FEBD patients (Chen et al., 2012). Contrary to these studies, Yatham et al.'s (2007) VBM study failed to find any significant differences between the FEBD and HC group after correcting for multiple comparisons. These few studies differed greatly in terms of sample characteristics and methodology, including their definition of FEBD (discussed below), making it difficult to interpret the results.

A handful of longitudinal neuroimaging studies have been conducted in FEBD. One study found significant within-group reductions in the anterior cingulate of a small sample of FEBD patients ($n = 8$; age range = 17–20) over an average of 2.5 years, which was similarly observed in their FE schizophrenia group (although this latter group had more widespread GM reductions) (Farrow et al., 2005). This is partially supported by Koo and colleagues (2008), who found specifically the subgenual region of the cingulate to decrease significantly over an average of 1.5 years, when compared to HCs. Kasai et al. (2003), however, failed to find any abnormal GM changes in their ROIs (superior temporal gyrus and amygdala–hippocampal complex), despite finding significant abnormalities in their FE schizophrenia group. Enlargement of total neocortical GM has been observed over a two-year period in FEBD in comparison to HCs, despite patients having smaller relative volumes at baseline (Nakamura et al., 2007). This is in the opposite direction to what is observed in established BD, and was suggested to be due to the possible neurotrophic effects of mood stabilisers. Notably, volumetric abnormalities in the FEBD group were less extensive than for the FE schizophrenia group, who showed typical reductions over time. One limitation of these studies is that they describe their patient group as having a first-episode affective disorder/psychosis (albeit approximately 95 per cent of the individuals had a BD diagnosis), where the line between manic and psychotic presentation was often poorly defined. Lastly, one recent study that specifically focused on adolescents (age range = 12–17 years) with FEBD found that this group failed to demonstrate the normal amygdala volume increases that were observed in their age-matched healthy counterparts (as well as adolescents with attention deficit hyperactivity disorder) over a one-year period (Bitter et al., 2011).

At Risk of Bipolar Disorders

To our knowledge, only one meta-analysis of the neuroimaging literature in individuals at high risk for BD, defined as genetic risk (i.e. Stage 0), has been conducted (Fusar-Poli et al., 2012a). This meta-analysis found no GM volumetric differences between HCs and high risk (HR) for BD participants for any of the ROIs analysed, including the thalamus, striatum, amygdala, hippocampus, pituitary gland and frontal lobe (Fusar-Poli et al., 2012a). However, in comparison to meta-analyses of psychosis literature, these analyses comprised small study numbers (i.e. ranging from 3 to 8), and there was an insufficient number for conducting whole-brain vertex-wise analyses.

Bechdolf and colleagues (2012) were one of the first groups to examine brain morphology in individuals with an at-risk mental state who later went on to develop BD. While their initial sample met criteria for UHR for psychosis, at one-year follow-up a subgroup ($n = 11$) met criteria for a primary diagnosis of bipolar I or II disorder. In this ROI study, while no significant group differences were found for ventricular or hippocampal volumes, amygdala and insula volumes were significantly reduced in the UHR-BD group at baseline, relative to HCs. There were no statistically significant group differences between UHR-BD and UHR-non-transition individuals (although investigators suggested this was due to low power and that UHR-BD patients appear to have greater reductions in these brain regions in comparison to the non-transition UHR group). Unfortunately there was no comparison with a UHR-P group, and there were no repeat scans conducted at follow-up.

To date, only one study has specifically focused on adolescents at clinical high risk of BD ($n = 30$; mean age = 15 years), defined as 'a distinct period of abnormally and persistently elevated, expansive or irritable mood associated with one or more manic or hypomanic symptoms in number and duration below criteria threshold to qualify for a diagnosis of bipolar episode' (Paillere Martinot et al., 2014: 463). Participants did not meet criteria for any psychiatric diagnosis at the time of assessment (although 8 of the UHR for BD group and 21 of the controls reported a history of either a depressive episode(s) or a first-/second-degree relative with BD). Frontal-limbic VBM analyses of GM volumes revealed a significant reduction in the anterior cingulate of UHR for BD patients relative to controls. In addition, patients displayed reduced FA in various WM tracts, including the corpus callosum, cingulum bundle and the longitudinal and uncinate fasciculi. These findings are generally in line with abnormalities observed in the later stages of BD.

While the neurodevelopmental trajectory of early-stage BD is presently unknown, Theodoridou et al. (2014) have initiated a multidisciplinary longitudinal study as part of the Zurich Program for Sustainable Development of Mental Health Services, aimed at developing a risk model to estimate conversion and identify cognitive and neurobiological predictors of functional outcome. The findings of this promising study will further our knowledge of Stage 1b for psychotic and bipolar illnesses.

Summary

Despite the dearth of early-stage BD research, given what we know of later illness stages of BD, amygdala abnormalities which do not appear to persist into adult BD may be a feature specific to Stage 2 (and possibly Stage 1b) of the illness, while WM hyperintensities may be a neurobiological feature of the illness which develops (or only becomes detectable) after Stage 2, regardless of whether onset is early in childhood or later in life. The literature regarding GM and WM is extremely mixed, with only reductions in volume of the cingulate, and compromised WM integrity, presenting as potential features of early-stage BD illness. Consistent with the literature on established illness stages, there continues to be overlap in the brain regions affected in FEBD and FEP, with the latter group overall presenting with more severe abnormalities. There have been too few studies into the UHR 1b stage of BD to make any summations at this time. Thus, key questions that remain are whether the neural abnormalities observed in FEBD have been present even prior to the first manic episode, and whether they are distinct from those of early-stage depression. In most of the studies reviewed here, FEBD individuals were in their mid-twenties to early thirties, almost always had at least one prior major depressive episode and were often previously/currently treated with antidepressants (and sometimes mood stabilisers and/or antipsychotics). Thus, more rigorously controlled studies in individuals who are within the adolescent/early-adult life stage and who are clearly identified as being in Stage 2 or in Stage 1b of the BD illness are warranted.

Depressive Disorders
First-Episode Depression

Cole et al. (2011) were the first to conduct a meta-analysis that focused on FE depression (primarily FEMDD; mean illness duration = 14.4 months), and found that patients (n = 191; mean age = 37.6 years) showed significantly reduced hippocampi (average of −4.25 per cent) relative to HCs. There were no moderating effects found for age, gender or illness duration. However, one limitation of this study is that hippocampal volume was the only ROI investigated. Zhao et al.'s (2014) voxel-wise meta-analysis found that their FEMDD group (n = 171; six studies) displayed significant volume reductions in the superior and middle frontal gyri, parahippocampus and hippocampus (extending to the amygdala), while increased volume was found for the thalamus, relative to HCs. All FEMDD participants (mean age = 29.3 years) were drug-naïve and had an average illness duration of 0.52 years. Conversely, a recent ROI-based (subcortical structures) meta-analysis comprising 583 FEMDD patients did not find any volumetric differences when compared to HCs, despite recurrent MDD patients displaying reduced hippocampal volumes (Schmaal et al., 2016). Interestingly, Schmaal and colleagues (2016) found that within the whole sample (mean age = 38.2), individuals with an illness onset age of ≤21 years had significantly smaller hippocampal volumes compared to HCs. Individuals with a later illness onset (i.e. >21 years) showed no volume differences for any of the ROIs when compared to HCs, or when compared to the earlier-onset group. The authors argued that it is unlikely the finding of volume loss in the earlier-onset group was entirely driven by the recurrent episode patients (approximately 57 per cent had recurrent episode MDD), given that this percentage value was not found to be a significant moderator. However, because Schmaal et al. (2016) did not analyse subcortical structures in the FEMDD group for adolescents and adults separately, it is difficult to draw conclusions from a neurodevelopmental clinical staging standpoint. More recently, however, Schmaal and colleagues (2017) examined cortical thickness and surface area in both adults ($n = 583$) and adolescents ($n = 80$) with FEMDD. Adults with FEMDD showed extensive thinning in the fusiform gyrus, anterior and posterior cingulate cortices, insula and orbitofrontal and superior frontal cortices. Adolescents with FEMDD, on the other hand, showed no cortical abnormalities/differences when compared to either the controls or FE adults.

A handful of cross-sectional VBM studies have been conducted in medication-naïve adults with FEMDD (mean age range = 35–48 years; mean illness duration range = 4–5 months). Qiu et al. (2014) found increased GM volumes of the paracentral lobule, superior frontal gyrus, cuneus and thalamus, as well as increased cortical thickness in several frontoparietal regions. Conversely, Lai and Wu's (2015) recent study showed FEMDD patients displayed significant GM reductions in the medial and superior frontal cortices, superior temporal gyrus and regions of the cerebellum relative to HCs. Several of these regions were also significantly reduced when compared to patients with FE panic disorder. Watanabe and colleagues (2015) observed volume reductions of the caudate and superior temporal gyrus, and further showed that caudate reductions were more pronounced in FEMDD patients who were Val/Met carriers of the catechol-O-methyltransferase (COMT) gene (involved in the degradation of dopamine). Ide et al. (2015) found volume reductions (of the prefrontal cortex) only after brain-derived neurotrophic factor genotype (Val66Met polymorphism) was entered into the analysis, where FEMDD Met carriers (but not Val/Val carriers) displayed reductions in comparison to HCs.

A recent meta-analysis on cross-sectional diffusion tensor imaging data from seven studies conducted in medication-naïve adults with FEMDD ($n = 174$ patients; mean age range = 21–44 years; mean illness duration range = 0.4–1.3 years) found FA reductions in the genu of the corpus callosum and anterior thalamic projections, relative to HCs (Jiang et al., 2017). A number of these studies, which used vertex-wise or regional parcellation approaches, warrant further discussion; Han et al. (2014) conducted a comprehensive study that examined several morphological parameters, including cortical thickness, cortical and subcortical volumes and WM integrity. Despite the breadth of analyses, only the anterior cingulate and corpus callosum were reduced in volume and FA respectively, in comparison to HCs. Conversely, Wang et al. (2014) found FA was increased in their FEMDD patients, in WM of the superior longitudinal fasciculus. This unexpected finding was suggested to reflect the putative regeneration of axonal fibres that may be an initial compensatory mechanism in response to recent illness onset. While these two studies comprised medication-naïve samples with comparable illness durations (mean = 5 months), age may be a moderating factor, as FEMDD patients in the latter study were on average ten years younger (mean age = 32 years) than patients in Han et al.'s (2014) study. Although it is possible that differences in analysis methods could explain the discrepant findings, a question that remains unanswered is whether the type and direction of WM abnormality (e.g. FA vs WM volume; increase vs decrease) is region-dependent, and if so what implications are there for the corresponding region that the fibre tracts connect with? Indeed, Long et al. (2015) recently examined WM structural connectivity networks in FE depression. They found that, in addition to patients displaying an abnormal topological organisation of the whole-brain network, two sub-networks that particularly involved connections with the orbitofrontal cortex were significantly increased in connectivity in comparison to HCs.

That is, patients had more connections extending from the orbitofrontal cortex to a number of other cortical regions (e.g. fusiform and inferior temporal gyri) as well as subcortical structures (e.g. insula and hippocampus).

These initial findings suggest disparate results across studies may be related to moderator variables, such as age of illness onset, effects of illness duration, genetic variation or other secondary factors related to the consequences of the illness.

At Risk of Depression

At present, there is no operationalised definition for, or clearly identified characteristics of, an at-risk mental state for depression. The majority of studies in this area have been conducted in individuals who have a genetic risk for depression (Stage 0), and very few explored structural neuroimaging parameters. Munn et al. (2007) used a twin cohort (aged 13–25 years) to examine amygdala volume between females with MDD and their unaffected female twin (both with a positive family history of depression) and also compared them to HC twins with no personal or family history of depression. They found no volumetric differences. However, although samples were matched for age, differences in stage of neurodevelopment were not factored into the analyses. A recent longitudinal study into adolescent development shows a sex-specific interaction between amygdala volume changes (from age 12 to 16) and prediction of depression in a risk-enriched (based on temperament) community cohort (Whittle et al., 2014). Specifically, for females, increased growth of the amygdala from early to mid adolescence was associated with the onset of depression, whereas the opposite was found for males. Such gender effects on trajectories of brain change have not been adequately addressed by most studies to date.

Hippocampal volume has been examined in individuals at risk for depression. Rao et al. (2010) found adolescents (mean age = 15 years) at high genetic risk had smaller hippocampal volumes than HCs, and similar volumes to adolescents with MDD. This was significant even after controlling for age, gender, ethnicity/race, pubertal status and socioeconomic status. Spalletta and colleagues (2014) showed that smaller hippocampal volumes in healthy males (but not females) from the general population were a significant predictor of subthreshold depressive symptoms (based on the Beck Depression Inventory (Beck et al., 1961)). Thus, future research should consider the sex-specific trajectories of change in amygdala and hippocampal volumes and how deviations from normal neurodevelopment may impact the prevalence of depression and other mental illnesses in young people.

In terms of cortical anomalies, cross-sectional research has shown individuals (age range = 6–54 years) at high familial risk of developing MDD display cortical thinning in regions of the frontal cortex, somatosensory and motor cortices, regions of the parietal and occipital cortices and the posterior temporal cortex (Peterson et al., 2009). In addition, cortical thickening was observed in the subgenual cortex, orbitofrontal cortex and both the anterior and posterior cingulate in high-risk participants compared to individuals with no family history (i.e. low risk) of depressive illness. A similar pattern of cortical GM volume abnormalities was also observed in these regions. While authors stated cortical thickness findings were similar when adults (≥18 years) and children (<18 years) were analysed separately, they did report that thinning was of slightly greater magnitude in children, particularly in the superior temporal/temporoparietal region. Given that the authors did not exclude or covary for individuals who had a lifetime history of MDD from these latter analyses of adults and children (25 per cent of the high-risk group; 11 per cent of the low-risk group), these results should be interpreted with caution.

In a longitudinal healthy community cohort study of children aged 5–22 years, it was found that individuals who presented with high levels of sub-syndromal anxious/depressed symptomatology at baseline had a slower rate of thinning in the ventromedial prefrontal cortex (gyrus rectus, orbitofrontal cortex and subgenual anterior cingulate) when compared to the individuals with low levels of symptomatology (Ducharme et al., 2014). The association of ventromedial prefrontal cortical thickness with sub-syndromal symptoms was significantly dependent on age; children <9 years with higher symptom scores displayed thinner cortical mantles, while adolescents/young adults aged >18 years with higher scores displayed thicker cortical mantles. A positive association between symptoms and thickness was also observed in the precuneus/posterior cingulate in the participants more than 18 years old. Given that throughout the life of the study no participant displayed symptoms above the threshold level for a diagnosed depressive disorder, it was suggested that, in the individuals that had higher subthreshold symptoms, the development of thicker cortices over the late adolescent period was potentially a protective mechanism. This study reflects the importance of examining trajectories of change over the adolescent period, particularly given the findings of Whittle et al. (2014) demonstrating that differences in trajectories predicted depression onset.

Summary

Given that adolescence is the highest-risk period for onset of depressive disorders in both males and females, the future consideration of age in FEMDD research, in combination with the length of time since initial onset, is critical for determining how the pathophysiology of depression may impact on and potentially alter the normal developmental brain changes that take place in adolescence and early adulthood. One limitation of FEMDD research to date is the inclusion of large age ranges and the lack of focus on youth. Despite this, the FEMDD literature is informative in terms of ruling out the confounding effects of medication, as the majority of studies comprised medication-naïve individuals; and for homing in on phenotypic unipolar depression, as comorbid mental illnesses were typically exclusion criteria in most studies.

Overall, evidence thus far is extremely mixed, with findings of both increases and decreases in GM volumes and WM integrity, which appear to be largely dependent on age. Limited preliminary evidence suggests that early-stage depression may be associated with hippocampal volume reductions, irrespective of age. Notably, the brain regions found to be abnormal in early-stage depression thus far appear to overlap with those implicated in schizophrenia-spectrum and bipolar disorders. Contrary to these latter research fields, trait versus state phenomena continue to be hotly debated in MDD, although support is mounting for specifically smaller hippocampal volume being a potential risk marker of the depressive illness. However, this area of research is in its infancy and it remains unknown whether the brain changes observed in chronic MDD (i.e. stages >2), namely WM hyperintensities and volume loss of the anterior cingulate and hippocampus, are present early on and, if so, whether they are pathophysiological in nature or are a potential secondary consequence of (or compensatory response to) the depressive illness. Needless to say, longitudinal studies are essential to further elucidate the nature of neural phenomena in FEMDD and their stability from the pre-onset phase. Moreover, future large-scale studies in youth who are within a broad 'clinical high-risk' window for developing a range of mental illnesses will be most informative (McGorry, 2014); for identifying whether certain brain changes are predictive of: (1) transition to a specific mental illness; (2) treatment responsiveness; and (3) risk of relapse/likelihood of remission.

Are there Neurobiological Remission and Relapse Signatures for a Given Mental Illness?

The clinical staging model has recently been considered as unidirectional (Hickie et al., 2013), whereas the original conceptualisation suggested bidirectionality (McGorry et al., 2007), whereby an individual could move to an earlier stage with remission/amelioration of symptoms (e.g. from Stage 2 to Stage 1b). From a phenotypic viewpoint, this may present itself as 'remission' of symptoms, and suggests that it is possible to return to an earlier illness stage. From a neurobiological perspective this would imply neuroplasticity and reversal or normalisation of abnormal neuropathology. There is some support for this notion. For example, Kempton and colleagues (2011) showed in their meta-analysis that MDD patients who were experiencing an active depressive episode had significantly smaller hippocampal volumes than the MDD patients who were in remission. Moreover, those in remission had hippocampal volumes comparable to HCs. Similarly, Bitter et al. (2011) found that adolescents with FEBD who were in remission at 12 months' follow-up had larger amygdala volumes at baseline in comparison to FEBD patients who did not achieve remission. In a more recent study of UHR for psychosis, Katagiri et al. (2015) identified that improvement in measures of WM integrity was associated with improvement in symptoms over a 12-month follow-up, providing some initial support for the notion of bidirectionality.

Similarly, it is unknown whether individuals with a diagnosed schizophrenia-spectrum disorder can, from a neurobiological standpoint, move backwards within the staging model. Limited research has focused on brain abnormalities associated with relapse and/or remission (for discussion, see Cropley & Pantelis, 2014). Andreasen and colleagues (2013), using data from the Iowa Longitudinal Study in FE schizophrenia (described earlier), showed that duration of relapse (mean = 1.43 years) had a significant impact on brain volume loss, specifically total cerebral volume, total frontal volume and WM of the frontal and temporal lobes, which was independent of the effects of antipsychotic treatment. However, they found no effect of the number of relapses (range = 1–4) on brain volumes. The authors did not report on the predictive value of abnormal baseline volumes on later illness outcomes/risk of relapse. Fung et al. (2014), however, specifically aimed to investigate the ability of MRI to predict remission at one-year follow-up in treatment-naïve FE schizophrenia patients. They found that for females but not for males, larger volumes of the thalamus and lentiform nuclei at baseline were significantly associated with remission at one year. While they adopted a conventional definition of 'remission' (Andreasen et al., 2005), more broadly there continues to be a lack of consensus on the definition of remission, which continues to make this area of research challenging.

Overall, despite the generally consistent finding of volume loss over time in schizophrenia-spectrum disorders, some preliminary evidence suggests that preservation and even restoration of GM tissue may be possible via certain neuroprotective interventions. For example, Eack et al. (2010) showed that two years of cognitive enhancement therapy significantly protected against GM volume loss of medial temporal lobe structures, namely the fusiform gyrus, hippocampus and parahippocampal gyrus, which were significantly reduced in the control (enriched supportive therapy) group at the two-year time point. Interestingly, amygdala volume significantly increased over time for the cognitive enhancement therapy group relative to the control group. Similarly, three months of aerobic exercise therapy (30 min cycling three times per week in a gym) has been shown to significantly increase volume of the hippocampus in a sample of men with chronic schizophrenia (Pajonk et al., 2010). Although these studies did not report on whether patients had achieved symptomatic or functional remission, it was found that both interventions and subsequent brain changes were significantly associated with improvements in cognition.

Given the limited neurobiological research into relapse and remission across all three major mental illness domains, we are unable to comment on whether distinct neurobiological signatures of these (often poorly defined) phenotypic profiles exist at this time. Nonetheless, this brief overview will hopefully provide food for thought for researchers who are planning future longitudinal studies.

Limitations and Caveats

It should be acknowledged that the evidence presented herein has been largely based on meta-analyses, many of which found significant heterogeneity between studies. Further, while the majority of studies have primarily reported volumetric decreases, volume increases have also been reported on occasion, adding complexity to the interpretation of findings. Due to the breadth of this topic and for the sake of brevity, we decided to focus on structural brain abnormalities as indicated from MRI. We decided not to present or discuss findings on whole-brain volumes, as this was unlikely to be useful for determining illness specificity. Nor did we evaluate the extensive functional MRI evidence, which is deserving of a separate chapter. In addition, other forms of neuroimaging, such as magnetic resonance spectroscopy (MRS), positron emission tomography (PET) and single photon emission computerised tomography (SPECT) are also informative and should be considered in future research, especially as some (e.g. SPECT) have been suggested to be more sensitive than MRI for detecting abnormalities (Zakzanis et al., 2000).

Exploration of all mental illness domains (i.e. personality, anxiety, addiction disorders) was beyond the scope of this review. Individual disorders within these other broad illness domains are quite diverse in their phenotypic presentations (for example, obsessive-compulsive disorder vs post-traumatic stress disorder) and as such these individual disorders have been thought to more readily and consistently be associated with specific neural anomalies. For example, abnormalities of the orbitofrontal cortex, until recently, were thought to be an inherent characteristic of obsessive-compulsive disorder, but several recent meta-analyses have failed to verify this (Eng et al., 2015; Radua & Mataix-Cols, 2009). Thus, with the premise that dysfunctional neural mechanisms underlie symptomatology, a shift from a holistic phenotypic classification of 'disorders' to a model whereby neurobiological markers can be mapped to specific symptomatology (for example, see Fontenelle et al., 2011), which is often *transdiagnostic*, may need to occur in the future. Indeed, a limitation of the current chapter is that we reviewed the broad illness domains without exploration into discrete subgroup populations. For example, there is some evidence to suggest that hippocampal volume loss may be specific to the schizophrenia illness, rather than the psychosis spectrum per se (Velakoulis et al., 2006). Similarly, biological subgroups were not considered; for example, a distinct subgroup of schizophrenia patients are suggested to display cortical muscarinic receptor deficiency (Scarr et al., 2009), while others suggest treatment-resistant patients have a non-dopamine-dependent form of the illness that may be related to elevated glutamate (Demjaha et al., 2014). Lastly, while we attempted to address the confounding issues of medication, a number of other potential confounders and moderators of brain volumetric changes were not taken into account, including substance and alcohol abuse (e.g. Lorenzetti et al., 2015; Yucel et al., 2008), comorbid mental illnesses, neuroradiological factors, environmental factors and early-life adversity, in particular childhood trauma (e.g. Kelly et al., 2013).

Summary and Clinical Implications

The large degree of overlap in abnormal neuropathology across the broad mental illness groups, which is no doubt partially due to *within-group* heterogeneity, makes the discovery of sets or networks of localised diagnosis-specific neural biomarkers unlikely. However, this is not to say that subtle distinctions in neural abnormalities do not exist, but rather challenges the usefulness of diagnostic categories in the context of brain imaging being applied within a clinical staging model. To date, only one research group has forgone traditional diagnostic classifications and adopted a clinical staging model to cross-sectionally investigate GM and WM differences between young people who are help-seeking/have attenuated syndrome (i.e. seeking help for anxiety, depressive, hypomanic or psychotic symptoms; Stage 1) and those with a discrete disorder/persistent or recurrent illness (Stage 2/3; comprising patients with BD, MDD and/or psychosis) (Lagopoulos et al., 2012; 2013). Lagopoulos and colleagues found that relative to HCs both illness groups had reduced GM in the insula, which appeared to be a stable deficit across illness stages (Lagopoulos et al., 2012). When compared to controls, Stage 1 additionally showed GM decreases in the amygdala and precuneus, while Stage 2/3 showed greater (yet disparate) GM reductions within distributed frontal regions. Indeed, direct comparison between the two illness groups revealed significantly greater GM loss in numerous frontal cortical regions and the cingulate cortex (Lagopoulos et al., 2012). Interestingly, the GM abnormalities observed in the amygdala and precuneus of Stage 1 participants were no longer detectable in the Stage 2/3 sample, suggestive of these being potentially stage-specific biomarkers of attenuated psychiatric (anxiety/depressive/hypomanic/psychotic) symptoms (which likely interact with neurodevelopmental life stage). In terms of WM, relative to HCs both the Stage 1 and Stage 2/3 groups displayed decreased FA in the left anterior corona radiata, although this was more extensive for the Stage 2/3 group who additionally displayed increased radial diffusivity in this same region (Lagopoulos et al., 2013). This pioneering work provides strong support for adopting not only a staging model in neuropsychiatry, but a model that is transdiagnostic in nature.

Much of the evidence to date highlights the need for longitudinal designs and a consideration of the 'age' of the sample population and how this relates to the normal trajectory of brain development (Gogtay et al., 2011; Pantelis et al., 2005; 2009; Paus, 2005). Collectively, neuroimaging evidence in psychiatry continues to support a systems neuroscience/neural networks approach (Frangou, 2014; Hulshoff Pol & Bullmore, 2013), which acknowledges that symptoms of mental illness and dysfunctions emerge from disturbances in structural and functional integrity within large-scale neural networks. It is proposed that to move the field forward, researchers should focus on differentiating between abnormalities in 'domain-general' superordinate networks (which are likely associated with general processing impairments that give rise to common clinical, cognitive and affective symptoms) and *microscale abnormalities* within these large-scale networks (which may well be disease-specific) (Frangou, 2014). Thus, a focus on identifying and characterising microscale circuits that are dysfunctional may have the greatest implications for clinical translation in the near future. In terms of moving towards personalising medicine in psychiatry, machine learning techniques (Kloppel et al., 2012), combined with multimodal imaging (e.g. Cocchi et al., 2014), appear most promising but require further investigation to address the issue of specificity when multiple-illness populations are pooled together (as opposed to differentiating patients from HC individuals).

The influence of genetics was touched on in the earlier section on FEMDD, which was included given the relatively limited research that has been conducted in early-stage depression. While a wider review of the literature linking genes to brain morphology in all three major mental illnesses was beyond the scope of this chapter, it is important to note that a wealth of neuroimaging literature has shown links between brain changes and genetics in all of these major psychiatric disorders, which attests to *interdisciplinary research* being a necessary way forward for this field (Ducharme et al., 2014). Thus, identifying neuroimaging-based intermediate phenotypes is more informative than simply investigating gene polymorphisms with behaviour, given that an intermediate phenotype (i.e. cell activity) is a heritable trait that is located on the pathogenesis pathway from genetic predisposition to psychopathology (Rasetti & Weinberger, 2011). These authors make the point that intermediate phenotypes are likely associated with a more basic and proximal aetiological process, and are therefore more amenable to genetic investigation (Rasetti & Weinberger, 2011). Similarly, other biological factors (e.g. pro-inflammatory cytokines in plasma) will be more informative if examined in the context of predicting later brain changes (Cannon et al., 2015).

Neuroimaging in psychiatry has great potential for aiding in the prediction of treatment response, although this area of research is still nascent (for discussion, see Kempton & McGuire, 2015). Meta-analysis of 20 studies in established depression found that decreased GM volume of the DLPFC, and decreased hippocampal volume, both (independently) reduced the likelihood of responding well to antidepressant medication (Fu et al., 2013). Another example is a cortical gyrification study in FEP, in which patients who were non-responsive to antipsychotic treatment had significant hypogyria (i.e. less cortical folding) of the insula, as well as frontal and temporal regions, when compared to FEP patients who responded well (Palaniyappan et al., 2013). Medication is typically a first-line treatment in individuals in Stages 2 and above, but often patients go through months (or even years) of trial and error with several iterations of differing medications to discover the optimal treatment. Thus, effective predictive tools of medication response could provide timely optimal treatment for individual patients and minimise illness burden.

The potential utility of neuroimaging extends beyond prediction of response to medication and may be useful for predicting response to psychological and cognitive therapies. Preliminary evidence suggests that larger volumes of the caudal anterior cingulate are associated with better response to cognitive behavioural therapy in individuals with MDD (Fujino et al., 2015). Keshavan and colleagues (2011) found that in early-course schizophrenia, greater global cortical reserve (i.e. larger GM and surface area; particularly of the temporal lobes) was predictive of a more rapid response to cognitive therapy in the first year of treatment (although this was only with respect to predicting social cognitive improvements). We have proposed that select cognitive abilities (e.g. set-shifting ability) appear to be preserved in the psychosis prodrome, but soon decline with illness progression (Pantelis et al., 2015). Therefore, tailoring treatment to target specific cognitive abilities would be best initiated at the UHR stage (i.e. Stages 1a and 1b), which is the time point at which the brain is changing dynamically and gains, particularly in relation to preserving/

strengthening *resilience* factors, will be most evident. Personalised MRI information may further guide treatment choice by aiding in the assessment of individuals' capacity for new learning based on the integrity of the underlying neural networks subserving specific cognitive domains.

Concluding Remarks

Broadly, neuroimaging data thus far support the behavioural and clinical literature attesting to a critical window for targeted intervention in the 'clinical at risk' phase. It is hoped that the evidence from longitudinal neuroimaging of early illness stages incites a sense of urgency for applying the right clinical treatment at this early illness stage. In addition, the initial knowledge that brain changes can occur in such a small time frame (i.e. within 12 months) suggests future research should aim to: (1) better characterise the trajectories of brain changes; (2) identify precipitators and mechanisms driving brain changes; and (3) identify what the 'right' treatment would be and how such treatment would affect the brain and illness outcomes.

There are still remaining questions around the clinical utility of neuroimaging methods. Are imaging methods too invasive or too expensive? Does the benefit outweigh the costs involved, including burden to patients? And lastly, the question posed in the title of this chapter: is it possible that certain mental illnesses have distinct neurodevelopmental trajectories? We conclude that it is possible that altered neurodevelopmental pathways could potentially identify an individual at risk of a specific disorder or developing specific psychiatric symptoms later in life; or, for individuals already suffering from an early-stage mental illness, neural abnormalities may be predictive of progressing to later and more severe illness stages – however, we are not there yet. It is likely that the monetary costs of scanning will become more affordable in the future. If future research is successful at uncovering neural biomarkers, both of disability and resilience, that are clinically useful for predicting illness outcomes and/or treatment response, then neuroimaging techniques may well be integrated into routine practice.

Acknowledgements

Professor C. Pantelis was supported by an NHMRC Senior Principal Research Fellowship (628386 and 1105825), and a Brain and Behavior Research Foundation (NARSAD) Distinguished Investigator Award (US; Grant ID: 18722).

References

Adler, C. M., DelBello, M. P., Jarvis, K., Levine, A., Adams, J., & Strakowski, S. M. (2007). Voxel-based study of structural changes in first-episode patients with bipolar disorder. *Biological Psychiatry*, **61**(6), 776–781.

Adolphs, R. (2001). The neurobiology of social cognition. *Current Opinion in Neurobiology*, **11**(2), 231–239.

Adriano, F., Caltagirone, C., & Spalletta, G. (2012). Hippocampal volume reduction in first-episode and chronic schizophrenia: a review and meta-analysis. *Neuroscientist*, **18**(2), 180–200.

Andreasen, N. C., Carpenter Jr, W. T., Kane, J. M., Lasser, R. A., Marder, S. R., & Weinberger, D. R. (2005). Remission in schizophrenia: proposed criteria and rationale for consensus. *American Journal of Psychiatry*, **162**(3), 441–449.

Andreasen, N. C., Liu, D., Ziebell, S., Vora, A., & Ho, B. C. (2013). Relapse duration, treatment intensity, and brain tissue loss in schizophrenia: a prospective longitudinal MRI study. *American Journal of Psychiatry,* **170**(6), 609–615.

Andreasen, N. C., Nopoulos, P., Magnotta, V., Pierson, R., Ziebell, S., & Ho, B. C. (2011). Progressive brain change in schizophrenia: a prospective longitudinal study of first-episode schizophrenia. *Biological Psychiatry,* **70**(7), 672–679.

Ansell, B. R., Dwyer, D. B., Wood, S. J., Bora, E., Brewer, W. J., Proffitt, T. M., ... Pantelis, C. (2014). Divergent effects of first-generation and second-generation antipsychotics on cortical thickness in first-episode psychosis. *Psychological Medicine,* **45**, 515–527.

Arnone, D., Cavanagh, J., Gerber, D., Lawrie, S. M., Ebmeier, K. P., & McIntosh, A. M. (2009). Magnetic resonance imaging studies in bipolar disorder and schizophrenia: meta-analysis. *British Journal of Psychiatry,* **195**(3), 194–201.

Atmaca, M., Ozdemir, H., & Yildirim, H. (2007). Corpus callosum areas in first-episode patients with bipolar disorder. *Psychological Medicine,* **37**(5), 699–704.

Bechdolf, A., Wood, S. J., Nelson, B., Velakoulis, D., Yucel, M., Takahashi, T., ... McGorry, P. D. (2012). Amygdala and insula volumes prior to illness onset in bipolar disorder: a magnetic resonance imaging study. *Psychiatry Research,* **201**(1), 34–39.

Beck, A. T., Ward, C. H., Mendelson, M., Mock, J., & Erbaugh, J. (1961). An inventory for measuring depression. *Archives of General Psychiatry,* **4**, 561–571.

Beyer, J. L., Young, R., Kuchibhatla, M., & Krishnan, K. R. (2009). Hyperintense MRI lesions in bipolar disorder: a meta-analysis and review. *International Review of Psychiatry,* **21**(4), 394–409.

Bitter, S. M., Mills, N. P., Adler, C. M., Strakowski, S. M., & DelBello, M. P. (2011). Progression of amygdala volumetric abnormalities in adolescents after their first manic episode. *Journal of the American Academy of Child and Adolescent Psychiatry,* **50**(10), 1017–1026.

Bloemen, O. J., de Koning, M. B., Schmitz, N., Nieman, D. H., Becker, H. E., de Haan, L., ... van Amelsvoort, T. A. (2010). White-matter markers for psychosis in a prospective ultra-high-risk cohort. *Psychological Medicine,* **40**(8), 1297–1304.

Bois, C., Whalley, H. C., McIntosh, A. M., & Lawrie, S. M. (2015). Structural magnetic resonance imaging markers of susceptibility and transition to schizophrenia: a review of familial and clinical high risk population studies. *Journal of Psychopharmacology,* **29**(2), 144–154.

Boos, H. B., Aleman, A., Cahn, W., Hulshoff Pol, H., & Kahn, R. S. (2007). Brain volumes in relatives of patients with schizophrenia: a meta-analysis. *Archives of General Psychiatry,* **64**(3), 297–304.

Bora, E., Fornito, A., Yucel, M., & Pantelis, C. (2010). Voxelwise meta-analysis of gray matter abnormalities in bipolar disorder. *Biological Psychiatry,* **67**(11), 1097–1105.

Bora, E., Harrison, B. J., Davey, C. G., Yucel, M., & Pantelis, C. (2012). Meta-analysis of volumetric abnormalities in cortico-striatal-pallidal-thalamic circuits in major depressive disorder. *Psychological Medicine,* **42**(4), 671–681.

Borgwardt, S. J., Riecher-Rossler, A., Dazzan, P., Chitnis, X., Aston, J., Drewe, M., ... McGuire, P. K. (2007). Regional gray matter volume abnormalities in the at risk mental state. *Biological Psychiatry,* **61**(10), 1148–1156.

Buschlen, J., Berger, G. E., Borgwardt, S. J., Aston, J., Gschwandtner, U., Pflueger, M. O., ... Riecher-Rossler, A. (2011). Pituitary volume increase during emerging psychosis. *Schizophrenia Research,* **125**(1), 41–48.

Campbell, S., & MacQueen, G. (2004). The role of the hippocampus in the pathophysiology of major depression. *Journal of Psychiatry and Neuroscience,* **29**(6), 417–426.

Cannon, T. D., Chung, Y., He, G., Sun, D., Jacobson, A., van Erp, T. G., ... Heinssen, R. (2015). Progressive reduction in cortical thickness as psychosis develops: a multisite longitudinal neuroimaging study of youth at elevated clinical risk. *Biological Psychiatry,* **77**(2), 147–157.

Cardoso de Almeida, J. R., & Phillips, M. L. (2013). Distinguishing between unipolar depression and bipolar depression: current and future clinical and neuroimaging perspectives. *Biological Psychiatry, 73*(2), 111–118.

Carletti, F., Woolley, J. B., Bhattacharyya, S., Perez-Iglesias, R., Fusar Poli, P., Valmaggia, L., . . . McGuire, P. K. (2012). Alterations in white matter evident before the onset of psychosis. *Schizophrenia Bulletin, 38*(6), 1170–1179.

Carpenter, W. T., Bustillo, J. R., Thaker, G. K., van Os, J., Krueger, R. F., & Green, M. J. (2009). The psychoses: cluster 3 of the proposed meta-structure for DSM-V and ICD-11. *Psychological Medicine, 39*(12), 2025–2042.

Chan, R. C., Di, X., McAlonan, G. M., & Gong, Q. Y. (2011). Brain anatomical abnormalities in high-risk individuals, first-episode, and chronic schizophrenia: an activation likelihood estimation meta-analysis of illness progression. *Schizophrenia Bulletin, 37*(1), 177–188.

Chen, Z., Cui, L., Li, M., Jiang, L., Deng, W., Ma, X., . . . Li, T. (2012). Voxel based morphometric and diffusion tensor imaging analysis in male bipolar patients with first-episode mania. *Progress in Neuro-Psychopharmacology and Biological Psychiatry, 36*(2), 231–238.

Clark, S. R., Schubert, K. O., & Baune, B. T. (2015). Towards indicated prevention of psychosis: using probabilistic assessments of transition risk in psychosis prodrome. *Journal of Neural Transmission, 122*(1), 155–169.

Cocchi, L., Harding, I. H., Lord, A., Pantelis, C., Yucel, M., & Zalesky, A. (2014). Disruption of structure–function coupling in the schizophrenia connectome. *NeuroImage: Clinical, 4*, 779–787.

Cole, J., Costafreda, S. G., McGuffin, P., & Fu, C. H. (2011). Hippocampal atrophy in first episode depression: a meta-analysis of magnetic resonance imaging studies. *Journal of Affective Disorders, 134*(1–3), 483–487.

Cooper, D., Barker, V., Radua, J., Fusar-Poli, P., & Lawrie, S. M. (2014). Multimodal voxel-based meta-analysis of structural and functional magnetic resonance imaging

studies in those at elevated genetic risk of developing schizophrenia. *Psychiatry Research, 221*(1), 69–77.

Cropley, V. L., & Pantelis, C. (2014). Using longitudinal imaging to map the 'relapse signature' of schizophrenia and other psychoses. *Epidemiology and Psychiatric Sciences, 23*(3), 219–225.

Davidson, L. L., & Heinrichs, R. W. (2003). Quantification of frontal and temporal lobe brain-imaging findings in schizophrenia: a meta-analysis. *Psychiatry Research, 122*(2), 69–87.

Dazzan, P., Soulsby, B., Mechelli, A., Wood, S. J., Velakoulis, D., Phillips, L. J., . . . Pantelis, C. (2012). Volumetric abnormalities predating the onset of schizophrenia and affective psychoses: an MRI study in subjects at ultrahigh risk of psychosis. *Schizophrenia Bulletin, 38*(5), 1083–1091.

De Peri, L., Crescini, A., Deste, G., Fusar-Poli, P., Sacchetti, E., & Vita, A. (2012). Brain structural abnormalities at the onset of schizophrenia and bipolar disorder: a meta-analysis of controlled magnetic resonance imaging studies. *Current Pharmaceutical Design, 18*(4), 486–494.

Demjaha, A., Egerton, A., Murray, R. M., Kapur, S., Howes, O. D., Stone, J. M., & McGuire, P. K. (2014). Antipsychotic treatment resistance in schizophrenia associated with elevated glutamate levels but normal dopamine function. *Biological Psychiatry, 75*(5), e11–e13.

Desmyter, S., van Heeringen, C., & Audenaert, K. (2011). Structural and functional neuroimaging studies of the suicidal brain. *Progress in Neuro-Psychopharmacology and Biological Psychiatry, 35*(4), 796–808.

Di, X., Chan, R. C., & Gong, Q. Y. (2009). White matter reduction in patients with schizophrenia as revealed by voxel-based morphometry: an activation likelihood estimation meta-analysis. *Progress in Neuro-Psychopharmacology and Biological Psychiatry, 33*(8), 1390–1394.

Du, M. Y., Wu, Q. Z., Yue, Q., Li, J., Liao, Y., Kuang, W. H., . . . Gong, Q. Y. (2012). Voxelwise meta-analysis of gray matter reduction in major depressive disorder.

Progress in Neuro-Psychopharmacology and Biological Psychiatry, **36**(1), 11–16.

Ducharme, S., Albaugh, M. D., Hudziak, J. J., Botteron, K. N., Nguyen, T. V., Truong, C., . . . Karama, S. (2014). Anxious/depressed symptoms are linked to right ventromedial prefrontal cortical thickness maturation in healthy children and young adults. *Cerebral Cortex,* **24**(11), 2941–2950.

Duman, R. S., Nakagawa, S., & Malberg, J. (2001). Regulation of adult neurogenesis by antidepressant treatment. *Neuropsychopharmacology,* **25**(6), 836–844.

Eack, S. M., Hogarty, G. E., Cho, R. Y., Prasad, K. M., Greenwald, D. P., Hogarty, S. S., & Keshavan, M. S. (2010). Neuroprotective effects of cognitive enhancement therapy against gray matter loss in early schizophrenia: results from a 2-year randomized controlled trial. *Archives of General Psychiatry,* **67**(7), 674–682.

Eichenbaum, H. (2004). Hippocampus: cognitive processes and neural representations that underlie declarative memory. *Neuron,* **44**(1), 109–120.

Ellison-Wright, I., & Bullmore, E. (2009). Meta-analysis of diffusion tensor imaging studies in schizophrenia. *Schizophrenia Research,* **108**(1–3), 3–10.

Ellison-Wright, I., & Bullmore, E. (2010). Anatomy of bipolar disorder and schizophrenia: a meta-analysis. *Schizophrenia Research,* **117**(1), 1–12.

Ellison-Wright, I., Glahn, D. C., Laird, A. R., Thelen, S. M., & Bullmore, E. (2008). The anatomy of first-episode and chronic schizophrenia: an anatomical likelihood estimation meta-analysis. *American Journal of Psychiatry,* **165**(8), 1015–1023.

Eng, G. K., Sim, K., & Chen, S. H. (2015). Meta-analytic investigations of structural grey matter, executive domain-related functional activations, and white matter diffusivity in obsessive compulsive disorder: an integrative review. *Neuroscience and Biobehavioral Reviews,* **52**, 233–257.

Farrow, T. F., Whitford, T. J., Williams, L. M., Gomes, L., & Harris, A. W. (2005).

Diagnosis-related regional gray matter loss over two years in first episode schizophrenia and bipolar disorder. *Biological Psychiatry,* **58**(9), 713–723.

Fontenelle, L. F., Oostermeijer, S., Harrison, B. J., Pantelis, C., & Yucel, M. (2011). Obsessive-compulsive disorder, impulse control disorders and drug addiction: common features and potential treatments. *Drugs,* **71**(7), 827–840.

Fornito, A., Yucel, M., Patti, J., Wood, S. J., & Pantelis, C. (2009). Mapping grey matter reductions in schizophrenia: an anatomical likelihood estimation analysis of voxel-based morphometry studies. *Schizophrenia Research,* **108**(1–3), 104–113.

Fornito, A., Yung, A. R., Wood, S. J., Phillips, L. J., Nelson, B., Cotton, S., . . . Yucel, M. (2008). Anatomic abnormalities of the anterior cingulate cortex before psychosis onset: an MRI study of ultra-high-risk individuals. *Biological Psychiatry,* **64**(9), 758–765.

Frangou, S. (2014). A systems neuroscience perspective of schizophrenia and bipolar disorder. *Schizophrenia Bulletin,* **40**(3), 523–531.

Frank, E., Nimgaonkar, V. L., Phillips, M. L., & Kupfer, D. J. (2015). All the world's a (clinical) stage: rethinking bipolar disorder from a longitudinal perspective. *Molecular Psychiatry,* **20**(1), 23–31.

Fu, C. H., Steiner, H., & Costafreda, S. G. (2013). Predictive neural biomarkers of clinical response in depression: a meta-analysis of functional and structural neuroimaging studies of pharmacological and psychological therapies. *Neurobiology of Disease,* **52**, 75–83.

Fujino, J., Yamasaki, N., Miyata, J., Sasaki, H., Matsukawa, N., Takemura, A., . . . Murai, T. (2015). Anterior cingulate volume predicts response to cognitive behavioral therapy in major depressive disorder. *Journal of Affective Disorders,* **174**, 397–399.

Fung, G., Cheung, C., Chen, E., Lam, C., Chiu, C., Law, C. W., . . . Chua, S. E. (2014). MRI predicts remission at 1 year in first-episode schizophrenia in females with larger striato-thalamic volumes. *Neuropsychobiology*, **69**(4), 243–248.

Fusar-Poli, P., Crossley, N., Woolley, J., Carletti, F., Perez-Iglesias, R., Broome, M., . . . McGuire, P. (2011). White matter alterations related to P300 abnormalities in individuals at high risk for psychosis: an MRI-EEG study. *Journal of Psychiatry and Neuroscience*, **36**(4), 239–248.

Fusar-Poli, P., Howes, O., Bechdolf, A., & Borgwardt, S. (2012a). Mapping vulnerability to bipolar disorder: a systematic review and meta-analysis of neuroimaging studies. *Journal of Psychiatry and Neuroscience*, *37*(3), 170–184.

Fusar-Poli, P., Radua, J., McGuire, P., & Borgwardt, S. (2012b). Neuroanatomical maps of psychosis onset: voxel-wise meta-analysis of antipsychotic-naive VBM studies. *Schizophrenia Bulletin*, *38*(6), 1297–1307.

Fusar-Poli, P., Smieskova, R., Kempton, M. J., Ho, B. C., Andreasen, N. C., & Borgwardt, S. (2013). Progressive brain changes in schizophrenia related to antipsychotic treatment? A meta-analysis of longitudinal MRI studies. *Neuroscience and Biobehavioral Reviews*, *37*(8), 1680–1691.

Fusar-Poli, P., Smieskova, R., Serafini, G., Politi, P., & Borgwardt, S. (2014). Neuroanatomical markers of genetic liability to psychosis and first episode psychosis: a voxelwise meta-analytical comparison. *World Journal of Biological Psychiatry*, *15*(3), 219–228.

Garner, B., Pariante, C. M., Wood, S. J., Velakoulis, D., Phillips, L., Soulsby, B., . . . Pantelis, C. (2005). Pituitary volume predicts future transition to psychosis in individuals at ultra-high risk of developing psychosis. *Biological Psychiatry*, *58*(5), 417–423.

Gogtay, N., Vyas, N. S., Testa, R., Wood, S. J., & Pantelis, C. (2011). Age of onset of schizophrenia: perspectives from structural neuroimaging studies. *Schizophrenia Bulletin*, *37*(3), 504–513.

Gupta, C. N., Calhoun, V. D., Rachakonda, S., Chen, J., Patel, V., Liu, J., . . . Turner, J. A. (2015). Patterns of gray matter abnormalities in schizophrenia based on an international mega-analysis. *Schizophrenia Bulletin*, **41**(5), 1133–1142.

Hahn, C., Lim, H. K., & Lee, C. U. (2014). Neuroimaging findings in late-onset schizophrenia and bipolar disorder. *Journal of Geriatric Psychiatry and Neurology*, **27**(1), 56–62.

Haijma, S. V., Van Haren, N., Cahn, W., Koolschijn, P. C., Hulshoff Pol, H. E., & Kahn, R. S. (2013). Brain volumes in schizophrenia: a meta-analysis in over 18 000 subjects. *Schizophrenia Bulletin*, **39**(5), 1129–1138.

Hajek, T., Kopecek, M., Hoschl, C., & Alda, M. (2012). Smaller hippocampal volumes in patients with bipolar disorder are masked by exposure to lithium: a meta-analysis. *Journal of Psychiatry and Neuroscience*, **37**(5), 333–343.

Hajek, T., Kopecek, M., Kozeny, J., Gunde, E., Alda, M., & Hoschl, C. (2009). Amygdala volumes in mood disorders: meta-analysis of magnetic resonance volumetry studies. *Journal of Affective Disorders*, **115**(3), 395–410.

Han, K. M., Choi, S., Jung, J., Na, K. S., Yoon, H. K., Lee, M. S., & Ham, B. J. (2014). Cortical thickness, cortical and subcortical volume, and white matter integrity in patients with their first episode of major depression. *Journal of Affective Disorders*, **155**, 42–48.

Heinze, K., Reniers, R. L., Nelson, B., Yung, A. R., Lin, A., Harrison, B. J., . . . Wood, S. J. (2015). Discrete alterations of brain network structural covariance in individuals at ultra-high risk for psychosis. *Biological Psychiatry*, **77**(11), 989–996.

Hibar, D. P., Westlye, L. T., van Erp, T. G., Rasmussen, J., Leonardo, C. D., Faskowitz, J., . . . Andreassen, O. A. (2016). Subcortical volumetric abnormalities in bipolar disorder. *Molecular Psychiatry*, **21**(12), 1710–1716.

Hickie, I. B., Scott, E. M., Hermens, D. F., Naismith, S. L., Guastella, A. J., Kaur, M., . . . McGorry, P. D. (2013). Applying clinical staging to young people who present for mental health care. *Early Intervention in Psychiatry*, *7*(1), 31–43.

Hikosaka, O. (2010). The habenula: from stress evasion to value-based decision-making. *Nature Reviews Neuroscience,* **11**(7), 503–513.

Hirschfeld, R. M., Lewis, L., & Vornik, L. A. (2003). Perceptions and impact of bipolar disorder: how far have we really come? Results of the national depressive and manic-depressive association 2000 survey of individuals with bipolar disorder. *Journal of Clinical Psychiatry,* **64**(2), 161–174.

Ho, B. C., Andreasen, N. C., Ziebell, S., Pierson, R., & Magnotta, V. (2011). Long-term antipsychotic treatment and brain volumes: a longitudinal study of first-episode schizophrenia. *Archives of General Psychiatry,* **68**(2), 128–137.

Houenou, J., Frommberger, J., Carde, S., Glasbrenner, M., Diener, C., Leboyer, M., & Wessa, M. (2011). Neuroimaging-based markers of bipolar disorder: evidence from two meta-analyses. *Journal of Affective Disorders,* **132**(3), 344–355.

Hulshoff Pol, H., & Bullmore, E. (2013). Neural networks in psychiatry. *European Neuropsychopharmacology,* **23**(1), 1–6.

Ide, S., Kakeda, S., Watanabe, K., Yoshimura, R., Abe, O., Hayashi, K., . . . Korogi, Y. (2015). Relationship between a BDNF gene polymorphism and the brain volume in treatment-naive patients with major depressive disorder: a VBM analysis of brain MRI. *Psychiatry Research,* **233**(2), 120–124.

Ivleva, E. I., Morris, D. W., Moates, A. F., Suppes, T., Thaker, G. K., & Tamminga, C. A. (2010). Genetics and intermediate phenotypes of the schizophrenia–bipolar disorder boundary. *Neuroscience and Biobehavioral Reviews,* **34**(6), 897–921.

Jenkins, L. M., Barba, A., Campbell, M., Lamar, M., Shankman, S. A., Leow, A. D., . . . Langenecker, S. A. (2016). Shared white matter alterations across emotional disorders: a voxel-based meta-analysis of fractional anisotropy. *NeuroImage: Clinical,* **12**, 1022–1034.

Jiang, J., Zhao, Y. J., Hu, X. Y., Du, M. Y., Chen, Z. Q., Wu, M., . . . Gong, Q. Y. (2017). Microstructural brain abnormalities in medication-free patients with major depressive disorder: a systematic review and meta-analysis of diffusion tensor imaging. *Journal of Psychiatry and Neuroscience,* **42**(3), 150–163.

Johnstone, E. C., Crow, T. J., Frith, C. D., Husband, J., & Kreel, L. (1976). Cerebral ventricular size and cognitive impairment in chronic schizophrenia. *Lancet,* **2**(7992), 924–926.

Judd, L. L., Akiskal, H. S., Schettler, P. J., Coryell, W., Endicott, J., Maser, J. D., . . . Keller, M. B. (2003). A prospective investigation of the natural history of the long-term weekly symptomatic status of bipolar II disorder. *Archives of General Psychiatry,* **60**(3), 261–269.

Judd, L. L., Akiskal, H. S., Schettler, P. J., Endicott, J., Maser, J., Solomon, D. A., . . . Keller, M. B. (2002). The long-term natural history of the weekly symptomatic status of bipolar I disorder. *Archives of General Psychiatry,* **59**(6), 530–537.

Kandel, E. R., Schwartz, J. H., & Jessell, T. M. (2000). *Principles of neural science* (4th ed.). New York: McGraw-Hill Health Professions Division.

Kasai, K., Shenton, M. E., Salisbury, D. F., Hirayasu, Y., Lee, C. U., Ciszewski, A. A., . . . McCarley, R. W. (2003). Progressive decrease of left superior temporal gyrus gray matter volume in patients with first-episode schizophrenia. *American Journal of Psychiatry,* **160**(1), 156–164.

Katagiri, N., Pantelis, C., Nemoto, T., Zalesky, A., Hori, M., Shimoji, K., . . . Mizuno, M. (2015). A longitudinal study investigating sub-threshold symptoms and white matter changes in individuals with an 'at risk mental state' (ARMS). *Schizophrenia Research,* **162**(1–3), 7–13.

Kelly, P. A., Viding, E., Wallace, G. L., Schaer, M., De Brito, S. A., Robustelli, B., & McCrory, E. J. (2013). Cortical thickness, surface area, and gyrification abnormalities in children exposed to maltreatment: neural markers of vulnerability? *Biological Psychiatry,* **74**(11), 845–852.

Kempton, M. J., Geddes, J. R., Ettinger, U., Williams, S. C., & Grasby, P. M. (2008). Meta-analysis, database, and meta-regression of 98 structural imaging studies in bipolar disorder. *Archives of General Psychiatry,* **65**(9), 1017–1032.

Kempton, M. J., & McGuire, P. (2015). How can neuroimaging facilitate the diagnosis and stratification of patients with psychosis? *European Neuropsychopharmacology,* **25**(5), 725–732.

Kempton, M. J., Salvador, Z., Munafo, M. R., Geddes, J. R., Simmons, A., Frangou, S., & Williams, S. C. (2011). Structural neuroimaging studies in major depressive disorder: meta-analysis and comparison with bipolar disorder. *Archives of General Psychiatry,* **68**(7), 675–690.

Kempton, M. J., Stahl, D., Williams, S. C., & DeLisi, L. E. (2010). Progressive lateral ventricular enlargement in schizophrenia: a meta-analysis of longitudinal MRI studies. *Schizophrenia Research,* **120**(1–3), 54–62.

Keshavan, M. S., Eack, S. M., Wojtalik, J. A., Prasad, K. M., Francis, A. N., Bhojraj, T. S., . . . Hogarty, S. S. (2011). A broad cortical reserve accelerates response to cognitive enhancement therapy in early course schizophrenia. *Schizophrenia Research,* **130**(1–3), 123–129.

Klauser, P., Zhou, J., Lim, J. K., Poh, J. S., Zheng, H., Tng, H. Y., . . . Chee, M. W. (2015). Lack of evidence for regional brain volume or cortical thickness abnormalities in youths at clinical high risk for psychosis: findings from the Longitudinal Youth at Risk Study. *Schizophrenia Bulletin,* **41**, 1285–1293.

Kloppel, S., Abdulkadir, A., Jack Jr, C. R., Koutsouleris, N., Mourao-Miranda, J., & Vemuri, P. (2012). Diagnostic neuroimaging across diseases. *NeuroImage,* **61**(2), 457–463.

Koo, M. S., Levitt, J. J., Salisbury, D. F., Nakamura, M., Shenton, M. E., & McCarley, R. W. (2008). A cross-sectional and longitudinal magnetic resonance imaging study of cingulate gyrus gray matter volume abnormalities in first-episode schizophrenia and first-episode affective psychosis. *Archives of General Psychiatry,* **65**(7), 746–760.

Koolschijn, P. C., van Haren, N. E., Lensvelt-Mulders, G. J., Hulshoff Pol, H. E., & Kahn, R. S. (2009). Brain volume abnormalities in major depressive disorder: a meta-analysis of

magnetic resonance imaging studies. *Human Brain Mapping,* **30**(11), 3719–3735.

Koutsouleris, N., Meisenzahl, E. M., Davatzikos, C., Bottlender, R., Frodl, T., Scheuerecker, J., . . . Gaser, C. (2009). Use of neuroanatomical pattern classification to identify subjects in at-risk mental states of psychosis and predict disease transition. *Archives of General Psychiatry,* **66**(7), 700–712.

Kozicky, J. M., Ha, T. H., Torres, I. J., Bond, D. J., Honer, W. G., Lam, R. W., & Yatham, L. N. (2013). Relationship between frontostriatal morphology and executive function deficits in bipolar I disorder following a first manic episode: data from the Systematic Treatment Optimization Program for Early Mania (STOP-EM). *Bipolar Disorders,* **15**(6), 657–668.

Lagopoulos, J., Hermens, D. F., Hatton, S. N., Battisti, R. A., Tobias-Webb, J., White, D., . . . Hickie, I. B. (2013). Microstructural white matter changes are correlated with the stage of psychiatric illness. *Translational Psychiatry,* **3**, e248.

Lagopoulos, J., Hermens, D. F., Naismith, S. L., Scott, E. M., & Hickie, I. B. (2012). Frontal lobe changes occur early in the course of affective disorders in young people. *BMC Psychiatry,* **12**, 4.

Lai, C. H. (2013). Gray matter volume in major depressive disorder: a meta-analysis of voxel-based morphometry studies. *Psychiatry Research,* **211**(1), 37–46.

Lai, C. H., & Wu, Y. T. (2015). The gray matter alterations in major depressive disorder and panic disorder: putative differences in the pathogenesis. *Journal of Affective Disorders,* **186**, 1–6.

Lesh, T. A., Tanase, C., Geib, B. R., Niendam, T. A., Yoon, J. H., Minzenberg, M. J., . . . Carter, C. S. (2015). A multimodal analysis of antipsychotic effects on brain structure and function in first-episode schizophrenia. *JAMA Psychiatry,* **72**(3), 226–234.

Liao, Y., Huang, X., Wu, Q., Yang, C., Kuang, W., Du, M., . . . Gong, Q. (2013). Is depression a disconnection syndrome? Meta-analysis of diffusion tensor imaging studies in patients with MDD. *Journal of Psychiatry and Neuroscience,* **38**(1), 49–56.

Lim, C. S., Baldessarini, R. J., Vieta, E., Yucel, M., Bora, E., & Sim, K. (2013). Longitudinal neuroimaging and neuropsychological changes in bipolar disorder patients: review of the evidence. *Neuroscience and Biobehavioral Reviews,* **37**(3), 418–435.

Lin, A., Reniers, R. L., & Wood, S. J. (2013). Clinical staging in severe mental disorder: evidence from neurocognition and neuroimaging. *British Journal of Psychiatry Supplement,* **54**, s11–s17.

Long, Z., Duan, X., Wang, Y., Liu, F., Zeng, L., Zhao, J. P., & Chen, H. (2015). Disrupted structural connectivity network in treatment-naive depression. *Progress in Neuro-Psychopharmacology and Biological Psychiatry,* **56**, 18–26.

Lorenzetti, V., Solowij, N., Whittle, S., Fornito, A., Lubman, D. I., Pantelis, C., & Yucel, M. (2015). Gross morphological brain changes with chronic, heavy cannabis use. *British Journal of Psychiatry,* **206**(1), 77–78.

Lyoo, I. K., Lee, H. K., Jung, J. H., Noam, G. G., & Renshaw, P. F. (2002). White matter hyperintensities on magnetic resonance imaging of the brain in children with psychiatric disorders. *Comprehensive Psychiatry,* **43**(5), 361–368.

McDonald, C., Zanelli, J., Rabe-Hesketh, S., Ellison-Wright, I., Sham, P., Kalidindi, S., ... Kennedy, N. (2004). Meta-analysis of magnetic resonance imaging brain morphometry studies in bipolar disorder. *Biological Psychiatry,* **56**(6), 411–417.

McGorry, P. D. (2014). Beyond psychosis risk: early clinical phenotypes in mental disorder and the subthreshold pathway to safe, timely and effective care. *Psychopathology,* **47**(5), 285–286.

McGorry, P., Keshavan, M., Goldstone, S., Amminger, P., Allott, K., Berk, M., ... Hickie, I. (2014). Biomarkers and clinical staging in psychiatry. *World Psychiatry,* **13**(3), 211–223.

McGorry, P. D., Purcell, R., Hickie, I. B., Yung, A. R., Pantelis, C., & Jackson, H. J. (2007). Clinical staging: a heuristic model for psychiatry and youth mental health. *Medical Journal of Australia,* **187**(7 Suppl.), S40–S42.

McIntosh, A. M., Owens, D. C., Moorhead, W. J., Whalley, H. C., Stanfield, A. C., Hall, J., ... Lawrie, S. M. (2011). Longitudinal volume reductions in people at high genetic risk of schizophrenia as they develop psychosis. *Biological Psychiatry,* **69**(10), 953–958.

Mills, N. P., Delbello, M. P., Adler, C. M., & Strakowski, S. M. (2005). MRI analysis of cerebellar vermal abnormalities in bipolar disorder. *American Journal of Psychiatry,* **162**(8), 1530–1532.

Mittal, V. A., Dean, D. J., Bernard, J. A., Orr, J. M., Pelletier-Baldelli, A., Carol, E. E., ... Millman, Z. B. (2014). Neurological soft signs predict abnormal cerebellar-thalamic tract development and negative symptoms in adolescents at high risk for psychosis: a longitudinal perspective. *Schizophrenia Bulletin,* **40**(6), 1204–1215.

Moore, G. J., Bebchuk, J. M., Wilds, I. B., Chen, G., & Menji, H. K. (2000). Lithium-induced increase in human brain grey matter. *Lancet,* **356**(9237), 1241–1242.

Moore, M. T., Nathan, D., Elliott, A. R., & Laubach, C. (1935). Encephalographic studies in mental disease: an analysis of 152 cases. *American Journal of Psychiatry,* **92**, 43–67.

Mueser, K. T., & McGurk, S. R. (2004). Schizophrenia. *Lancet,* **363**(9426), 2063–2072.

Munn, M. A., Alexopoulos, J., Nishino, T., Babb, C. M., Flake, L. A., Singer, T., ... Botteron, K. N. (2007). Amygdala volume analysis in female twins with major depression. *Biological Psychiatry,* **62**(5), 415–422.

Nakamura, M., Salisbury, D. F., Hirayasu, Y., Bouix, S., Pohl, K. M., Yoshida, T., ... McCarley, R. W. (2007). Neocortical gray matter volume in first-episode schizophrenia and first-episode affective psychosis: a cross-sectional and longitudinal MRI study. *Biological Psychiatry,* **62**(7), 773–783.

Nelson, B., Yuen, H. P., Wood, S. J., Lin, A., Spiliotacopoulos, D., Bruxner, A., ... Yung, A. R. (2013). Long-term follow-up of a group at ultra high risk ('prodromal') for psychosis: the PACE 400 study. *JAMA Psychiatry,* **70**(8), 793–802.

Nelson, M. D., Saykin, A. J., Flashman, L. A., & Riordan, H. J. (1998). Hippocampal volume reduction in schizophrenia as assessed by magnetic resonance imaging: a meta-analytic study. *Archives of General Psychiatry,* **55**(5), 433–440.

Nordholm, D., Krogh, J., Mondelli, V., Dazzan, P., Pariante, C., & Nordentoft, M. (2013). Pituitary gland volume in patients with schizophrenia, subjects at ultra high-risk of developing psychosis and healthy controls: a systematic review and meta-analysis. *Psychoneuroendocrinology,* **38**(11), 2394–2404.

Olabi, B., Ellison-Wright, I., McIntosh, A. M., Wood, S. J., Bullmore, E., & Lawrie, S. M. (2011). Are there progressive brain changes in schizophrenia? A meta-analysis of structural magnetic resonance imaging studies. *Biological Psychiatry,* **70**(1), 88–96.

Orru, G., Pettersson-Yeo, W., Marquand, A. F., Sartori, G., & Mechelli, A. (2012). Using support vector machine to identify imaging biomarkers of neurological and psychiatric disease: a critical review. *Neuroscience and Biobehavioral Reviews,* **36**(4), 1140–1152.

Paillere Martinot, M. L., Lemaitre, H., Artiges, E., Miranda, R., Goodman, R., Penttila, J., . . . Martinot, J. L. (2014). White-matter microstructure and gray-matter volumes in adolescents with subthreshold bipolar symptoms. *Molecular Psychiatry,* **19**(4), 462–470.

Pajonk, F. G., Wobrock, T., Gruber, O., Scherk, H., Berner, D., Kaizl, I., . . . Falkai, P. (2010). Hippocampal plasticity in response to exercise in schizophrenia. *Archives of General Psychiatry,* **67**(2), 133–143.

Palaniyappan, L., Marques, T. R., Taylor, H., Handley, R., Mondelli, V., Bonaccorso, S., . . . Dazzan, P. (2013). Cortical folding defects as markers of poor treatment response in first-episode psychosis. *JAMA Psychiatry,* **70**(10), 1031–1040.

Pantelis, C., Velakoulis, D., McGorry, P. D., Wood, S. J., Suckling, J., Phillips, L. J., . . . McGuire, P. K. (2003). Neuroanatomical abnormalities before and after onset of psychosis: a cross-sectional and longitudinal MRI comparison. *Lancet,* **361**(9354), 281–288.

Pantelis, C., Wannan, C., Bartholomeusz, C. F., Allott, K., & McGorry, P. (2015). Cognitive intervention in early psychosis: preserving abilities versus remediating deficits. *Current Opinion in Behavioral Sciences,* **4**, 63–72.

Pantelis, C., Yucel, M., Bora, E., Fornito, A., Testa, R., Brewer, W. J., . . . Wood, S. J. (2009). Neurobiological markers of illness onset in psychosis and schizophrenia: the search for a moving target. *Neuropsychology Review,* **19**(3), 385–398.

Pantelis, C., Yucel, M., Wood, S. J., Brewer, W. J., Fornito, A., Berger, G., . . . Velakoulis, D. (2008). Neurobiological endophenotypes of psychosis and schizophrenia: are there biological markers of illness onset? In H. J. Jackson & P. McGorry (Eds), *Recognition and management of early psychosis: a preventative approach* (2nd ed.). Cambridge: Cambridge University Press pp. 61–80.

Pantelis, C., Yucel, M., Wood, S. J., Velakoulis, D., Sun, D., Berger, G., . . . McGorry, P. D. (2005). Structural brain imaging evidence for multiple pathological processes at different stages of brain development in schizophrenia. *Schizophrenia Bulletin,* **31**(3), 672–696.

Paus, T. (2005). Mapping brain maturation and cognitive development during adolescence. *Trends in Cognitive Sciences,* **9**(2), 60–68.

Peterson, B. S., Warner, V., Bansal, R., Zhu, H., Hao, X., Liu, J., . . . Weissman, M. M. (2009). Cortical thinning in persons at increased familial risk for major depression. *Proceedings of the National Academy of Sciences of the United States of America,* **106**(15), 6273–6278.

Pfeifer, J. C., Welge, J., Strakowski, S. M., Adler, C. M., & DelBello, M. P. (2008). Meta-analysis of amygdala volumes in children and adolescents with bipolar disorder. *Journal of the American Academy of Child and Adolescent Psychiatry,* **47**(11), 1289–1298.

Phillips, L. J., Velakoulis, D., Pantelis, C., Wood, S., Yuen, H. P., Yung, A. R., . . . McGorry, P. D. (2002). Non-reduction in hippocampal volume is associated with higher risk of psychosis. *Schizophrenia Research,* **58**(2–3), 145–158.

Qiu, L., Lui, S., Kuang, W., Huang, X., Li, J., Li, J., . . . Gong, Q. (2014). Regional increases of cortical thickness in untreated, first-episode major depressive disorder. *Translational Psychiatry*, 4, e378.

Radua, J., Borgwardt, S., Crescini, A., Mataix-Cols, D., Meyer-Lindenberg, A., McGuire, P. K., & Fusar-Poli, P. (2012). Multimodal meta-analysis of structural and functional brain changes in first episode psychosis and the effects of antipsychotic medication. *Neuroscience and Biobehavioral Reviews*, 36(10), 2325–2333.

Radua, J., & Mataix-Cols, D. (2009). Voxel-wise meta-analysis of grey matter changes in obsessive-compulsive disorder. *British Journal of Psychiatry*, 195(5), 393–402.

Rao, U., Chen, L. A., Bidesi, A. S., Shad, M. U., Thomas, M. A., & Hammen, C. L. (2010). Hippocampal changes associated with early-life adversity and vulnerability to depression. *Biological Psychiatry*, 67(4), 357–364.

Rasetti, R., & Weinberger, D. R. (2011). Intermediate phenotypes in psychiatric disorders. *Current Opinion in Genetics and Development*, 21(3), 340–348.

Rosso, I. M., Killgore, W. D., Cintron, C. M., Gruber, S. A., Tohen, M., & Yurgelun-Todd, D. A. (2007). Reduced amygdala volumes in first-episode bipolar disorder and correlation with cerebral white matter. *Biological Psychiatry*, 61(6), 743–749.

Sachdev, P., Wen, W., Chen, X., & Brodaty, H. (2007). Progression of white matter hyperintensities in elderly individuals over 3 years. *Neurology*, 68(3), 214–222.

Sacher, J., Neumann, J., Funfstuck, T., Soliman, A., Villringer, A., & Schroeter, M. L. (2012). Mapping the depressed brain: a meta-analysis of structural and functional alterations in major depressive disorder. *Journal of Affective Disorders*, 140(2), 142–148.

Scarr, E., Cowie, T. F., Kanellakis, S., Sundram, S., Pantelis, C., & Dean, B. (2009). Decreased cortical muscarinic receptors define a subgroup of subjects with schizophrenia. *Molecular Psychiatry*, 14(11), 1017–1023.

Schmaal, L., Hibar, D. P., Samann, P. G., Hall, G. B., Baune, B. T., Jahanshad, N., . . . Veltman, D. J. (2017). Cortical abnormalities in adults and adolescents with major depression based on brain scans from 20 cohorts worldwide in the ENIGMA Major Depressive Disorder Working Group. *Molecular Psychiatry*, 22, 900–909.

Schmaal, L., Veltman, D. J., van Erp, T. G., Samann, P. G., Frodl, T., Jahanshad, N., . . . Hibar, D. P. (2016). Subcortical brain alterations in major depressive disorder: findings from the ENIGMA Major Depressive Disorder working group. *Molecular Psychiatry*, 21, 806–812.

Schnack, H. G., Nieuwenhuis, M., van Haren, N. E., Abramovic, L., Scheewe, T. W., Brouwer, R. M., . . . Kahn, R. S. (2014). Can structural MRI aid in clinical classification? A machine learning study in two independent samples of patients with schizophrenia, bipolar disorder and healthy subjects. *NeuroImage*, 84, 299–306.

Selvaraj, S., Arnone, D., Job, D., Stanfield, A., Farrow, T. F., Nugent, A. C., . . . McIntosh, A. M. (2012). Grey matter differences in bipolar disorder: a meta-analysis of voxel-based morphometry studies. *Bipolar Disorders*, 14(2), 135–145.

Shaw, P., Kabani, N. J., Lerch, J. P., Eckstrand, K., Lenroot, R., Gogtay, N., . . . Wise, S. P. (2008). Neurodevelopmental trajectories of the human cerebral cortex. *Journal of Neuroscience*, 28(14), 3586–3594.

Shenton, M. E., Dickey, C. C., Frumin, M., & McCarley, R. W. (2001). A review of MRI findings in schizophrenia. *Schizophrenia Research*, 49(1–2), 1–52.

Shepherd, A. M., Laurens, K. R., Matheson, S. L., Carr, V. J., & Green, M. J. (2012). Systematic meta-review and quality assessment of the structural brain alterations in schizophrenia. *Neuroscience and Biobehavioral Reviews*, 36(4), 1342–1356.

Simon, A. E., Borgwardt, S., Riecher-Rossler, A., Velthorst, E., de Haan, L., & Fusar-Poli, P. (2013). Moving beyond transition outcomes: meta-analysis of remission rates in individuals at high clinical risk for psychosis. *Psychiatry Research*, 209(3), 266–272.

Smieskova, R., Fusar-Poli, P., Allen, P., Bendfeldt, K., Stieglitz, R. D., Drewe, J., . . . Borgwardt, S. J. (2010). Neuroimaging predictors of transition to psychosis: a systematic review and meta-analysis. *Neuroscience and Biobehavioral Reviews,* 34(8), 1207–1222.

Spalletta, G., Piras, F., Caltagirone, C., & Fagioli, S. (2014). Hippocampal multimodal structural changes and subclinical depression in healthy individuals. *Journal of Affective Disorders,* 152–154, 105–112.

Steen, R. G., Mull, C., McClure, R., Hamer, R. M., & Lieberman, J. A. (2006). Brain volume in first-episode schizophrenia: systematic review and meta-analysis of magnetic resonance imaging studies. *British Journal of Psychiatry,* 188, 510–518.

Sun, D., Phillips, L., Velakoulis, D., Yung, A., McGorry, P. D., Wood, S. J., . . . Pantelis, C. (2009a). Progressive brain structural changes mapped as psychosis develops in 'at risk' individuals. *Schizophrenia Research,* 108(1–3), 85–92.

Sun, D., Stuart, G. W., Jenkinson, M., Wood, S. J., McGorry, P. D., Velakoulis, D., . . . Pantelis, C. (2009b). Brain surface contraction mapped in first-episode schizophrenia: a longitudinal magnetic resonance imaging study. *Molecular Psychiatry,* 14(10), 976–986.

Takahashi, T., Wood, S. J., Soulsby, B., McGorry, P. D., Tanino, R., Suzuki, M., . . . Pantelis, C. (2009a). Follow-up MRI study of the insular cortex in first-episode psychosis and chronic schizophrenia. *Schizophrenia Research,* 108(1–3), 49–56.

Takahashi, T., Wood, S. J., Yung, A. R., Phillips, L. J., Soulsby, B., McGorry, P. D., . . . Pantelis, C. (2009b). Insular cortex gray matter changes in individuals at ultra-high-risk of developing psychosis. *Schizophrenia Research,* 111(1–3), 94–102.

Takahashi, T., Wood, S. J., Yung, A. R., Soulsby, B., McGorry, P. D., Suzuki, M., . . . Pantelis, C. (2009c). Progressive gray matter reduction of the superior temporal gyrus during transition to psychosis. *Archives of General Psychiatry,* 66(4), 366–376.

Takahashi, T., Wood, S. J., Yung, A. R., Walterfang, M., Phillips, L. J., Soulsby, B., . . . Pantelis, C. (2010). Superior temporal gyrus volume in antipsychotic-naive people at risk

of psychosis. *British Journal of Psychiatry,* 196(3), 206–211.

Theodoridou, A., Heekeren, K., Dvorsky, D., Metzler, S., Franscini, M., Haker, H., . . . Rossler, W. (2014). Early recognition of high risk of bipolar disorder and psychosis: an overview of the ZInEP 'early recognition' study. *Frontiers in Public Health,* 2, 166.

van Erp, T. G., Hibar, D. P., Rasmussen, J. M., Glahn, D. C., Pearlson, G. D., Andreassen, O. A., . . . Turner, J. A. (2016). Subcortical brain volume abnormalities in 2028 individuals with schizophrenia and 2540 healthy controls via the ENIGMA consortium. *Molecular Psychiatry,* 21(4), 547–553.

Velakoulis, D., Wood, S. J., Wong, M. T., McGorry, P. D., Yung, A., Phillips, L., . . . Pantelis, C. (2006). Hippocampal and amygdala volumes according to psychosis stage and diagnosis: a magnetic resonance imaging study of chronic schizophrenia, first-episode psychosis, and ultra-high-risk individuals. *Archives of General Psychiatry,* 63(2), 139–149.

Vita, A., & de Peri, L. (2007). Hippocampal and amygdala volume reductions in first-episode schizophrenia. *British Journal of Psychiatry,* 190, 271.

Vita, A., de Peri, L., Deste, G., & Sacchetti, E. (2012). Progressive loss of cortical gray matter in schizophrenia: a meta-analysis and meta-regression of longitudinal MRI studies. *Translational Psychiatry,* 2, e190.

Vita, A., de Peri, L., & Sacchetti, E. (2009). Gray matter, white matter, brain, and intracranial volumes in first-episode bipolar disorder: a meta-analysis of magnetic resonance imaging studies. *Bipolar Disorders,* 11(8), 807–814.

Vita, A., de Peri, L., Silenzi, C., & Dieci, M. (2006). Brain morphology in first-episode schizophrenia: a meta-analysis of quantitative magnetic resonance imaging studies. *Schizophrenia Research,* 82(1), 75–88.

Wall, P. M., & Messier, C. (2001). The hippocampal formation: orbitomedial prefrontal cortex circuit in the attentional control of active memory. *Behavioural Brain Research,* 127(1–2), 99–117.

Walter, A., Studerus, E., Smieskova, R., Kuster, P., Aston, J., Lang, U. E., . . . Borgwardt, S. (2012). Hippocampal volume in subjects at high risk of psychosis: a longitudinal MRI study. *Schizophrenia Research*, **142**(1–3), 217–222.

Walterfang, M., McGuire, P. K., Yung, A. R., Phillips, L. J., Velakoulis, D., Wood, S. J., . . . Pantelis, C. (2008a). White matter volume changes in people who develop psychosis. *British Journal of Psychiatry*, **193**(3), 210–215.

Walterfang, M., Wood, S. J., Velakoulis, D., & Pantelis, C. (2006). Neuropathological, neurogenetic and neuroimaging evidence for white matter pathology in schizophrenia. *Neuroscience and Biobehavioral Reviews*, **30**(7), 918–948.

Walterfang, M., Yung, A., Wood, A. G., Reutens, D. C., Phillips, L., Wood, S. J., . . . Pantelis, C. (2008b). Corpus callosum shape alterations in individuals prior to the onset of psychosis. *Schizophrenia Research*, **103**(1–3), 1–10.

Wang, Y., Xu, C., Zhang, A., Zuo, X. N., Gao, Q., Li, X., . . . Zhang, K. (2014). White matter abnormalities in medication-naive adult patients with major depressive disorder: tract-based spatial statistical analysis. *Neuro Endocrinology Letters*, **35**(8), 697–702.

Watanabe, K., Kakeda, S., Yoshimura, R., Abe, O., Ide, S., Hayashi, K., . . . Korogi, Y. (2015). Relationship between the catechol-O-methyl transferase Val108/158Met genotype and brain volume in treatment-naive major depressive disorder: voxel-based morphometry analysis. *Psychiatry Research*, **233**(3), 481–487.

Whittle, S., Lichter, R., Dennison, M., Vijayakumar, N., Schwartz, O., Byrne, M. L., . . . Allen, N. B. (2014). Structural brain development and depression onset during adolescence: a prospective longitudinal study. *American Journal of Psychiatry*, **171**(5), 564–571.

Witthaus, H., Mendes, U., Brune, M., Ozgurdal, S., Bohner, G., Gudlowski, Y., . . . Juckel, G. (2010). Hippocampal subdivision and amygdalar volumes in patients in an at-risk mental state for schizophrenia. *Journal of Psychiatry and Neuroscience*, **35**(1), 33–40.

Wood, S. J., Kennedy, D., Phillips, L. J., Seal, M. L., Yucel, M., Nelson, B., . . . Pantelis, C. (2010). Hippocampal pathology in individuals at ultra-high risk for psychosis: a multi-modal magnetic resonance study. *NeuroImage*, **52**(1), 62–68.

Wood, S. J., Yung, A. R., McGorry, P. D., & Pantelis, C. (2011). Neuroimaging and treatment evidence for clinical staging in psychotic disorders: from the at-risk mental state to chronic schizophrenia. *Biological Psychiatry*, **70**(7), 619–625.

World Federation for Mental Health (2012). *Depression: a global crisis*. Occoquan, VA: World Federation for Mental Health.

Wright, I. C., Rabe-Hesketh, S., Woodruff, P. W., David, A. S., Murray, R. M., & Bullmore, E. T. (2000). Meta-analysis of regional brain volumes in schizophrenia. *American Journal of Psychiatry*, **157**(1), 16–25.

Yao, L., Lui, S., Liao, Y., Du, M. Y., Hu, N., Thomas, J. A., & Gong, Q. Y. (2013). White matter deficits in first episode schizophrenia: an activation likelihood estimation meta-analysis. *Progress in Neuro-Psychopharmacology and Biological Psychiatry*, **45**, 100–106.

Yatham, L. N., Lyoo, I. K., Liddle, P., Renshaw, P. F., Wan, D., Lam, R. W., & Hwang, J. (2007). A magnetic resonance imaging study of mood stabilizer- and neuroleptic-naive first-episode mania. *Bipolar Disorders*, **9**(7), 693–697.

Yucel, M., Solowij, N., Respondek, C., Whittle, S., Fornito, A., Pantelis, C., & Lubman, D. I. (2008). Regional brain abnormalities associated with long-term heavy cannabis use. *Archives of General Psychiatry*, **65**(6), 694–701.

Zakzanis, K. K., Poulin, P., Hansen, K. T., & Jolic, D. (2000). Searching the schizophrenic brain for temporal lobe deficits: a systematic review and meta-analysis. *Psychological Medicine*, **30**(3), 491–504.

Zanetti, M. V., Schaufelberger, M. S., de Castro, C. C., Menezes, P. R., Scazufca, M., McGuire, P. K., . . . Busatto, G. F. (2008). White-matter hyperintensities in first-episode psychosis. *British Journal of Psychiatry*, **193**(1), 25–30.

Zhao, Y. J., Du, M. Y., Huang, X. Q., Lui, S., Chen, Z. Q., Liu, J., . . . Gong, Q. Y. (2014). Brain grey matter abnormalities in medication-free patients with major depressive disorder: a meta-analysis. *Psychological Medicine,* **44**(14), 2927–2937.

Zhuo, C., Liu, M., Wang, L., Tian, H., & Tang, J. (2016). Diffusion tensor MR imaging evaluation of callosal abnormalities in schizophrenia: a meta-analysis. *PLoS One,* **11**(8), e0161406.

Ziermans, T. B., Schothorst, P. F., Schnack, H. G., Koolschijn, P. C., Kahn, R. S., van Engeland, H., & Durston, S. (2012). Progressive structural brain changes during development of psychosis. *Schizophrenia Bulletin,* **38**(3), 519–530.

Zipursky, R. B., Reilly, T. J., & Murray, R. M. (2013). The myth of schizophrenia as a progressive brain disease. *Schizophrenia Bulletin,* **39**(6), 1363–1372.

Chapter

7

Staging of Cognition in Psychiatric Illness

Kelly Allott

Introduction

Disturbances in cognitive functioning, such as poor concentration and memory, slowed speed of information processing, or difficulty organising one's thoughts are commonly experienced during an acute episode of most mental illnesses. In many cases, such cognitive disturbances improve with symptom alleviation, indicating they are 'state-based' disturbances that co-occur with psychiatric symptoms. However, extensive research indicates that 'trait-based' and/or 'progressive/scar' impairments are also frequently present in many psychiatric disorders (Allott et al., 2016; David et al., 2008). Cognitive abilities are of interest because they are measureable characteristics of an individual that reflect the integrity of underlying neurobiology and are fundamental for behaviours of daily functioning, thus having clear implications for prognosis and treatment. Accordingly, there has been focused investigation into the characteristics of cognition and development of cognitive interventions for psychiatric disorders (Millan et al., 2012). An online literature search shows that psychotic disorders (especially schizophrenia) have clearly received the most investigation, but increasingly, cognition research is emerging across the full spectrum of mental health conditions (Table 7.1).

Cognition has been proposed as a potentially important biomarker in the staging model of psychiatric illness (Kapczinski et al., 2014; Lin et al., 2013; McGorry et al., 2014; Pantelis et al., 2015; Wood et al., 2013). While the presenting psychiatric symptoms and diagnosis are central for guiding treatment, the cognitive functioning of a person with mental illness may provide additional clues with regards to the underlying pathophysiology, aetiology and severity of illness (Allott et al., 2013; Keefe, 1995). Furthermore, independent of symptomatic state, cognitive impairments are robustly associated with functional outcomes and disability in psychiatric disorders across the lifespan (Andreou & Bozikas, 2013; Depp et al., 2012; Fett et al., 2011; Lee et al., 2013b; Rosa et al., 2014). Thus, regardless of diagnosis, in conjunction with an examination of other clinical factors, cognitive assessment is a useful clinical tool that may shed light on diagnostic or functional prognosis and the likely effectiveness of particular interventions, and so subsequently guide clinical care. It is important to note that cognition does not operate independently from other neurobiological or psychological factors and it is the interaction of these factors in one individual over time that leads to the clinical presentation (Nolen-Hoeksema & Watkins, 2011). Within the scope of this chapter, however, examination of cognition in psychiatric disorders within the staging framework may help to further inform and refine the staging model. Specifically, the following questions arise. Can cognitive profiles differentiate or predict psychiatric subgroups or stages in people presenting with mental health difficulties? What is the trajectory of cognition in mental illness? How does the trajectory of cognition

Table 7.1 Number of publications relating to neuropsychology, neurocognition and social cognition in different psychiatric disorders

Disorder[a]	Neuropsych*	Percentage of schizophrenia	Neurocogniti*	Percentage of schizophrenia	Social cogniti*	Percentage of schizophrenia
Schizophrenia	18,555	100.0	4021	100.0	1125	100.0
Schizophreniform disorder	5874	31.7	1956	48.6	272	24.2
Schizoaffective disorder	6149	33.1	2023	50.3	300	26.7
Delusional disorder	791	4.3	310	7.7	41	3.6
Bipolar disorder	5529	29.8	1165	29.0	143	12.7
Major depressi*	5570	30.0	429	10.7	73	6.5
Obsessive-compulsive disorder	2658	14.3	286	7.1	24	2.1
Post-traumatic stress disorder	1753	9.4	194	4.8	41	3.6
Social anxiety disorder	1036	5.6	94	2.3	137	12.2
Social phobia	261	1.4	12	0.3	17	1.5
Panic disorder	1024	5.5	52	1.3	2	0.2
Generali* anxiety disorder	776	4.2	45	1.1	14	1.2
Anorexia nervosa	801	4.3	89	2.2	43	3.8
Bulimia nervosa	393	2.1	27	0.7	12	1.1

'Cognition' was not included as a search term as it overlaps significantly with cognitive styles/processes. The search was conducted in PubMed only, given the table is for illustrative purposes; the 'all fields' search field was used. * denotes truncated search terms to identify various word endings (e.g., depression and depressive for depressi*).
[a] Selective disorders included.

relate to the course of mental health difficulties? Does the severity and course of cognitive impairments affect or predict pharmacological and psychological treatment response? Does the severity and course of cognitive impairments relate to functional outcomes at different stages of mental illness? Can cognitive interventions alter the course of illness? Although not easy to answer (and not all of them will be addressed here), these are important questions for the field. It is also important to be cognisant of the imbalance in the evidence-base across psychiatric disorders, as highlighted in Table 7.1. With these issues in mind, the aim of this chapter is to explore how the clinical staging model might help to organise and explain the existing evidence on cognition during the onset and evolution of mental illness and evaluate the evidence for staging of cognition. Key cognitive research findings will be organised according to the putative clinical stages as outlined in Chapter 2. Most of the existing research has examined cognition in separate diagnostic groups, but mixed or transdiagnostic studies will be included where possible in an attempt to draw on commonalities across psychopathology. This chapter will focus on psychiatric disorders that have been diagnosed in adolescence or adulthood. Personality disorders will not be reviewed in detail and substance use disorders are also not reviewed, given space limitations and likely different mechanisms of cognitive impairment associated with substance-related neurotoxicity.

Definition of Cognition and Cognitive Dysfunction

Cognitive functions are the interrelated unconscious and conscious mental activities of a person that are not directly observed, but inferred from behaviour (Lezak et al., 2004; Millan et al., 2012). They encompass receptive functions, memory and learning, thinking skills and expressive functions. For the current chapter, the term 'cognition' includes both neurocognition and social cognition that has been examined via objective measures rather than self-report. Metacognition (awareness or knowledge of one's thinking or cognition) can also be included under the rubric of cognition, but is beyond the scope of this chapter. Cognition research in major psychiatric disorders has been dominated by a focus on neurocognition (Table 7.1), which can be defined as the fundamental mental operations underlying goal-directed behaviour, such as attention and vigilance, working memory, processing speed, learning and memory, language and visual functions, executive functions, and global intellectual functions, including intelligence. Social cognition, a related but independent construct to neurocognition, has received increasing investigation in the psychiatry field (Table 7.1). Social cognition involves the perception, processing and interpretation of people's intentions, feelings and thoughts (Adolphs, 2009; Fiske & Taylor, 2013; Pinkham et al., 2014). The domains that have received the most investigation in psychiatry include emotion processing, theory of mind or mentalising, social perception/ knowledge and attributional style. Table 7.2 lists the key cognitive domains, a brief definition of each and commonly used measures.

Broadly speaking, cognitive dysfunction may be conceptualised as deficits or biases. Deficits are evident when an individual's performance is significantly below a demographic- ally matched normative sample (e.g. >1–1.5 standard deviations below the mean) or below what is expected based on the individual's estimated premorbid intellectual functioning. For example, an individual with an estimated premorbid IQ of 95 (average range) performs well below average on a verbal memory task, reflecting a deficit in verbal memory. Biases are not associated with accuracy in performance, but are the tendency to process information in a

Table 7.2 Definitions of cognitive domains and example tasks used to assess them

Cognitive domains	Definition	Example tests or batteries used to assess domain
Neurocognition		
Intelligence/IQ	'General' intellectual ability subserved by a multiplicity of cognitive functions, examined by a range of tests that provide a composite IQ (intelligence quotient) score. Mean IQ in the general population is 100, with a standard deviation of 15. Premorbid IQ can be estimated based on a graded word reading task	• National Adult Reading Test (NART) • Wechsler Test of Adult Reading • Wide Range Achievement Test (WRAT) – Reading subtest • Wechsler Intelligence Scale for Children (WISC) • Wechsler Adult Intelligence Scale (WAIS) • Wechsler Abbreviated Scale of Intelligence (WASI)
Language abilities	Ability to perceive and understand/comprehend the meaning of words and sentences/prose and use or express oneself with language. Also includes acquired general knowledge	• Vocabulary test from Wechsler Scales • Information test from Wechsler Scales • Comprehension from Wechsler Scales
Visuospatial/non-verbal abilities	Ability to perceive, integrate and analyse visual information. Includes spatial and constructional abilities. For example, copying a picture, putting together a puzzle, finding what is missing from a picture or completing a visual puzzle (e.g. Rubik's cube)	• Rey-Osterrieth Complex Figure Test – Copy • Block Design from Wechsler Scales • Matrix Reasoning from Wechsler Scales[1] • Picture Completion from Wechsler Scales[1] • Raven's Progressive Matrices[1]
Attention	Several capacities relating to the reception and processing of information (in lay terms referred to as 'concentration'), including: • attention *span* refers to how much information can be held in the mind at once • *focused* or *selective* attention is the capacity to focus on important information while ignoring or suppressing awareness of competing information (non-relevant information/distractions) • *sustained* attention or *vigilance* is the capacity to maintain attention or concentration over a period of time • *divided* attention is the ability to respond to more than one stimuli or task at a time • attention *shifting* is the capacity to alternate focus	• Digit Span from Wechsler Scales • Spatial Span from Wechsler Scales • Continuous Performance Test • Trail Making Test – Part B[1,2] • Test of Everyday Attention (TEA)

143

Table 7.2 (cont.)

Cognitive domains	Definition	Example tests or batteries used to assess domain
Working memory	Capacity to mentally hold and manipulate verbal or visual information (e.g. working out how much change you are owed)	• Digit Span from Wechsler Scales • Letter–Number Sequencing from Wechsler Scales • Spatial Span from Wechsler Memory Scale • N-back tasks
Speed of information processing	Speed with which one can 'take in' and process information. May also involve the speed with which one can complete a motor task, referred to as psychomotor speed	• Trail Making Test – Part A • Symbol–Digit Coding from the Wechsler Scales • Stroop Task (part A and B)
Verbal learning and memory	Ability to learn and remember information that is presented verbally or in words (e.g. a conversation, a telephone number). Includes immediate and delayed recall and recognition	• Rey Auditory Verbal Learning Test • California Verbal Learning Test • Logical Memory from the Wechsler Memory Scale • Verbal Paired Associate Learning
Visual learning and memory	Ability to learn and remember information that is presented visually or in pictures/figures (e.g. route on a map, the scene of a crime). Includes immediate and delayed recall and recognition	• Rey–Osterrieth Complex Figure Test – Recall • Visual Reproduction from the Wechsler Memory Scale • Benton Visual Retention Test
Verbal fluency	Ease, speed and quantity of verbal production	• Controlled Oral Word Association (e.g. FAS)[1,2] • Semantic (e.g. animal) fluency[1,2]
Executive functions	Executive functions involve the capacity for engagement in independent, purposeful and self-serving behaviour. They relate to *how* an individual goes about performing goal-directed behaviours and *how* they engage with *novel* tasks and situations. Executive functions is the rubric for a number of 'higher-level' cognitive abilities including flexibility/set-shifting, inhibition, planning, organisation, reasoning, and problem-solving	• Wisconsin Card Sorting Test • Stroop Colour–Word (interference) task • Similarities from Wechsler Scales • Tower of Hanoi/London • Twenty Questions Task • Porteus Mazes • Go/No-Go Task • Behavioural Assessment of the Dysexecutive Syndrome (BADS) • Delis–Kaplan Executive Function System (D-KEFS)

Social cognition

Theory of mind	Involves the ability to infer the mental states of others, including their intentions, dispositions and beliefs. Also referred to as mentalising or mental state attribution	• Hinting Task • Reading the Mind in the Eyes Task • Picture Sequencing Task • False Belief Stories Task • The Awareness of Social Inferences Test (TASIT) – Parts 2 and 3 • Faux Pas Test
Emotion processing	Ability to perceive, interpret and use emotions – conveyed via face, body and speech. Includes the ability to discriminate between and recognise specific emotions, as well as understand and manage emotions	• Bell Lysaker Emotion Recognition Task (BLERT) • Penn Emotion Recognition Test (ER-40) • Diagnostic Assessment of Nonverbal Accuracy (DANVA) • Facial Emotion Identification Test (FEIT) • Facial Emotion Discrimination Test (FEDT) • The Awareness of Social Inferences Test (TASIT) – Part 1
Social perception and knowledge	Social perception is the ability to perceive and interpret social cues from social contextual information and communicative (verbal, non-verbal) gestures. Social knowledge is the awareness of the roles, rules and goals that characterise social situations and guide social interactions	• Social Cue Recognition Test • Situational Features Recognition Test • Profile of Nonverbal Sensitivity (PONS) • Interpersonal Perception Task (IPT-15) • Trustworthiness Task • Relationships Across Domains (RAD)
Attributional style	How an individual tends to explain the causes for positive and negative events or interactions. Includes external personal attributions (i.e. event is caused by others), external situational attributions (i.e. event is caused by situational factors), and internal attributions (i.e. event is caused by oneself). As opposed to other domains, this domain is a measure of *bias* or *tendency*, rather than a deficit (or not) in performance	• Ambiguous Intentions Hostility Questionnaire (AIHQ) • Adult Nowicki–Strickland Internal External Scale • Attributional Style Questionnaire • Internal, Personal and Situational Attributions Questionnaire (IPSAQ)

[1] Sometimes classified as an executive functioning task.
[2] Sometimes classified as a processing speed task.
Sources: Lezak et al., 2004; Pinkham et al., 2014; Snyder et al., 2015b.

way that favours certain types of emotional valence or meaning. For example, the tendency to attend to negative information in depression or threatening information in anxiety disorders (Mathews & MacLeod, 2005). Given the vast literature in these two areas and space limitations, the current chapter will primarily focus on cognitive deficits.

Stage 0: Increased Risk of Mental Illness, but Asymptomatic

Three lines of evidence support the importance of cognitive function as a risk marker for the later development of psychiatric illness. The first comes from studies of neurodevelopmental conditions diagnosed at birth or in childhood, where cognitive impairment is a core feature. Epidemiological research shows that 30–40 per cent of individuals with intellectual disability (ID; defined as an IQ below 70 and associated impairment in adaptive functioning evident from early childhood) experience at least one psychiatric disorder later in life (Cooper et al., 2007; Morgan et al., 2008). Psychotic disorders are especially implicated such that people with ID are at 3–5 times greater risk of experiencing a psychotic disorder than the general population (Morgan et al., 2008). Furthermore, having an ID is associated with an earlier age of first contact with mental health services and a more severe psychiatric presentation relative to those with no history of ID (Morgan et al., 2008). Given intelligence is on a continuum, it is not surprising that an IQ within the borderline range (~70–80) is also associated with an increased risk of mental illness (Morgan et al., 2008). One population-based study showed that borderline IQ was associated with more than twice the risk (OR = 2.37) of experiencing any psychiatric diagnosis relative to individuals with an average IQ, but risks were highest (OR > 3.3) for antisocial personality disorder and non-affective psychotic disorders (Gigi et al., 2014). Furthermore, population-based longitudinal research shows a significant association between neurodevelopmental disorders diagnosed in childhood (such as autism spectrum, dyslexia and dyspraxia) and a nearly twofold risk of psychotic experiences in adolescence; this relationship was found to be partially mediated by IQ assessed at age 9–11 years (Khandaker et al., 2014). Together these findings indicate that early aberrant neurodevelopmental processes play a role in psychiatric illnesses, particularly psychosis (Owen, 2012).

The second line of evidence comes from large birth or conscript cohort studies that have examined the cognitive functioning of individuals before they experience first onset of psychiatric disorder. Again, most studies have examined IQ, with a lower premorbid IQ being associated with a subsequent diagnosis of a range of psychiatric disorders, including psychotic disorders, anxiety disorders and major depressive disorder (MDD) (Batty et al., 2005; David et al., 2008; Koenen et al., 2009; Reichenberg et al., 2002; Zammit et al., 2004). A review of pre-trauma risk factors for the development of post-traumatic stress disorder (PTSD) identified ten studies that had examined cognition (ranging from IQ to specific cognitive domains) prior to experiencing trauma; all ten studies found that lower pre-trauma cognitive performance was predictive of the development of PTSD symptomatology (DiGangi et al., 2013).

An exception to these findings appears to be in the case of bipolar disorder, where there has either been no relationship found between premorbid IQ and bipolar disorder (Reichenberg et al., 2002; Zammit et al., 2004), or higher IQ being a risk for onset of non-psychotic bipolar disorder (Gale et al., 2013; Koenen et al., 2009). There is also evidence showing that higher motor and expressive language abilities in childhood are associated with the onset of mania in young adulthood (Cannon et al., 2002). Another study found that the risk for bipolar disorder increased as a function of increased performance on an arithmetic task, but decreased performance on a visuospatial reasoning task (Tiihonen et al., 2005). Interestingly, in a longitudinal Swedish cohort study, MacCabe et al. (2010) found that scholastic grades of two or more standard deviations above average were associated with almost four times the risk of developing bipolar disorder than average grades; the lowest grades were associated with an almost twofold increased risk. Contrastingly, highest school grades were associated with a decreased risk for schizophrenia (MacCabe et al., 2010). Although not a prospective cohort study, a meta-analysis of estimated premorbid IQ in individuals with anorexia nervosa is worth highlighting, as it also showed superior estimated premorbid ($d = 0.72$) IQ relative to the normative population (Lopez et al., 2010).

Focusing on psychotic disorders, a premorbid deficit in IQ (assessed as early as age three) of approximately 0.5 standard deviations below healthy controls has been consistently found in studies of people who develop schizophrenia (Khandaker et al., 2011; Reichenberg et al., 2010; Woodberry et al., 2008) and −0.33 standard deviation unit difference in schizophreniform disorder (Cannon et al., 2002). In their meta-analysis of longitudinal population-based studies, Khandaker et al. (2011) identified a linear relationship between IQ deficit in the premorbid period and future risk of schizophrenia, whereby risk increased by 3.7 per cent for every point decrease in IQ (see also Kendler et al., 2015). Furthermore, greater IQ decrement was associated with earlier age of onset (Khandaker et al., 2011). Lower IQ does not appear to be a by-product of insidious prodromal symptoms, as studies have confirmed the association between lower IQ assessed early and the onset of schizophrenia many years later (Kendler et al., 2015; Reichenberg et al., 2010; Tiihonen et al., 2005). There is also evidence showing that a decline (or lack of development) in IQ or verbal ability during adolescence is an independent risk factor for later development of schizophrenia and other psychotic disorders, but not bipolar, depression or anxiety disorder (MacCabe et al., 2013; Reichenberg et al., 2005). Recent evidence indicates decline in verbal IQ (evident as early as age 11) and risk for psychosis may be associated with 22q11.2 deletion syndrome (Vorstman et al., 2015). Together, these findings suggest a static continuity of developmental risk (with likely shared genetic aetiology) in association with premorbid IQ, possibly followed by further relative or actual cognitive deterioration prior to onset of full-threshold psychotic disorder.

The third line of evidence comes from studies of individuals considered at genetic or familial high risk of psychiatric illness. This is based on evidence showing similar but milder cognitive deficits in unaffected first-degree relatives of people with a psychiatric illness, including psychotic and non-psychotic disorders (Weiser et al., 2008). Evidence that cognitive impairments are greater in multiplex (more than one affected sibling) versus simplex (one affected sibling) sibships further supports the premise that there is some degree of heritability that cuts across psychiatric disorders (Faraone et al., 2000; Weiser et al., 2008). The evidence is strongest and impairments are largest in relatives of people with schizophrenia (Bora et al., 2014; Sitskoorn et al., 2004; Snitz et al., 2006; Weiser et al., 2008), including unaffected co-twins from twin pairs discordant for schizophrenia (Cannon et al., 2000). According to four meta-analyses, multiple neurocognitive domains are implicated, but the most affected are attention (including vigilance), processing speed, executive functions and verbal memory, with effect sizes ranging from small to large ($d = 0.17$–0.81) (Bora et al., 2014; Dickinson et al., 2007; Sitskoorn et al., 2004; Snitz et al., 2006). Social cognition, particularly in the domains of theory of mind, emotion recognition and social perception, was also found to be impaired to a moderate degree ($d = 0.37$–0.48) in two meta-analyses of first-degree relatives of people with schizophrenia (Bora & Pantelis, 2013; Lavoie et al., 2013).

Milder neurocognitive deficits have also been reported in healthy first-degree relatives of people with bipolar disorder. Findings have been less consistent than in schizophrenia, but verbal learning and memory and executive functioning appear most reliably impaired, with effect sizes in the small to medium range ($d = \leq 0.56$) (Arts et al., 2008; Balanza-Martinez et al., 2008; Bora et al., 2009a). Furthermore, verbal fluency and IQ appear relatively spared in first-degree relatives of people with bipolar disorder (Balanza-Martinez et al., 2008; Bora et al., 2009a). The findings regarding processing speed are equivocal (Balanza-Martinez et al., 2008; Bora et al., 2009a; Glahn et al., 2010). One study found deficits in face emotion recognition in youths with a first-degree relative with bipolar disorder (Brotman et al., 2008), although another found no evidence for social cognition impairments in relatives, including emotion recognition and theory of mind (Whitney et al., 2013).

Two studies of offspring at genetic risk for depression have found no significant impairment in neurocognitive function relative to healthy controls (Klimes-Dougan et al., 2006; Micco et al., 2009), whereas two relatively recent studies have found executive functioning impairments in asymptomatic offspring at risk for depression (Belleau et al., 2013; Hughes et al., 2013). With respect to anxiety disorders, executive functioning impairments have been found in first-degree relatives of people with obsessive-compulsive disorder (OCD) (Cavedini et al., 2010; Viswanath et al., 2009), but neurocognitive impairments have not been observed in relatives of people with panic disorder (Micco et al., 2009). Finally, medium impairments in set-shifting ($d = 0.49$) and central coherence ($d = 0.51–0.55$) are evident in first-degree relatives of people with eating disorders (Kanakam & Treasure, 2013). A recent twin study suggests weak central coherence (detail-focused, rather than global processing) may have a stronger genetic basis than set-shifting (Kanakam et al., 2013).

Stage 1a and 1b: Distress (with or without Subthreshold Specificity)

Significant neurocognitive and social cognitive deficits have been established in individuals who are considered at clinical high risk (CHR) or ultra-high risk (UHR) for psychosis, henceforth referred to as 'at risk'. In addition to compromised IQ as described in the previous section, several reviews have identified widespread small to moderate neurocognitive deficits (effect size (ES) = 0.16–0.71) in at-risk individuals relative to healthy controls (aged 15–29), particularly in the domains of verbal and visual memory, working memory, verbal fluency, olfactory identification and social cognition (Bora et al., 2014; Brewer et al., 2006; Fusar-Poli et al., 2012; Giuliano et al., 2012; Hauser et al., 2017; Pukrop & Klosterkotter, 2010). A recent meta-analysis of social cognition in at-risk individuals (mean age 15–26 years) found medium-sized impairment in global social cognition ($g = -0.48$), with effects ranging from large to small in the specific domains of attributional bias ($g = -0.71$), emotion processing ($g = -0.45$), theory of mind ($g = -0.43$) and social perception ($g = -0.38$) (Lee et al., 2015).

Four meta-analyses revealed that neurocognitive deficits in several domains were larger (ES = 0.23–0.84) in at-risk individuals who later developed a full-threshold schizophrenia-spectrum disorder relative to those who did not (Bora et al., 2014; Fusar-Poli et al., 2012; Giuliano et al., 2012; Hauser et al., 2017). Additionally, using multivariate neurocognitive pattern classification for the individualised prediction of psychosis in at-risk individuals

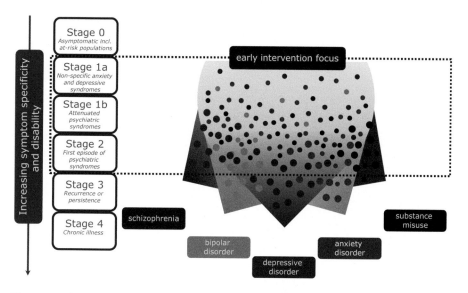

Figure 2.1 Clinical staging model depicting the progression of mental illness whereby early clinical phenotypes are broad and non-specific, with clearer syndromes emerging in more advanced stages, coinciding with increased disability. Reprinted from *The Lancet*, Vol. 381, McGorry, P. & van Os, J., Redeeming diagnosis in psychiatry: timing versus specificity, 343–345, Copyright 2013, with permission from Elsevier.

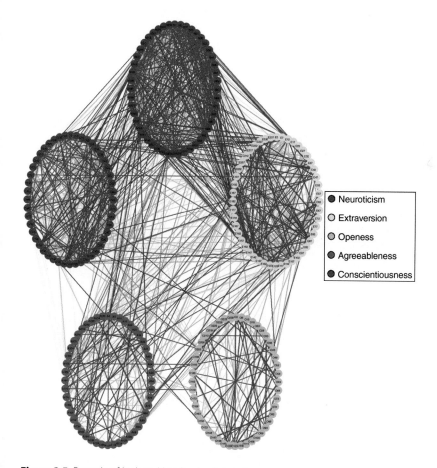

Figure 3.5 Example of high and low levels of clustering.

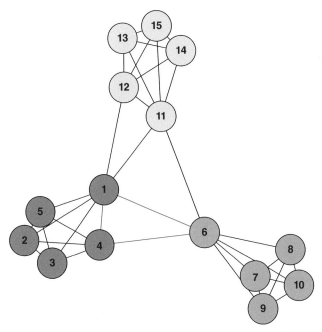

Figure 3.6 An example of a network with communities and bridge symptoms.

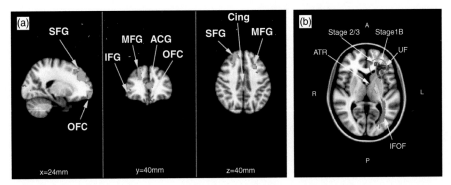

Figure 5.6 (a) Grey matter volume changes in Stage 1 versus Stage 2+ subjects (regions of grey matter loss are in green). SFG = superior frontal gyrus; OFC = orbitofrontal cortex; IFG = inferior frontal gyrus; MFG = middle frontal gyrus; ACG = anterior cingulate gyrus; Cing = cingulate, from Lagopoulos et al. (2012). (b) Graphical overlay of the fractional anisotropy results for Stage 1b (red) and Stage 2+ (blue) subjects along with the coregistered fibre tracts for anterior thalamic radiation (ATR), inferior fronto-occipital fasciculus (IFOF) and uncinate fasciculus (UF), from Lagopoulos et al. (2013).

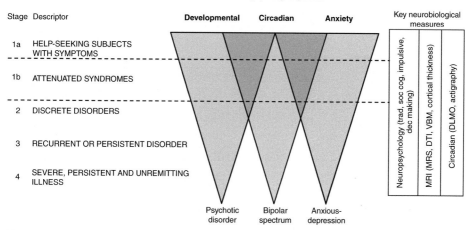

Figure 5.9 Clinical staging model for post-pubertal onset and course of major mental disorders: developmental, circadian or anxiety pathophysiological pathways progress from non-specific to discrete syndromes. Trad, traditional; soc cog, social cognition; dec, decision; MRI, magnetic resonance imaging; MRS, magnetic resonance spectroscopy; DTI, diffusion tensor imaging; VBM, voxel-based morphometry; DLMO, dim light melatonin onset.

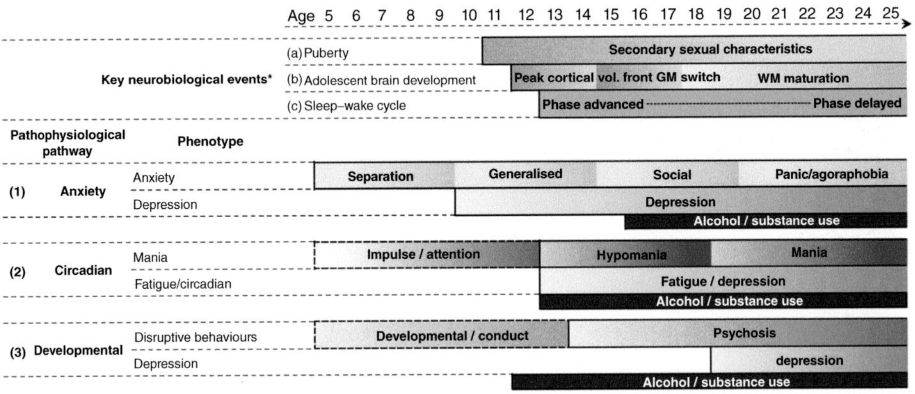

Figure 5.10 Pathophysiological pathways to early-onset depressive disorders. There are at least three common trajectories that lead to depression in the teenage and early-adult years. These are characterised by (1) 'anxiety–central nervous system reactivity'; (2) 'circadian and 24-hour sleep–wake cycle dysfunction'; and (3) 'developmental brain abnormalities'. The six corresponding phenotypic patterns have distinct ages of onset and characteristics. From age 8–10 years onwards these processes are transformed by key neurobiological phenomena: (a) puberty, (b) adolescent brain development and (c) sleep–wake cycle. From Hickie et al. (2013b).

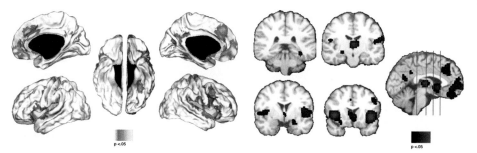

Figure 6.2 Extent of cortical and subcortical GM loss in schizophrenia-spectrum disorders. Regions showing significant GM reductions in patients with schizophrenia across all 37 studies included in the anatomical likelihood estimation analysis (Fornito et al., 2009). The left hemisphere is on the right side of the brain images; statistics are displayed on brain templates. (Image reproduced with permission).

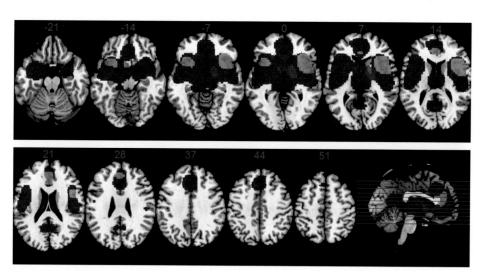

Figure 6.3 Regions of GM change in people with BD and people with schizophrenia. Regions of GM decreases in bipolar subjects compared with controls (yellow), regions of GM decreases in schizophrenia subjects compared with controls (red) and regions of GM increases in schizophrenia subjects compared with controls (purple), displayed on a brain template (Ellison-Wright & Bullmore, 2010). The left side of the image represents the left side of the brain. (Image reproduced with permission).

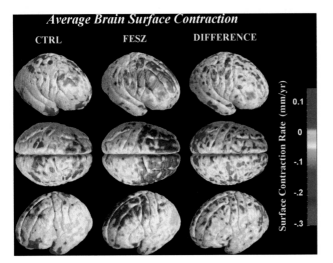

Figure 6.4 Average brain surface contraction in FE psychosis. Displayed are the average rates of brain surface contraction (mm per year) in control individuals (CTRL), first-episode schizophrenia patients (FESZ) and the absolute difference between the two groups. Negative values (warm colours) denote surface contraction (Sun et al., 2009b; image reproduced with permission).

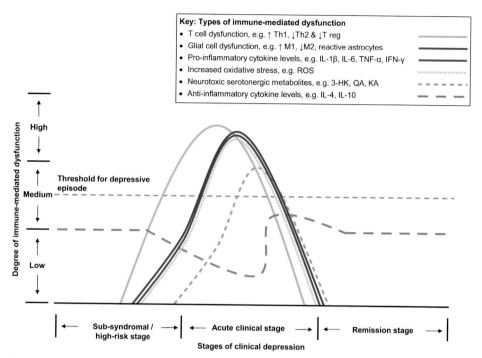

Figure 8.4 Dynamic changes of the immune response during stages of clinical depression until recovery. This figure represents an acute clinical depressive episode with full remission in the context of the three phases of the phase-specific neuroimmune model of clinical depression: sub-syndromal, acute clinical and remission stages as shown on the x-axis show the relevant phases; the y-axis shows the degree of immune-mediated dysfunction. The shaded lines represent the various types of immune-mediated dysfunction. The horizontal grey dashed line indicates an immune dysfunction threshold line whereby a clinically significant depressive episode is diagnosable. 3-HK, 3-hydroxykynurenine; IFN, interferon; IL, interleukin; KA, kynurenic acid; QA, quinolinic acid; ROS, reactive oxygen species; T reg, T regulatory cell; Th, T helper; TNF, tumour necrosis factor.

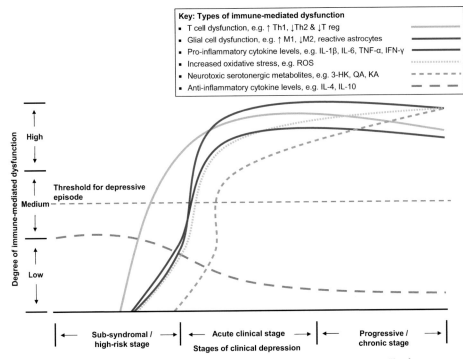

Figure 8.5 Progressive immune changes during a progressive course of clinical depression. This figure represents a chronic and progressive major depressive episode. The x-axis shows the relevant phases (sub-syndromal/high-risk stage, acute clinical stage, progressive/chronic stage); the y-axis shows the degree of immune-mediated dysfunction. The shaded lines represent the various types of immune-mediated dysfunction. The horizontal grey dashed line indicates an immune dysfunction threshold line whereby a clinically significant depressive episode is diagnosable. 3-HK, 3-hydroxykynurenine; IFN, interferon; IL. interleukin; KA, kynurenic acid; QA, quinolinic acid; ROS, reactive oxygen species; T reg, T regulatory cell; Th, T helper; TNF, tumour necrosis factor.

(via machine learning techniques), classification accuracy was found to be 91 per cent for converters and 89 per cent for non-converters (Koutsouleris et al., 2012). Impaired executive functioning (verbal fluency, cognitive flexibility) and verbal learning were most predictive of psychosis transition using this method (Koutsouleris et al., 2012). There is also emerging evidence that social cognition (especially theory of mind and emotion recognition) may be a useful marker of psychosis transition (Allott et al., 2014; Bora & Pantelis, 2013; Kim et al., 2011; Lee et al., 2015), but few studies have been conducted to date.

The cognitive impairments in the at-risk phase of psychotic illness are milder than those observed in full-threshold disorder, which suggests there is further progression of impairment pre- or peri-onset (Giuliano et al., 2012), although it remains unclear exactly when this occurs. A recent meta-analysis of longitudinal studies concluded that there is currently limited evidence for progression of neurocognitive impairment after psychosis onset (Bora & Murray, 2014), although this conclusion is restricted by the methodology of studies included in the review (e.g. many lacked a healthy comparison group, variable timing and number of prospective follow-up assessments, few studies examined the same individuals from UHR to first-episode psychosis (FEP)). Pertinently, regardless of later transition status, neurocognitive impairments in at-risk individuals are predictive of poorer functional outcomes, and therefore require clinical consideration in individuals identified as 'at risk' (Bora et al., 2014; Lin et al., 2011; Niendam et al., 2006).

Contrary to psychotic disorders, whether neurocognitive deficits are evident prior to the onset of bipolar disorder or first-episode mania remains less clear, as defining the risk syndrome or prodromal phase of bipolar disorder has been challenging and a relatively recent development in the field (Bechdolf et al., 2014; Conus et al., 2008; Correll et al., 2007; Olvet et al., 2013). Preliminary evidence suggests that specific neurocognitive deficits may be present in at-risk young people who later develop a bipolar spectrum disorder compared to healthy controls (Metzler et al., 2015; Meyer et al., 2004; Olvet et al., 2010; Ratheesh et al., 2013). Significant prodromal impairments have been found in global and verbal IQ (Ratheesh et al., 2013), performance IQ (Meyer et al., 2004; Ratheesh et al., 2013) and executive functioning (Meyer et al., 2004). Opposing results were reported on a task of attention and processing speed (Meyer et al., 2004; Ratheesh et al., 2013). It is important to note that these findings may not be specific to bipolar risk, as the neurocognitive performance of at-risk participants who transitioned to bipolar disorder did not differ from other at-risk individuals who did not transition to bipolar disorder (Ratheesh et al., 2013), nor in those who transitioned to psychotic disorder (Olvet et al., 2010).

For similar reasons to bipolar disorder, at-risk mood and anxiety disorder research (including examination of cognition) is scarce (Hetrick et al., 2008). Depressive and anxiety symptoms are common in at-risk for psychosis samples (Svirskis et al., 2005), but recent research suggests that these comorbid symptoms are not associated with increased neurocognitive impairments (Lim et al., 2015). Depressive symptoms were shown to be significantly correlated with neurocognitive functioning in individuals at risk for psychosis (but not in FEP patients), suggesting a mental state-driven relationship (Ohmuro et al., 2015). One population study found mild premorbid deficits in psychomotor speed and attention in children who later developed MDD (Cannon et al., 2006), whereas another study found no impairment in executive functioning in adolescents who later developed MDD (Meyer et al., 2004). There has been no research on cognitive functioning in individuals at risk for eating disorders (Kanakam & Treasure, 2013).

Stage 2: First Treated Episode

Population-level research has shown that, relative to their peers who do not have a psychiatric diagnosis, significant neurocognitive impairments are evident in male adolescents (aged 16–17) diagnosed with a range of psychiatric disorders (Weiser et al., 2004). The degree of impairment varies between psychiatric disorders, with the largest neurocognitive impairments observed in psychotic and antisocial personality disorders (ES = 1.01–1.15), moderate impairments in other personality disorders, major affective disorders, PTSD and substance abuse (ES = 0.62–0.69), and smaller impairments in minor affective, anxiety and adjustment disorders (ES = 0.33–0.41). These data are remarkably similar to studies of clinical samples described below.

In people with FEP (aged 15–33), compared to healthy controls, significant medium to large impairments (d = 0.64–1.20) are present across all cognitive domains examined, including IQ and social cognition, with the most severe deficits observed in verbal memory and information processing speed (Mesholam-Gately et al., 2009; Rajji et al., 2009). Age appears to moderate the pattern and degree of cognitive impairment in first-episode schizophrenia, with earlier age of onset associated with poorer neurocognition (and some differences in domains impacted), which is likely associated with the neurodevelopmental vulnerability in younger individuals relative to older individuals and possible differing aetiological factors, particularly when comparing to onset after the age of 45 (Rajji et al., 2009). Large deficits in social cognition are also found in FEP, including theory of mind (d = 1.0) (Bora & Pantelis, 2013) and emotion recognition, particularly for negative emotions (Amminger et al., 2012; Edwards et al., 2001). Neurocognitive impairments in FEP have been conceptualised as trait markers of illness, as longitudinal studies show there is minimal evidence for decline over the first five (Bora & Murray, 2014) to ten years (Bozikas & Andreou, 2011; Hoff et al., 2005) following a first treated psychotic episode. Preliminary findings also point to relative stability in social cognition from early through to later stages of psychosis (Comparelli et al., 2013; Green et al., 2012).

Cognitive ability in early course bipolar disorder has received much less investigation (Table 7.1). Nevertheless, there is growing evidence of significant impairments during acute and euthymic phases following a first treated bipolar disorder, prompting several reviews (mean age = 19–37) (Bora & Pantelis, 2015; Daglas et al., 2015; Lee et al., 2014; Martino et al., 2015). Relatively consistent small to large deficits in attention and working memory (ES = 0.34–0.80) are reported (Bora & Pantelis, 2015; Daglas et al., 2015; Lee et al., 2014; Martino et al., 2015), with small to medium deficits also observed in psychomotor speed, cognitive flexibility and verbal learning and memory (ES = 0.30–0.63) (Bora & Pantelis, 2015; Lee et al., 2014). Verbal fluency, reasoning and response inhibition (ES = 0.31–44) appear to be the least impacted in the early euthymic phase of illness (Bora & Pantelis, 2015; Daglas et al., 2015; Lee et al., 2014) and findings are inconsistent in relation to non-verbal memory (Bora & Pantelis, 2015; Lee et al., 2014). Overall, the breadth and severity of neurocognitive impairment in early bipolar disorder is smaller than in FEP, particularly in IQ, verbal memory and verbal fluency (Bora & Pantelis, 2015; Trotta et al., 2015). Two recent 12-month follow-up studies found selective improvements in processing speed, while other domains remained stably impaired in first-episode patients relative to healthy controls (Daglas et al., 2016; Torres et al., 2014). The stability and trajectory of impairments following first-episode bipolar disorder is an important area for ongoing study.

A meta-analysis of neurocognition in first-episode MDD in adults (mean age 39) found significant small to medium impairments in psychomotor speed (Hedges' $g = 0.48$), attention (Hedges' $g = 0.36$), visual learning and memory (Hedges' $g = 0.53$) and several domains of executive functioning (attentional switching, cognitive flexibility, verbal fluency: Hedges' $g = 0.22$–0.59) (Lee et al., 2012). No impairments were found in working memory and verbal learning and memory (Lee et al., 2012). Furthermore, psychomotor speed, working memory and general memory functioning were associated with clinical state, suggesting that at least some aspects of neurocognitive functioning in MDD are state-related. Consistent with normal neurocognitive functioning, age was a moderating factor, with older age being associated with poorer performance in first-episode MDD (Lee et al., 2012). As most first-episode studies (and depression studies in general) have been conducted in adults, Baune et al. (2014) conducted a systematic review of studies specifically with youth (aged 12–25), although notably most participants were not in remission. Of the seven cross-sectional studies included, the most consistent deficits were in working memory and psychomotor speed, while there was no evidence for impairment in attention and verbal learning and memory, and equivocal evidence in executive functioning, verbal fluency and visual memory (Baune et al., 2014). Two of the included studies involved first-episode MDD samples, showing selective impairments in executive functions and a bias towards sad stimuli (fewer errors) (Klimkeit et al., 2011; Kyte et al., 2005). One cross-sectional study comparing adolescents with current or remitted MDD with healthy controls suggested executive functioning impairments were state- and not trait-based (Maalouf et al., 2011), whereas a 12-month longitudinal study found that executive functioning impairments persisted despite symptomatic remission following first-episode MDD (Schmid & Hammar, 2013). Other research suggests that neurocognitive deficits are milder in adults with first-episode relative to recurrent MDD, although accentuated impairments (in verbal memory) were evident by the second depressive episode (Talarowska et al., 2015). As with bipolar disorder, much more research is needed to characterise cognitive dysfunction in terms of age of onset, separating out trait- from state-related impairments, and whether there is progression of cognitive impairment early in the course of MDD (Allott et al., 2016).

Studies on cognitive functioning in the first treated episode of an anxiety disorder are lacking, but there is some research in youth specifically, which captures the period in which onset and prevalence is common (Castaneda et al., 2008). A review of young adults (mean age range 18–36) found deficits were most evident in executive functioning, visual memory and attention (Castaneda et al., 2011). These findings were replicated in a large study of youth (aged 7–17 years) with OCD, with executive functioning (especially set-shifting) and non-verbal memory impairments found in up to 65 per cent of participants (Lewin et al., 2014). Impairments were not associated with OCD severity, suggesting they are possible trait markers. Few studies have been conducted in young people with other types of anxiety disorders, although there is some evidence for selective impairments in panic disorder, social phobia (social anxiety disorder), and PTSD, and equivocal evidence in generalised anxiety disorder (GAD) or specific phobia (Castaneda et al., 2008; 2011; Tempesta et al., 2013). A study of emotion recognition in a mixed anxiety disorder sample of non-medicated adolescents found that those with an anxiety disorder were poorer at recognising anger and better at recognising neutral affect than healthy controls (Jarros et al., 2012).

Similarly, the literature on cognitive functioning in youth with eating disorders is small. A population-level study of adolescents (mean age 17) with various eating disorders versus healthy and psychiatric controls showed impaired performance on measures of executive functioning, including global processing (central coherence) and set-shifting (mental flexibility), but better performance on measures of visual attention and vigilance (Allen et al., 2013). However, a recent meta-analysis of nine studies on set-shifting ability in adolescents (mean age range 14–19) with anorexia nervosa found no significant difference from the performance of healthy controls ($d = 0.01–0.2$) (Lang et al., 2014b), which contrasts with adult populations (Wu et al., 2014). This suggests there may be progressive or 'scar' impairments in association with chronicity (Treasure et al., 2015), although longitudinal research is needed to confirm this.

Stage 3 to Stage 4: Recurrence, Persistence or Treatment Resistance

Adults with schizophrenia (aged 18–57 years) who have experienced multiple episodes, hospitalisations and/or prolonged treatment exposure consistently perform below healthy controls on all examined domains of neurocognition ($d = 0.46–1.41$) (Heinrichs & Zakzanis, 1998). The largest impairments are found in verbal memory and processing speed (Dickinson et al., 2007; Heinrichs & Zakzanis, 1998); degree of impairment in processing speed is moderated by age, with younger patients (with shorter illness duration) performing better, although the effect size is still large and unrelated to medication or symptom status (Dickinson et al., 2007). A similar pattern and magnitude of deficits was reported in a meta-analysis of older people (aged 48–78) with chronic schizophrenia (0.46–1.57 SDs below healthy controls) (Irani et al., 2011). A comparable picture emerges in meta-analyses of social cognition in established psychotic illness (mean age range 35–36), with large impairments found in the domains of theory of mind (ES = 0.80–1.23) (Bora et al., 2009c; Savla et al., 2013; Sprong et al., 2007), emotion perception – including identification and differentiation (ES = 0.89–0.91) and processing (ES = 0.88) (Kohler et al., 2010; Savla et al., 2013) and social perception (ES = 1.04) (Savla et al., 2013). A medium deficit in social knowledge (ES = 0.54) was also found (Savla et al., 2013). The evidence for externalising or personalising attributional bias is negligible (ES = 0.02–0.17), but few studies have investigated this domain (Savla et al., 2013).

Notably, the effect sizes reported in these meta-analyses of chronic patients are broadly similar to those with FEP (Mesholam-Gately et al., 2009), suggesting that cognitive impairments are a core and relatively stable feature of psychotic illness, which are present during symptom remission and do not generally progress with illness chronicity. Reviews of longitudinal studies of neurocognition in established psychotic disorder support this notion, where impairments remain relatively stable for up to six years in both adults and older people with chronic schizophrenia (Irani et al., 2011; Szoke et al., 2008). However, this 'stability' in cognition contrasts with healthy individuals who tend to improve in neurocognition and IQ with repeated assessments over time (either due to practice effects or genuine gains in acquired knowledge and cognitive function), indicating a possible developmental 'arrest' (rather than decline) in people with schizophrenia (Hedman et al., 2013; Szoke et al., 2008). Nevertheless, there is some evidence to suggest that neurocognitive decline (greater than what is observed with normal ageing) may be evident in schizophrenia patients who experience prolonged institutionalisation (Rajji & Mulsant, 2008) or who are over the age of 65 (Harvey, 2014). It is likely that progressive decline occurs in subgroups of individuals with psychotic disorders, but parsing out these subgroups remains an important area of ongoing investigation.

Significant neurocognitive impairments (generally in the moderate to large range) are also well documented in adults with euthymic bipolar I disorder, as reviewed by multiple authors (Arts et al., 2008; Bora et al., 2009a; Bourne et al., 2013; Daban et al., 2006; Kurtz & Gerraty, 2009; Olley et al., 2005; Robinson et al., 2006; Torres et al., 2007). A similar degree of neurocognitive impairment is also observed in euthymic later-life (mean age 58–71) bipolar disorder (Samame et al., 2013). Earlier reviews suggested that verbal learning and memory, executive functioning, attention and processing speed were the most consistently impaired domains, with relative preservation of verbal abilities and intelligence (Arts et al., 2008; Bora et al., 2009a; Daban et al., 2006; Robinson et al., 2006; Torres et al., 2007). However, a more recent meta-analysis that included a broader range of measures and studies (mean age = 22–77) found generalised medium to large neurocognitive impairment across all domains examined (ES = 0.47–0.71), again with the exception of crystallised verbal ability (ES = 0.11) (Mann-Wrobel et al., 2011). Likewise, milder but significant neurocognitive impairments (d = 0.29–0.55) are observed in bipolar II disorder (Bora et al., 2011; Sole et al., 2011). Impairments in social cognition are also evident in adult euthymic bipolar disorder (mean age range 19–50), with moderate to large deficits found in theory of mind (ES = 0.79) (Samame et al., 2012) and small to moderate impairments in emotion recognition (ES = 0.35–0.46) (Kohler et al., 2011; Samame et al., 2012).

The impairments in well-established bipolar disorder appear to be greater than in first-episode illness (Lee et al., 2014), which may suggest a progressive process in association with persistent illness. Cross-sectional studies lend support for this notion, showing a relationship between the degree of neurocognitive dysfunction and number of mood episodes, as well as illness duration (Bourne et al., 2013; Elshahawi et al., 2011; Lopez-Jaramillo et al., 2010; Robinson & Ferrier, 2006). However, the direction of the relationship is uncertain – it may be that subgroups with more severe bipolar disorder and the type and dose of pharmacotherapy prescribed may influence the degree of neurocognitive impairments. Emerging evidence from longitudinal studies (mean follow-up of 4.6 years) suggests that deficits remain relatively stable, questioning a progressive course (Samame et al., 2014; Strejilevich et al., 2015). Clearly, more longitudinal research from early in the course of illness that includes healthy controls is needed to inform these findings. Although the cognitive deficits in bipolar disorder are relatively widespread, they are generally not as severe as those observed in psychotic disorders (Bora et al., 2009a; Bourne et al., 2013; Daban et al., 2006; Lee et al., 2013a; Mann-Wrobel et al., 2011; Stefanopoulou et al., 2009). Indeed, the presence of psychotic symptoms is an important determinant of poorer cognition in both bipolar disorder and MDD and needs to be taken into account in interpreting findings (Bora et al., 2010; Reichenberg et al., 2009; Simonsen et al., 2011).

Small to moderate neurocognitive deficits (ES = 0.33–0.65) are observed in adults with established MDD relative to healthy controls, especially in the domains of executive function, but also in verbal and visual memory, attention and processing speed (Austin et al., 2001; Douglas & Porter, 2009; Rock et al., 2014; Snyder, 2013). Meta-analyses have also revealed moderate generalised impairment (d = 0.55) in emotion recognition in MDD (Demenescu et al., 2010; Kohler et al., 2011), although the most recent meta-analysis suggests that impairments may be smaller (Hedges' g = 0.17–0.42) and specific to the recognition of anger, disgust, fear, happiness and surprise, but not sadness (Dalili et al., 2015). In line with this, evidence also suggests a tendency for a negative response bias to sadness, whereby positive, neutral or ambiguous facial expressions tend to be evaluated as more sad (Bourke et al., 2010). Findings in MDD have tended to indicate that neurocognitive impairments are state-dependent because they are often found to resolve with symptom improvement (Douglas & Porter, 2009). Indeed, evidence suggests there is a significant association between depressive symptom severity and neurocognitive impairment (Austin et al., 2001; Douglas & Porter, 2009; McClintock et al., 2010; McDermott & Ebmeier, 2009; Snyder, 2013). Nevertheless, a meta-analysis found that the severity of symptoms only accounted for approximately 10 per cent of variance in neurocognitive performance (McDermott & Ebmeier, 2009), suggesting that mental state is only one part of the observed deficits. Indeed longitudinal studies have found that past average depression severity was a better predictor of neurocognitive impairment than current symptoms (Dotson et al., 2008; Sarapas et al., 2012). Fewer studies have been conducted in remitted patients, but a body of emerging evidence suggests that trait- or 'scar'-related neurocognitive deficits are a likely feature of MDD, particularly in the domains of executive functioning and attention (Austin et al., 2001; Douglas & Porter, 2009; Hasselbalch et al., 2011; Rock et al., 2014; Snyder, 2013). Recent meta-analyses have reported neurocognitive impairments in the small to moderate range (ES = 0.22–0.61) in patients in remission from MDD (Bora et al., 2013; Rock et al., 2014). Age of onset appears to be an important moderator, with later age of onset associated with more severe neurocognitive impairment (Bora et al., 2013). To better characterise the possible progressive nature of neurocognitive dysfunction in association with MDD, the likely important moderating role of factors such as age, medication status, duration of illness and number of episodes requires further investigation via well-designed longitudinal studies (Hasselbalch et al., 2011; McClintock et al., 2010; McDermott & Ebmeier, 2009; Snyder, 2013).

Cognitive functioning in adults with established anxiety disorders has been examined to a lesser degree than other disorders (with the exception of PTSD; Table 7.1), and as in youth populations, results vary depending on the specific anxiety disorder examined. One population-level study comparing adults (aged 20–64) with at least one current anxiety disorder to healthy controls found that those with any anxiety disorder, OCD, or panic disorder had impaired executive functioning (especially set-shifting) and verbal memory, and those with social phobia (social anxiety disorder) displayed verbal memory dysfunction (Airaksinen et al., 2005). Specific phobia and GAD were not associated with neurocognitive impairments (Airaksinen et al., 2005). Two recent meta-analyses of 113 (Abramovitch et al., 2013) and 88 (Shin et al., 2014) studies on neurocognitive functioning in adult OCD (mean age = 24–49) found significant small to large impairments in almost all domains of neurocognition relative to healthy controls, with the largest impairments observed in non-verbal/visuospatial memory (ES = 0.62–0.76), executive functioning (ES = 0.44–0.52) and processing speed (ES = 0.44–0.52) (Abramovitch et al., 2013; Shin et al., 2014). A more recent meta-analysis of 110 studies confirmed that most domains of executive functioning are impaired to a moderate degree in OCD (Snyder et al., 2015a). Due to the psychopathological heterogeneity in OCD, another meta-analysis examined the neurocognitive functioning of obsessive-compulsive 'washers' versus 'checkers', finding that the checkers performed significantly worse than washers in most neurocognitive domains, but particularly in executive functioning (Leopold & Backenstrass, 2015). In all meta-analyses most deficits were not associated with symptom severity, including depressive symptoms (Abramovitch et al., 2013; Leopold & Backenstrass, 2015; Shin et al., 2014; Snyder et al., 2015a), but longitudinal studies are required to clarify whether impairments are stable illness characteristics. Panic disorder (with or without agoraphobia) has been much less studied, but at present two reviews suggest there is limited evidence for neurocognitive deficits, perhaps with the exception of immediate (short-term) memory (Alves et al., 2013; O'Sullivan & Newman, 2014). There are also relatively few studies of social anxiety disorder (social phobia) and findings are mixed, with no consistent evidence for specific neurocognitive impairments (O'Toole & Pedersen, 2011; Sutterby & Bedwell, 2012). There is evidence of an association between GAD and cognitive impairment in middle to late life, but the direction of the relationship and mechanisms remain under-studied (Beaudreau & O'Hara 2008).

A meta-analysis of 60 studies of neurocognitive function in adult PTSD (mean age 44) found impairments across all neurocognitive domains ranging from small to medium (d = 0.29–0.62), with the largest deficits found in verbal learning and memory (d = 0.46–0.62), information processing speed (d = 0.59), attention/working memory (d = 0.50), executive functioning (d = 0.45) and language (d = 0.43) (Scott et al., 2015). The type of trauma (military, interpersonal, state persecution/terror, mixed) and psychiatric or substance-use comorbidity did not significantly impact the findings. However, the severity of PTSD symptoms was associated with the severity of verbal learning impairment (but no other domains), and treatment-seeking individuals had more severe impairments overall than community or mixed samples (Scott et al., 2015). Another meta-analysis found that severity of co-occurring depressive symptoms was associated with degree of executive functioning impairment in PTSD (Polak et al., 2012). It may be concluded from these findings that neurocognitive impairment, particularly in verbal learning and executive functioning, is a consequence of PTSD-related symptomatology. However, there is evidence to suggest that pre-trauma neurocognitive functioning is a significant predictor of PTSD, as discussed earlier (DiGangi et al., 2013; Scott et al., 2015). As with all other anxiety disorders, further longitudinal work is needed to determine whether there is progression of neurocognitive impairment in association with illness severity and persistence.

Regarding social cognition, systematic reviews report emotion recognition impairments in anxiety disorders in general (d = 0.35) (Demenescu et al., 2010), with greatest impairments in OCD (d = 0.55) (Daros et al., 2014) and PTSD (d = 1.6) (Plana et al., 2014). A recent review also found large deficits in theory of mind in PTSD (d = 1.13) (Plana et al., 2014), as well as attributional biases in social phobia (d = 0.53–1.15) (Plana et al., 2014). In general, however, these findings are based on few studies, with significant gaps in knowledge across the spectrum of anxiety disorders as well as in social cognitive domains.

During the acute phase (e.g. starvation, purging, binge eating, malnutrition), a range of neurocognitive impairments appear evident in anorexia nervosa, but the evidence is less convincing in bulimia nervosa (Kanakam & Treasure, 2013; Van den Eynde et al., 2011; Zakzanis et al., 2010). Nevertheless, specific deficits in set-shifting and central coherence are evident across the spectrum of eating disorders (Kanakam & Treasure, 2013; Lang et al., 2014a; Wu et al., 2014). Meta-analytic findings show small to medium effects for inefficient set-shifting in anorexia nervosa (g = 0.44), binge eating disorder (g = 0.53) and bulimia nervosa (g = 0.50) (Wu et al., 2014). Interestingly, restricting-type anorexia is significantly impaired (g = 0.51), whereas binge/purge-type anorexia is not (g = 0.18). There was no difference in effect sizes between adolescent and adult samples, suggesting set-shifting impairments are evident early in the illness course (Wu et al., 2014). Meta-analysis has also revealed robust evidence for weak central coherence in both anorexia (d = 0.58–0.63) and bulimia (d = 0.28–0.84) nervosa (Lang et al., 2014a). Lower body mass index (BMI) has been associated with poorer premorbid IQ and neurocognitive functioning in anorexia nervosa (Lopez et al., 2010; Zakzanis et al., 2010), suggesting a possible role of both premorbid and postmorbid cognition in relation to illness severity. The current IQ of people with anorexia nervosa is found to be significantly higher than that of the general population (d = 0.40) (Lopez et al., 2010), but it is lower than estimated premorbid IQ, possibly indicating IQ decline or 'arrest' in association with the illness or reflecting poorer visuospatial abilities (as customary current IQ measurement includes visuospatial ability, whereas premorbid IQ measurement does not). Whether impaired set-shifting and weak central coherence are trait markers of eating disorders requires further research; however, preliminary studies in people who have recovered from eating disorders suggest attenuated impairments in set-shifting ($d = 0.33$–0.35) and moderate effects for weak central coherence ($d = 0.42$–0.62) (Kanakam & Treasure, 2013; Lang et al., 2014a). Social cognition in acute anorexia nervosa has received growing investigation, with a meta-analysis finding medium impairments in emotion recognition ($d = 0.51$) and growing evidence for impaired theory of mind (Oldershaw et al., 2011). A review of social cognition in five bulimia nervosa studies found minimal evidence for impairments in theory of mind or emotion processing (DeJong et al., 2013). Again, the question of whether impairments are purely state-related or reflect underlying trait or 'scar' features of eating disorders requires further study.

Discussion and Future Directions

In this chapter, a review of the literature on cognitive functioning in major adult psychiatric disorders within the clinical staging model has been presented. Table 7.3 provides a summary of these findings. Clearly there has been a dominance of research in schizophrenia and other psychotic disorders across all stages and a much larger focus on neurocognition than social cognition (also see Table 7.1). Broadly speaking, the findings on neurocognition

Table 7.3 Evidence for neurocognitive and social cognitive impairments in major psychiatric disorders according to clinical stage

Disorder	Neurocognition				Social cognition			
	0	1a–1b	2	3–4	0	1a–1b	2	3–4
Schizophrenia and psychotic disorders	++	++	+++	+++	++	++	+++	+++
Bipolar disorder	–/+*	–/+	++	++	?	?	?	++
MDD	–/+	–/+	+	++	?	?	?	+
OCD	–/+	?	+	++	?	?	?	++
PTSD	+	?	+	++	?	?	?	++
Social anxiety disorder (social phobia)	–/+	?	–/+	–/+	–/+	?	?	+
Panic disorder	–	?	–/+	–/+	–/+	?	?	–/+
GAD	?	?	–/+	–/+	?	?	?	?
Anorexia nervosa	–/+*	?	–/+	++	?	?	?	+
Bulimia nervosa	+	?	–/+	++	?	?	?	–/+

GAD, generalised anxiety disorder; MDD, major depressive disorder; OCD, obsessive-compulsive disorder; PTSD, post-traumatic stress disorder; –, deficits essentially absent; –/+, equivocal, variable findings; +, specific mild deficits; ++, moderate deficits; +++, large and widespread deficits; ?, unknown, research lacking.
* Higher cognitive (i.e. IQ) functioning predictive of later illness, but evidence for selective impairments in first-degree relatives.

according to the stages of psychiatric illness suggest that cognitive impairments reflect both neurodevelopmental trait vulnerabilities and progressive illness-related deficits in major psychiatric illness. Neurocognitive impairment, especially lower IQ, is a risk factor for most psychiatric disorders, conferring the greatest risk for psychotic disorders. An exception is the finding that higher (verbal) IQ may be a risk factor for both bipolar disorder and anorexia nervosa, although these disorders may still present with specific premorbid deficits. From a transdiagnostic perspective, because IQ is considered a relatively stable individual characteristic that can be reliably measured from early childhood (Neisser et al., 1996) it appears to be a useful measure of premorbid risk for later psychiatric disorder. The evidence for social cognition is much less advanced, although is beginning to parallel the neurocognitive findings in the psychotic disorders, but research is lacking in Stages 0–2 in all other psychiatric disorders.

While keeping in mind the significant gaps in the literature, there appears to be some evidence for specificity in the pattern and severity of cognitive dysfunction between diagnostic categories. Schizophrenia and other psychotic disorders are associated with the most severe and widespread cognitive impairment at all stages, in which most progression of impairment occurs prior to the first treated episode (Stage 2). Collectively, findings show a pattern of both cognitive lag (failure to develop normally) and progressive decline occurring predominantly between premorbid and first-episode psychosis phases, followed by relative stability of deficits. While more subtle and less widespread neurocognitive impairments are evident prior to the onset of major mood disorders, further progression of impairment appears evident during or shortly after the onset of these disorders. Moderate neurocognitive deficits are found after the onset of full-threshold bipolar illness and, as for schizophrenia-spectrum disorders, are being increasingly recognised as core illness features. However, their role as specific early risk markers remains undetermined, since few studies have focused on the premorbid and subthreshold stages. Evidence suggests there may be further progression of impairment in the more chronic stages (3–4) of major mood disorders, but a number of factors that are under-studied to date need to be considered, including the presence of psychotic symptoms, effects of medication, substance use and severity of mood episodes. Furthermore, separating out state from trait/scar cognitive impairments is a critical area for further research, particularly in MDD (Allott et al., 2016).

The research in anxiety disorders is most developed in OCD and PTSD, where neurocognitive impairment is both an early risk marker and apparent persistent feature of full-threshold disorder. Stages 3–4 are associated with larger neurocognitive impairments than Stage 2, possibly suggesting progression with chronicity, but this evidence is based primarily on cross-sectional studies, calling for well-designed longitudinal research. The profile of cognitive impairment shares similarities with eating disorders (e.g. poor executive functioning, especially set-shifting; visual-spatial impairments), suggesting these disorders may have shared neuropathology (Lang et al., 2014a). An interesting finding was that although several neurocognitive domains are found to be affected in psychotic, mood and severe anxiety disorders (especially executive functions, processing speed, attention/working memory and learning and memory), impairments appear relatively circumscribed in eating disorders. Poor set-shifting and weak central coherence are well-established findings, at least in symptomatic phases of both anorexia and bulimia nervosa, but much more work is needed regarding the stability or progression of these impairments in association with phases of remission and illness chronicity. In fact, it remains unclear whether progression of cognitive impairment occurs with illness chronicity in most of the disorders reviewed.

Although state-related neurocognitive deficits are relatively well established in major depression, anxiety and eating disorders, the research is much less advanced in early illness and remission stages, precluding any firm assertions regarding vulnerability and progression. To precisely determine the timing and pattern of cognitive deterioration as well as the value of using cognitive functions as more specific biomarkers of syndromal pathways, more longitudinal studies are required to serially compare cognitive functioning of the same at-risk samples before and after development of full-threshold psychiatric disorders. This issue is critical not only for determining trait-related impairments, but whether cognitive impairment worsens with progression through each stage.

Aside from the considerations discussed, a very important caveat to the findings presented in this chapter is that of clinical and cognitive heterogeneity; an inherent characteristic of psychiatric conditions, particularly in the earlier stages of illness. Validating the clinical staging model will be constrained by the data fed into it (Lin et al., 2013). As described, most of the research on cognition has focused on impairments in specific diagnostic categories, with evidence supporting some dissociation between them in cognitive profiles. However, a limitation to this approach is the underlying assumption of 'one-size-fits-all' when in fact there is significant clinical heterogeneity *within* diagnostic categories (Bora et al., 2009b), as well as high psychiatric comorbidity (Kessler et al., 2005). For example, up to 25 per cent of people with psychotic disorders and 40 per cent with bipolar disorder have 'normal' (i.e. indistinguishable from healthy controls) neurocognitive functioning (Holthausen et al., 2002; Palmer et al., 1997; Strejilevich et al., 2015; Uren et al., 2017). Moreover, an affective disorder with psychotic symptoms is associated with poorer cognition compared to an affective disorder without psychosis (Bora et al., 2007; Martinez-Aran et al., 2004). As already discussed, the cognitive impairments varied according to OCD and anorexia nervosa phenotype (Leopold & Backenstrass, 2015; Wu et al., 2014). There is also evidence that specific subgroups within diagnostic categories (e.g. psychotic disorders) may experience more severe neurocognitive impairments, including a deteriorating course (e.g. Arango et al., 2014; Barder et al., 2013; de Garcia Dominguez et al., 2009; Irani et al., 2011; Reinares et al., 2013; Seaton et al., 2001). This within-diagnostic heterogeneity limits broad-based assumptions about prognosis and, consequently, the guidance and effectiveness of treatment approaches within psychiatric disorders. Illustrating this point further, in a study of youth with mixed psychiatric presentations, structural equation modelling revealed that baseline neurocognition was the best predictor of 6–48-month social-occupational outcome, and diagnosis did not improve the model (Lee et al., 2013b). Thus, statistical approaches such as cluster analysis and latent class analysis conducted on the cognitive functioning of large samples of mixed psychiatric patients at different stages of illness may help homogenise subgroups and elucidate shared cognitive profiles that are associated with illness stage outside of traditional diagnostic categories. Indeed, one study that has taken this approach found that in a mixed diagnostic sample of young people aged 18–30, those classified as Stages 2/3 performed significantly worse than healthy controls, particularly in verbal memory and executive functioning, and those classified as Stage 1b performed intermediately between healthy controls and Stages 2/3 (Hermens et al., 2013). The findings remained largely unchanged in a sensitivity analysis that excluded those with psychosis (Hermens et al., 2013). As stressed in the introduction to this chapter, of course cognition cannot be considered in isolation. Sophisticated multivariate approaches such as machine learning are allowing increased specificity in predicting illness outcomes (Koutsouleris et al., 2012; Shen et al., 2014), and will be highly informative to the staging of psychiatric disorders in the years to come (Orru et al., 2012).

The brain systems that develop through adolescence and early adulthood are likely to be most relevant to the clinical staging model due to the common age of onset of adult psychiatric disorders coinciding with this neurodevelopmentally dynamic and vulnerable period, when higher-level cognitive functions are still developing (Allott et al., 2013; Pantelis et al., 2015; Paus et al., 2008; Wood et al., 2011). In this respect, subdomains of executive functioning may be of particular transdiagnostic interest and there is clear evidence for a broad range of executive functioning impairments in most of the psychiatric disorders as described herein (Goschke, 2014; Nolen-Hoeksema & Watkins, 2011; Snyder et al., 2015b). Thus, transdiagnostic and longitudinal investigation of the pattern, severity and trajectory of executive functioning impairments may be especially informative in the context of the staging model. Normal development of social cognition is not fully understood, but similarly appears to be a promising area of focus in early psychiatric illness. Relative to other cognitive domains executive functions and social cognition are especially critical for adaptive social and occupational functioning and for engaging in psychosocial treatments such as cognitive behavioural therapy. Thus, they may be especially valuable areas of further study in understanding prognosis and tailoring treatment across the spectrum of psychiatric illness.

Due to space limitations the implications of cognitive findings for treatment were not presented. Needless to say, research into the cognitive predictors of treatment response at different illness stages is also likely to be especially useful within the clinical staging model as this information will inform treatment choices, which lies at the heart of the utility of the model. Furthermore, the evidence for an assumption inherent to the staging model – that cognitive treatments should be more effective in earlier stages – is lacking, although recent research in psychosis and depression provides some support for this (Bowie et al., 2014; Fisher et al., 2013; Motter et al., 2016; Pantelis et al., 2015).

In conclusion, research in the field of psychotic disorders and increasingly other mental illnesses has underscored the important role of cognition in illness pathophysiology, aetiology, recovery and functional outcomes, which has placed cognition as an important consideration in clinical formulation and treatment. Information obtained from a cognitive (neuropsychological) assessment can be used in treatment planning, evaluating the efficacy or effects (positive or negative) of the treatment, and in certain cases differential diagnosis. In addition, it may be possible to differentiate which deficits are state-dependent and which are more fundamental trait abnormalities or vulnerability markers. These investigations could have considerable implications for prevention and clinical management of psychiatric disorders, as cognitive deficits are significant factors in affecting an individual's ability to function socially and occupationally in everyday life.

References

Abramovitch, A., Abramowitz, J. S., & Mittelman, A. (2013). The neuropsychology of adult obsessive-compulsive disorder: a meta-analysis. *Clinical Psychology Review*, 33(8), 1163–1171.

Adolphs, R. (2009). The social brain: neural basis of social knowledge. *Annual Review of Psychology*, **60**, 693–716.

Airaksinen, E., Larsson, M., & Forsell, Y. (2005). Neuropsychological functions in anxiety disorders in population-based samples: evidence of episodic memory dysfunction. *Journal of Psychiatric Research*, **39**(2), 207–214.

Allen, K. L., Byrne, S. M., Hii, H., van Eekelen, A., Mattes, E., & Foster, J. K. (2013). Neurocognitive functioning in adolescents with eating disorders: a population-based study. *Cognitive Neuropsychiatry,* **18**(5), 355–375.

Allott, K., Fisher, C. A., Amminger, G. P., Goodall, J., & Hetrick, S. (2016). Characterizing neurocognitive impairment in young people with major depression: state, trait, or scar? *Brain and Behavior,* **6**(10), e00527.

Allott, K., Proffitt, T.-M., McGorry, P. D., Pantelis, C., Wood, S. J., Cumner, M., & Brewer, W. J. (2013). Clinical neuropsychology within adolescent and young-adult psychiatry: conceptualizing theory and practice. *Applied Neuropsychology: Child,* **2**(1), 47–63.

Allott, K., Schafer, M. R., Thompson, A., Nelson, B., Bendall, S., Bartholomeusz, C. F., . . . Amminger, G. P. (2014). Emotion recognition as a predictor of transition to a psychotic disorder in ultra-high risk participants. *Schizophrenia Research,* **153**(1–3), 25–31.

Alves, M. R. P., Pereira, V. M., Machado, S., Nardi, A. E., & Silva, A. (2013). Cognitive functions in patients with panic disorder: a literature review. *Revista Brasileira De Psiquiatria,* **35**(2), 193–200.

Amminger, G. P., Schafer, M. R., Papageorgiou, K., Klier, C. M., Schlogelhofer, M., Mossaheb, N., . . . McGorry, P. D. (2012). Emotion recognition in individuals at clinical high-risk for schizophrenia. *Schizophrenia Bulletin,* **38**(5), 1030–1039.

Andreou, C., & Bozikas, V. P. (2013). The predictive significance of neurocognitive factors for functional outcome in bipolar disorder. *Current Opinion in Psychiatry,* **26**(1), 54–59.

Arango, C., Fraguas, D., & Parellada, M. (2014). Differential neurodevelopmental trajectories in patients with early-onset bipolar and schizophrenia disorders. *Schizophrenia Bulletin,* **40**(Suppl. 2), S138–S146.

Arts, B., Jabben, N., Krabbendam, L., & van Os, J. (2008). Meta-analyses of cognitive functioning in euthymic bipolar patients and their first-degree relatives. *Psychological Medicine,* **38**(6), 771–785.

Austin, M. P., Mitchell, P., & Goodwin, G. M. (2001). Cognitive deficits in depression: possible implications for functional neuropathology. *British Journal of Psychiatry,* **178**, 200–206.

Balanza-Martinez, V., Rubio, C., Selva-Vera, G., Martinez-Aran, A., Sanchez-Moreno, J., Salazar-Fraile, J., . . . Tabares-Seisdedos, R. (2008). Neurocognitive endophenotypes (endophenocognitypes) from studies of relatives of bipolar disorder subjects: a systematic review. *Neuroscience and Biobehavioral Reviews,* **32**(8), 1426–1438.

Barder, H. E., Sundet, K., Rund, B. R., Evensen, J., Haahr, U., Hegelstad, W. T., . . . Friis, S. (2013). Neurocognitive development in first episode psychosis 5 years follow-up: associations between illness severity and cognitive course. *Schizophrenia Research,* **149**(1–3), 63–69.

Batty, G. D., Mortensen, E. L., & Osler, M. (2005). Childhood IQ in relation to later psychiatric disorder: evidence from a Danish birth cohort study. *British Journal of Psychiatry,* **187**, 180–181.

Baune, B. T., Fuhr, M., Air, T., & Hering, C. (2014). Neuropsychological functioning in adolescents and young adults with major depressive disorder: a review. *Psychiatry Research,* **218**, 261–271.

Beaudreau, S. A., & O'Hara, R. (2008). Late-life anxiety and cognitive impairment: a review. *American Journal of Geriatric Psychiatry,* **16**(10), 790–803.

Bechdolf, A., Ratheesh, A., Cotton, S. M., Nelson, B., Chanen, A. M., Betts, J., . . . McGorry, P. D. (2014). The predictive validity of bipolar at-risk (prodromal) criteria in help-seeking adolescents and young adults: a prospective study. *Bipolar Disorders,* **16**(5), 493–504.

Belleau, E. L., Phillips, M. L., Birmaher, B., Axelson, D. A., & Ladouceur, C. D. (2013). Aberrant executive attention in unaffected youth at familial risk for mood disorders. *Journal of Affective Disorders,* **147**(1–3), 397–400.

Bora, E., Harrison, B. J., Yucel, M., & Pantelis, C. (2013). Cognitive impairment in euthymic major depressive disorder: a meta-analysis. *Psychological Medicine,* **43**(10), 2017–2026.

Bora, E., Lin, A., Wood, S. J., Yung, A. R., McGorry, P. D., & Pantelis, C. (2014). Cognitive deficits in youth with familial and clinical high risk to psychosis: a systematic review and meta-analysis. *Acta Psychiatrica Scandinavica*, **130**(1), 1–15.

Bora, E., & Murray, R. M. (2014). Meta-analysis of cognitive deficits in ultra-high risk to psychosis and first-episode psychosis: do the cognitive deficits progress over, or after, the onset of psychosis? *Schizophrenia Bulletin*, **40**, 744–755.

Bora, E., & Pantelis, C. (2013). Theory of mind impairments in first-episode psychosis, individuals at ultra-high risk for psychosis and in first-degree relatives of schizophrenia: systematic review and meta-analysis. *Schizophrenia Research*, **144**(1–3), 31–36.

Bora, E., & Pantelis, C. (2015). Meta-analysis of cognitive impairment in first-episode bipolar disorder: comparison with first-episode schizophrenia and healthy controls. *Schizophrenia Bulletin*, **41**(5), 1095–1104.

Bora, E., Vahip, S., Akdeniz, F., Gonul, A. S., Eryavuz, A., Ogut, M., & Alkan, M. (2007). The effect of previous psychotic mood episodes on cognitive impairment in euthymic bipolar patients. *Bipolar Disorders*, **9**(5), 468–477.

Bora, E., Yucel, M., & Pantelis, C. (2009a). Cognitive endophenotypes of bipolar disorder: a meta-analysis of neuropsychological deficits in euthymic patients and their first-degree relatives. *Journal of Affective Disorders*, **113**, 1–20.

Bora, E., Yucel, M., & Pantelis, C. (2009b). Cognitive functioning in schizophrenia, schizoaffective disorder and affective psychoses: meta-analytic study. *British Journal of Psychiatry*, **195**(6), 475–482.

Bora, E., Yucel, M., & Pantelis, C. (2009c). Theory of mind impairment in schizophrenia: meta-analysis. *Schizophrenia Research*, **109**(1–3), 1–9.

Bora, E., Yucel, M., & Pantelis, C. (2010). Cognitive impairment in affective psychoses: a meta-analysis. *Schizophrenia Bulletin*, **36**(1), 112–125.

Bora, E., Yucel, M., Pantelis, C., & Berk, M. (2011). Meta-analytic review of neurocognition in bipolar II disorder. *Acta Psychiatrica Scandinavica*, **123**(3), 165–174.

Bourke, C., Douglas, K., & Porter, R. (2010). Processing of facial emotion expression in major depression: a review. *Australian and New Zealand Journal of Psychiatry*, **44**(8), 681–696.

Bourne, C., Aydemir, O., Balanza-Martinez, V., Bora, E., Brissos, S., Cavanagh, J. T. O., . . . Goodwin, G. M. (2013). Neuropsychological testing of cognitive impairment in euthymic bipolar disorder: an individual patient data meta-analysis. *Acta Psychiatrica Scandinavica*, **128**(3), 149–162.

Bowie, C. R., Grossman, M., Gupta, M., Oyewumi, L. K., & Harvey, P. D. (2014). Cognitive remediation in schizophrenia: efficacy and effectiveness in patients with early versus long-term course of illness. *Early Intervention in Psychiatry*, **8**, 32–38.

Bozikas, V. P., & Andreou, C. (2011). Longitudinal studies of cognition in first episode psychosis: a systematic review of the literature. *Australian and New Zealand Journal of Psychiatry*, **45**(2), 93–108.

Brewer, W. J., Wood, S. J., Phillips, L. J., Francey, S. M., Pantelis, C., Yung, A. R., . . . McGorry, P. D. (2006). Generalized and specific cognitive performance in clinical high-risk cohorts: a review highlighting potential vulnerability markers for psychosis. *Schizophrenia Bulletin*, **32**(3), 538–555.

Brotman, M. A., Guyer, A. E., Lawson, E. S., Horsey, S. E., Rich, B. A., Dickstein, D. P., . . . Leibenluft, E. (2008). Facial emotion labeling deficits in children and adolescents at risk for bipolar disorder. *American Journal of Psychiatry*, **165**(3), 385–389.

Cannon, M., Caspi, A., Moffitt, T. E., Harrington, H., Taylor, A., Murray, R. M., & Poulton, R. (2002). Evidence for early-childhood, pan-developmental impairment specific to schizophreniform disorder: results from a longitudinal birth cohort. *Archives of General Psychiatry*, **59**(5), 449–456.

Cannon, M., Moffitt, T. E., Caspi, A., Murray, R. M., Harrington, H., & Poulton, R. (2006). Neuropsychological performance at the age of 13 years and adult schizophreniform disorder: prospective birth cohort study. *British Journal of Psychiatry,* **189**, 463–464.

Cannon, T. D., Huttunen, M. O., Lonnqvist, J., Tuulio-Henriksson, A., Pirkola, T., Glahn, D., ... Koskenvuo, M. (2000). The inheritance of neuropsychological dysfunction in twins discordant for schizophrenia. *American Journal of Human Genetics,* **67**, 369–382.

Castaneda, A. E., Suvisaari, J., Marttunen, M., Perala, J., Saarni, S. I., Aalto-Setala, T., ... Tuulio-Henriksson, A. (2011). Cognitive functioning in a population-based sample of young adults with anxiety disorders. *European Psychiatry,* **26**(6), 346–353.

Castaneda, A. E., Tuulio-Henriksson, A., Marttunen, M., Suvisaari, J., & Lonnqvist, J. (2008). A review on cognitive impairments in depressive and anxiety disorders with a focus on young adults. *Journal of Affective Disorders,* **106**(1–2), 1–27.

Cavedini, P., Zorzi, C., Piccinni, M., Cavallini, M. C., & Bellodi, L. (2010). Executive dysfunctions in obsessive-compulsive patients and unaffected relatives: searching for a new intermediate phenotype. *Biological Psychiatry,* **67**(12), 1178–1184.

Comparelli, A., Corigliano, V., De Carolis, A., Mancinelli, I., Trovini, G., Ottavi, G., ... Girardi, P. (2013). Emotion recognition impairment is present early and is stable throughout the course of schizophrenia. *Schizophrenia Research,* **143**(1), 65–69.

Conus, P., Ward, J., Hallam, K. T., Lucas, N., Macneil, C., McGorry, P. D., & Berk, M. (2008). The proximal prodrome to first episode mania: a new target for early intervention. *Bipolar Disorders,* **10**(5), 555–565.

Cooper, S. A., Smiley, E., Morrison, J., Williamson, A., & Allan, L. (2007). Mental ill-health in adults with intellectual disabilities: prevalence and associated factors. *British Journal of Psychiatry,* **190**, 27–35.

Correll, C. U., Penzner, J. B., Lencz, T., Auther, A., Smith, C. W., Malhotra, A. K., ... Cornblatt, B. A. (2007). Early identification and high-risk strategies for bipolar disorder. *Bipolar Disorders,* **9**(4), 324–338.

Daban, C., Martinez-Aran, A., Torrent, C., Tabares-Seisdedos, R., Balanza-Martinez, V., Salazar-Fraile, J. S., ... Vieta, E. (2006). Specificity of cognitive deficits in bipolar disorder versus schizophrenia: a systematic review. *Psychotherapy and Psychosomatics,* **75**(2), 72–84.

Daglas, R., Allott, K., Yucel, M., Pantelis, C., Macneil, C. A., Berk, M., & Cotton, S. M. (2016). The trajectory of cognitive functioning following first episode mania: a 12-month follow-up study. *Australian and New Zealand Journal of Psychiatry,* **50**(12), 1186–1197.

Daglas, R., Yucel, M., Cotton, S., Allott, K., Hetrick, S., & Berk, M. (2015). Cognitive impairment in first-episode mania: a systematic review of the evidence in the acute and remission phases of the illness. *International Journal of Bipolar Disorders,* **3**, 9.

Dalili, M. N., Penton-Voak, I. S., Harmer, C. J., & Munafo, M. R. (2015). Meta-analysis of emotion recognition deficits in major depressive disorder. *Psychological Medicine,* **45**(6), 1135–1144.

Daros, A. R., Zakzanis, K. K., & Rector, N. A. (2014). A quantitative analysis of facial emotion recognition in obsessive-compulsive disorder. *Psychiatry Research,* **215**(3), 514–521.

David, A. S., Zammit, S., Lewis, G., Dalman, C., & Allebeck, P. (2008). Impairments in cognition across the spectrum of psychiatric disorders: evidence from a Swedish conscript cohort. *Schizophrenia Bulletin,* **34**(6), 1035–1041.

de Garcia Dominguez, M., Viechtbauer, W., Simons, C. J. P., van Os, J., & Krabbendam, L. (2009). Are psychotic psychopathology and neurocognition orthogonal? A systematic review of their associations. *Psychological Bulletin,* **135**(1), 157–171.

DeJong, H., van den Eynde, F., Broadbent, H., Kenyon, M. D., Lavender, A., Startup, H., & Schmidt, U. (2013). Social cognition in bulimia nervosa: a systematic review. *European Psychiatry,* **28**(1), 1–6.

Demenescu, L. R., Kortekaas, R., den Boer, J. A., & Aleman, A. (2010). Impaired attribution of emotion to facial expressions in anxiety and major depression. *PLoS One,* 5(12), e15058.

Depp, C. A., Mausbach, B. T., Harmell, A. L., Savla, G. N., Bowie, C. R., Harvey, P. D., & Patterson, T. L. (2012). Meta-analysis of the association between cognitive abilities and everyday functioning in bipolar disorder. *Bipolar Disorders,* 14(3), 217–226.

Dickinson, D., Ramsey, M. E., & Gold, J. M. (2007). Overlooking the obvious: a meta-analytic comparison of digit symbol coding tasks and other cognitive measures in schizophrenia. *Archives of General Psychiatry,* 64, 532–542.

DiGangi, J. A., Gomez, D., Mendoza, L., Jason, L. A., Keys, C. B., & Koenen, K. C. (2013). Pretrauma risk factors for posttraumatic stress disorder: a systematic review of the literature. *Clinical Psychology Review,* 33(6), 728–744.

Dotson, V. M., Resnick, S. M., & Zonderman, A. B. (2008). Differential association of concurrent, baseline, and average depressive symptoms with cognitive decline in older adults. *American Journal of Geriatric Psychiatry,* 16(4), 318–330.

Douglas, K. M., & Porter, R. J. (2009). Longitudinal assessment of neuropsychological function in major depression. *Australian and New Zealand Journal of Psychiatry,* 43(12), 1105–1117.

Edwards, J., Pattison, P. E., Jackson, H. J., & Wales, R. J. (2001). Facial affect and affective prosody recognition in first-episode schizophrenia. *Schizophrenia Research,* 48, 235–253.

Elshahawi, H. H., Essawi, H., Rabie, M. A., Mansour, M., Beshry, Z. A., & Mansour, A. N. (2011). Cognitive functions among euthymic bipolar I patients after a single manic episode versus recurrent episodes. *Journal of Affective Disorders,* 130(1–2), 180–191.

Faraone, S. V., Seidman, L. J., Kremen, W. S., Toomey, R., Pepple, J. R., & Tsuang, M. T. (2000). Neuropsychologic functioning among the nonpsychotic relatives of schizophrenic patients: the effect of genetic loading. *Biological Psychiatry,* 48, 120–126.

Fett, A. K., Viechtbauer, W., Dominguez, M. D., Penn, D. L., van Os, J., & Krabbendam, L. (2011). The relationship between neurocognition and social cognition with functional outcomes in schizophrenia: a meta-analysis. *Neuroscience and Biobehavioral Reviews,* 35(3), 573–588.

Fisher, M., Loewy, R., Hardy, K., Schlosser, D., & Vinogradov, S. (2013). Cognitive interventions targeting brain plasticity in the prodromal and early phases of schizophrenia. *Annual Review of Clinical Psychology,* 9, 435–463.

Fiske, S. T., & Taylor, S. E. (2013). *Social cognition: from brains to culture* (2nd ed.). London: Sage.

Fusar-Poli, P., Deste, G., Smieskova, R., Barlati, S., Yung, A. R., Howes, O., . . . Borgwardt, S. (2012). Cognitive functioning in prodromal psychosis: a meta-analysis. *Archives of General Psychiatry,* 69(6), 562–571.

Gale, C. R., Batty, G. D., McIntosh, A. M., Porteous, D. J., Deary, I. J., & Rasmussen, F. (2013). Is bipolar disorder more common in highly intelligent people? A cohort study of a million men. *Molecular Psychiatry,* 18(2), 190–194.

Gigi, K., Werbeloff, N., Goldberg, S., Portuguese, S., Reichenberg, A., Fruchter, E., & Weiser, M. (2014). Borderline intellectual functioning is associated with poor social functioning, increased rates of psychiatric diagnosis and drug use: a cross sectional population based study. *European Neuropsychopharmacology,* 24(11), 1793–1797.

Giuliano, A. J., Li, H. J., Mesholam-Gately, R. I., Sorenson, S. M., Woodberry, K. A., & Seidman, L. J. (2012). Neurocognition in the psychosis risk syndrome: a quantitative and qualitative review. *Current Pharmaceutical Design,* 18(4), 399–415.

Glahn, D. C., Almasy, L., Barguil, M., Hare, E., Peralta, J. M., Kent, J. W., . . . Escamilla, M. A. (2010). Neurocognitive endophenotypes for bipolar disorder identified in multiplex multigenerational families. *Archives of General Psychiatry,* 67(2), 168–177.

Goschke, T. (2014). Dysfunctions of decision-making and cognitive control as transdiagnostic mechanisms of mental disorders: advances, gaps, and needs in current research. *International Journal of Methods in Psychiatric Research,* **23** (Suppl. 1), 41–57.

Green, M. F., Bearden, C. E., Cannon, T. D., Fiske, A. P., Hellemann, G. S., Horan, W. P., . . . Nuechterlein, K. H. (2012). Social cognition in schizophrenia, part 1: performance across phase of illness. *Schizophrenia Bulletin,* **38**(4), 854–864.

Harvey, P. D. (2014). What is the evidence for changes in cognition and functioning over the lifespan in patients with schizophrenia? *Journal of Clinical Psychiatry,* **75**, 34–38.

Hasselbalch, B. J., Knorr, U., & Kessing, L. V. (2011). Cognitive impairment in the remitted state of unipolar depressive disorder: a systematic review. *Journal of Affective Disorders,* **134**(1–3), 20–31.

Hauser, M., Zhang, J. P., Sheridan, E. M., Burdick, K. E., Mogil, R., Kane, J. M., . . . Correll, C. U. (2017). Neuropsychological test performance to enhance identification of subjects at clinical high risk for psychosis and to be most promising for predictive algorithms for conversion to psychosis: a meta-analysis. *Journal of Clinical Psychiatry,* **78**(1), E28–E40.

Hedman, A. M., van Haren, N. E. M., van Baal, C. G. M., Kahn, R. S., & Pol, H. E. H. (2013). IQ change over time in schizophrenia and healthy individuals: a meta-analysis. *Schizophrenia Research,* **146**(1–3), 201–208.

Heinrichs, R. W., & Zakzanis, K. K. (1998). Neurocognitive deficit in schizophrenia: a quantitative review of the evidence. *Neuropsychology,* **12**(3), 426–445.

Hermens, D. F., Naismith, S. L., Lagopoulos, J., Lee, R. S., Guastella, A. J., Scott, E. M., & Hickie, I. B. (2013). Neuropsychological profile according to the clinical stage of young persons presenting for mental health care. *BMC Psychology,* **1**(1), 8.

Hetrick, S. E., Parker, A. G., Hickie, I. B., Purcell, R., Yung, A. R., & McGorry, P. D. (2008). Early identification and intervention in depressive disorders: towards a clinical staging model. *Psychotherapy and Psychosomatics,* **77**(5), 263–270.

Hoff, A. L., Svetina, C., Shields, G., Stewart, J., & DeLisi, L. E. (2005). Ten year longitudinal study of neuropsychological functioning subsequent to a first episode of schizophrenia. *Schizophrenia Research,* **78**(1), 27–34.

Holthausen, E. A., Wiersma, D., Sitskoorn, M. M., Hijman, R., Dingemans, P. M., Schene, A. H., & van den Bosch, R. J. (2002). Schizophrenic patients without neuropsychological deficits: subgroup, disease severity or cognitive compensation? *Psychiatry Research,* **112**, 1–11.

Hughes, C., Roman, G., Hart, M. J., & Ensor, R. (2013). Does maternal depression predict young children's executive function? A 4-year longitudinal study. *Journal of Child Psychology and Psychiatry,* **54**(2), 169–177.

Irani, F., Kalkstein, S., Moberg, E. A., & Moberg, P. J. (2011). Neuropsychological performance in older patients with schizophrenia: a meta-analysis of cross-sectional and longitudinal studies. *Schizophrenia Bulletin,* **37**(6), 1318–1326.

Jarros, R. B., Salum, G. A., da Silva, C. T. B., Toazza, R., Costa, M. D., de Salles, J. F., & Manfro, G. G. (2012). Anxiety disorders in adolescence are associated with impaired facial expression recognition to negative valence. *Journal of Psychiatric Research,* **46**(2), 147–151.

Kanakam, N., Raoult, C., Collier, D., & Treasure, J. (2013). Set shifting and central coherence as neurocognitive endophenotypes in eating disorders: a preliminary investigation in twins. *World Journal of Biological Psychiatry,* **14**(6), 464–475.

Kanakam, N., & Treasure, J. (2013). A review of cognitive neuropsychiatry in the taxonomy of eating disorders: state, trait, or genetic? *Cognitive Neuropsychiatry,* **18**(1–2), 83–114.

Kapczinski, F., Magalhaes, P. V., Balanza-Martinez, V., Dias, V. V., Frangou, S., Gama, C. S., . . . Berk, M. (2014). Staging systems in bipolar disorder: an International Society for Bipolar Disorders Task Force Report. *Acta Psychiatrica Scandinavica,* **130**(5), 354–363.

Keefe, R. S. E. (1995). The contribution of neuropsychology to psychiatry. *American Journal of Psychiatry,* **152**(1), 6–15.

Kendler, K. S., Ohlsson, H., Sundquist, J., & Sundquist, K. (2015). IQ and schizophrenia in a Swedish national sample: their causal relationship and the interaction of IQ with genetic risk. *American Journal of Psychiatry,* **172**(3), 259–265.

Kessler, R. C., Chiu, W. T., Demler, O., Merikangas, K. R., & Walters, E. E. (2005). Prevalence, severity, and comorbidity of 12-month DSM-IV disorders in the National Comorbidity Survey Replication. *Archives of General Psychiatry,* **62**(6), 617–627.

Khandaker, G. M., Barnett, J. H., White, I. R., & Jones, P. B. (2011). A quantitative meta-analysis of population-based studies of premorbid intelligence and schizophrenia. *Schizophrenia Research,* **132**(2–3), 220–227.

Khandaker, G. M., Stochl, J., Zammit, S., Lewis, G., & Jones, P. B. (2014). A population-based longitudinal study of childhood neurodevelopmental disorders, IQ and subsequent risk of psychotic experiences in adolescence. *Psychological Medicine,* **44**(15), 3229–3238.

Kim, H. S., Shin, N. Y., Jang, J. H., Kim, E., Shim, G., Park, H. Y., . . . Kwon, J. S. (2011). Social cognition and neurocognition as predictors of conversion to psychosis in individuals at ultra-high risk. *Schizophrenia Research,* **130**(1–3), 170–175.

Klimes-Dougan, B., Ronsaville, D., Wiggs, E. A., & Martinez, P. E. (2006). Neuropsychological functioning in adolescent children of mothers with a history of bipolar or major depressive disorders. *Biological Psychiatry,* **60**(9), 957–965.

Klimkeit, E. I., Tonge, B., Bradshaw, J. L., Melvin, G. A., & Gould, K. (2011). Neuropsychological deficits in adolescent unipolar depression. *Archives of Clinical Neuropsychology,* **26**(7), 662–676.

Koenen, K. C., Moffitt, T. E., Roberts, A. L., Martin, L. T., Kubzansky, L., Harrington, H., . . . Caspi, A. (2009). Childhood IQ and adult mental disorders: a test of the cognitive reserve hypothesis. *American Journal of Psychiatry,* **166**(1), 50–57.

Kohler, C. G., Hoffman, L. J., Eastman, L. B., Healey, K., & Moberg, P. J. (2011). Facial emotion perception in depression and bipolar disorder: a quantitative review. *Psychiatry Research,* **188**(3), 303–309.

Kohler, C. G., Walker, J. B., Martin, E. A., Healey, K. M., & Moberg, P. J. (2010). Facial emotion perception in schizophrenia: a meta-analytic review. *Schizophrenia Bulletin,* **36**(5), 1009–1019.

Koutsouleris, N., Davatzikos, C., Bottlender, R., Patschurek-Kliche, K., Scheuerecker, J., Decker, P., . . . Meisenzahl, E. M. (2012). Early recognition and disease prediction in the at-risk mental states for psychosis using neurocognitive pattern classification. *Schizophrenia Bulletin,* **38**(6), 1200–1215.

Kurtz, M. M., & Gerraty, R. T. (2009). A meta-analytic investigation of neurocognitive deficits in bipolar illness: profile and effects of clinical state. *Neuropsychology,* **23**(5), 551–562.

Kyte, Z. A., Goodyer, I. M., & Sahakian, B. J. (2005). Selected executive skills in adolescents with recent first episode major depression. *Journal of Child Psychology and Psychiatry,* **46**(9), 995–1005.

Lang, K., Lopez, C., Stahl, D., Tchanturia, K., & Treasure, J. (2014a). Central coherence in eating disorders: an updated systematic review and meta-analysis. *World Journal of Biological Psychiatry,* **15**(8), 586–598.

Lang, K., Stahl, D., Espie, J., Treasure, J., & Tchanturia, K. (2014b). Set shifting in children and adolescents with anorexia nervosa: an exploratory systematic review and meta-analysis. *International Journal of Eating Disorders,* **47**(4), 394–399.

Lavoie, M. A., Plana, I., Lacroix, J. B., Godmaire-Duhaime, F., Jackson, P. L., & Achim, A. M. (2013). Social cognition in first-degree relatives of people with schizophrenia: a meta-analysis. *Psychiatry Research,* **209**(2), 129–135.

Lee, J., Altshuler, L., Glahn, D. C., Miklowitz, D. J., Ochsner, K., & Green, M. F. (2013a). Social and nonsocial cognition in bipolar disorder and schizophrenia: relative levels of impairment. *American Journal of Psychiatry,* **170**(3), 334–341.

Lee, R. S., Hermens, D. F., Porter, M. A., & Redoblado-Hodge, M. A. (2012). A meta-analysis of cognitive deficits in first-episode major depressive disorder. *Journal of Affective Disorders,* **140**(2), 113–124.

Lee, R. S., Hermens, D. F., Redoblado-Hodge, M. A., Naismith, S. L., Porter, M. A., Kaur, M., . . . Hickie, I. B. (2013b). Neuropsychological and socio-occupational functioning in young psychiatric outpatients: a longitudinal investigation. *PLoS One,* **8**(3), e58176.

Lee, R. S., Hermens, D. F., Scott, J., Redoblado-Hodge, M. A., Naismith, S. L., Lagopoulos, J., . . . Hickie, I. B. (2014). A meta-analysis of neuropsychological functioning in first-episode bipolar disorders. *Journal of Psychiatric Research,* **57**, 1–11.

Lee, T. Y., Hong, S. B., Shin, N. Y., & Kwon, J. S. (2015). Social cognitive functioning in prodromal psychosis: a meta-analysis. *Schizophrenia Research,* **164**(1–3), 28–34.

Leopold, R., & Backenstrass, M. (2015). Neuropsychological differences between obsessive-compulsive washers and checkers: a systematic review and meta-analysis. *Journal of Anxiety Disorders,* **30**, 48–58.

Lewin, A. B., Larson, M. J., Park, J. M., McGuire, J. F., Murphy, T. K., & Storch, E. A. (2014). Neuropsychological functioning in youth with obsessive compulsive disorder: an examination of executive function and memory impairment. *Psychiatry Research,* **216**(1), 108–115.

Lezak, M. D., Howieson, D. B., & Loring, D. W. (2004). *Neuropsychological assessment* (4th ed.). New York: Oxford University Press.

Lim, J., Rekhi, G., Rapisarda, A., Lam, M., Kraus, M., Keefe, R. S., & Lee, J. (2015). Impact of psychiatric comorbidity in individuals at ultra high risk of psychosis: findings from the Longitudinal Youth at Risk Study (LYRIKS). *Schizophrenia Research,* **164**, 8–14.

Lin, A., Reniers, R. L. E. P., & Wood, S. J. (2013). Clinical staging in severe mental disorder: evidence from neurocognition and neuroimaging. *British Journal of Psychiatry,* **202**(Suppl. 54), s11–s17.

Lin, A., Wood, S. J., Nelson, B., Brewer, W. J., Spiliotacopoulos, D., Bruxner, A., . . . Yung, A. R. (2011). Neurocognitive predictors of functional outcome two to 13 years after identification as ultra-high risk for psychosis. *Schizophrenia Research,* **132**, 1–7.

Lopez, C., Stahl, D., & Tchanturia, K. (2010). Estimated intelligence quotient in anorexia nervosa: a systematic review and meta-analysis of the literature. *Annals of General Psychiatry,* **9**, 40.

Lopez-Jaramillo, C., Lopera-Vasquez, J., Gallo, A., Ospina-Duque, J., Bell, V., Torrent, C., . . . Vieta, E. (2010). Effects of recurrence on the cognitive performance of patients with bipolar I disorder: implications for relapse prevention and treatment adherence. *Bipolar Disorders,* **12**(5), 557–567.

Maalouf, F. T., Brent, D., Clark, L., Tavitian, L., McHugh, R. M., Sahakian, B. J., & Phillips, M. L. (2011). Neurocognitive impairment in adolescent major depressive disorder: state vs. trait illness markers. *Journal of Affective Disorders,* **133**(3), 625–632.

MacCabe, J. H., Lambe, M. P., Cnattingius, S., Sham, P. C., David, A. S., Reichenberg, A., . . . Hultman, C. M. (2010). Excellent school performance at age 16 and risk of adult bipolar disorder: national cohort study. *British Journal of Psychiatry,* **196**, 109–115.

MacCabe, J. H., Wicks, S., Lofving, S., David, A. S., Berndtsson, A., Gustafsson, J. E., . . . Dalman, C. (2013). Decline in cognitive performance between ages 13 and 18 years and the risk for psychosis in adulthood: a Swedish longitudinal cohort study in males. *JAMA Psychiatry,* **70**(3), 261–270.

Mann-Wrobel, M. C., Carreno, J. T., & Dickinson, D. (2011). Meta-analysis of neuropsychological functioning in euthymic bipolar disorder: an update and investigation of moderator variables. *Bipolar Disorders,* **13**(4), 334–342.

Martinez-Aran, A., Vieta, E., Reinares, M., Colom, F., Torrent, C., Sanchez-Moreno, J., . . . Salamero, M. (2004). Cognitive function across manic or hypomanic, depressed, and euthymic states in bipolar disorder. *American Journal of Psychiatry,* **161**, 262–270.

Martino, D. J., Samame, C., Ibanez, A., & Strejilevich, S. A. (2015). Neurocognitive functioning in the premorbid stage and in the first episode of bipolar disorder: a systematic review. *Psychiatry Research*, **226**(1), 23–30.

Mathews, A., & MacLeod, C. (2005). Cognitive vulnerability to emotional disorders. *Annual Review in Clinical Psychology*, **1**, 167–195.

McClintock, S. A., Husain, M. M., Greer, T. L., & Cullum, C. M. (2010). Association between depression severity and neurocognitive function in major depressive disorder: a review and synthesis. *Neuropsychology*, **24**(1), 9–34.

McDermott, L. M., & Ebmeier, K. P. (2009). A meta-analysis of depression severity and cognitive function. *Journal of Affective Disorders*, **119**(1–3), 1–8.

McGorry, P. D., Keshavan, M., Goldstone, S., Amminger, P., Allott, K., Berk, M., . . . Hickie, I. (2014). Biomarkers and clinical staging in psychiatry. *World Psychiatry*, **13**, 211–223.

Mesholam-Gately, R., Giuliano, A. J., Faraone, S. V., Goff, K. P., & Seidman, L. J. (2009). Neurocognition in first-episode schizophrenia: a meta-analytic review. *Neuropsychology*, **23**(3), 315–336.

Metzler, S., Dvorsky, D., Wyss, C., Muller, M., Gerstenberg, M., Traber-Walker, N., . . . Heekeren, K. (2015). Changes in neurocognitive functioning during transition to manifest disease: comparison of individuals at risk for schizophrenic and bipolar affective psychoses. *Psychological Medicine*, **45**(10), 2123–2134.

Meyer, S. E., Carlson, G. A., Wiggs, E. A., Martinez, P. E., Ronsaville, D. S., Klimes-Dougan, B., . . . Radke-Yarrow, M. (2004). A prospective study of the association among impaired executive functioning, childhood attentional problems, and the development of bipolar disorder. *Development and Psychopathology*, **16**(2), 461–476.

Micco, J. A., Henin, A., Biederman, J., Rosenbaum, J. F., Petty, C., Rindlaub, L. A., . . . Hirshfeld-Becker, D. R. (2009). Executive functioning in offspring at risk for depression and anxiety. *Depression and Anxiety*, **26**(9), 780–790.

Millan, M. J., Agid, Y., Brüne, M., Bullmore, E. T., Carter, C. S., Clayton, N. S., . . . Young, L. J. (2012). Cognitive dysfunction in psychiatric disorders: characteristics, causes and the quest for improved therapy. *Nature Reviews Drug Discovery*, **11**, 141–168.

Morgan, V. A., Leonard, H., Bourke, J., & Jablensky, A. (2008). Intellectual disability co-occurring with schizophrenia and other psychiatric illness: population-based study. *British Journal of Psychiatry*, **193**(5), 364–372.

Motter, J. N., Pimontel, M. A., Rindskopf, D., Devanand, D. P., Doraiswamy, P. M., & Sneed, J. R. (2016). Computerized cognitive training and functional recovery in major depressive disorder: a meta-analysis. *Journal of Affective Disorders*, **189**, 184–191.

Neisser, U., Boodoo, G., Bouchard, T. J., Boykin, A. W., Brody, N., Ceci, S. J., . . . Urbina, S. (1996). Intelligence: knowns and unknowns. *American Psychologist*, **51**(2), 77–101.

Niendam, T. A., Bearden, C. E., Johnson, J. K., McKinley, M., Loewy, R., O'Brien, M., . . . Cannon, T. D. (2006). Neurocognitive performance and functional disability in the psychosis prodrome. *Schizophrenia Research*, **84**(1), 100–111.

Nolen-Hoeksema, S., & Watkins, E. R. (2011). A heuristic for developing transdiagnostic models of psychopathology: explaining multifinality and divergent trajectories. *Perspectives on Psychological Science*, **6**(6), 589–609.

O'Sullivan, K., & Newman, E. F. (2014). Neuropsychological impairments in panic disorder: a systematic review. *Journal of Affective Disorders*, **167**, 268–284.

O'Toole, M. S., & Pedersen, A. D. (2011). A systematic review of neuropsychological performance in social anxiety disorder. *Nordic Journal of Psychiatry*, **65**(3), 147–161.

Ohmuro, N., Matsumoto, K., Katsura, M., Obara, C., Kikuchi, T., Hamaie, Y., . . . Matsuoka, H. (2015). The association between cognitive deficits and depressive symptoms in at-risk mental state: a comparison with first-episode psychosis. *Schizophrenia Research*, **162**(1–3), 67–73.

Oldershaw, A., Hambrook, D., Stahl, D., Tchanturia, K., Treasure, J., & Schmidt, U. (2011). The socio-emotional processing stream in anorexia nervosa. *Neuroscience and Biobehavioral Reviews,* **35**(3), 970–988.

Olley, A., Malhi, G. S., Mitchell, P. B., Batchelor, J., Lagopoulos, J., & Austin, M. P. (2005). When euthymia is just not good enough: the neuropsychology of bipolar disorder. *Journal of Nervous and Mental Disease,* **193**(5), 323–330.

Olvet, D. M., Burdick, K. E., & Cornblatt, B. A. (2013). Assessing the potential to use neurocognition to predict who is at risk for developing bipolar disorder: a review of the literature. *Cognitive Neuropsychiatry,* **18**(1–2), 129–145.

Olvet, D. M., Stearns, W. H., McLaughlin, D., Auther, A. M., Correll, C. U., & Cornblatt, B. A. (2010). Comparing clinical and neurocognitive features of the schizophrenia prodrome to the bipolar prodrome. *Schizophrenia Research,* **123**(1), 59–63.

Orru, G., Pettersson-Yeo, W., Marquand, A. F., Sartori, G., & Mechelli, A. (2012). Using support vector machine to identify imaging biomarkers of neurological and psychiatric disease: a critical review. *Neuroscience and Biobehavioral Reviews,* **36**(4), 1140–1152.

Owen, M. J. (2012). Intellectual disability and major psychiatric disorders: a continuum of neurodevelopmental causality. *British Journal of Psychiatry,* **200**(4), 268–269.

Palmer, B. W., Heaton, R. K., Paulsen, J. S., Kuck, J., Braff, D., Harris, M. J., . . . Jeste, D. V. (1997). Is it possible to be schizophrenic yet neuropsychologically normal? *Neuropsychology,* **11**(3), 437–446.

Pantelis, C., Wannan, C., Bartholomeusz, C. F., Allott, K., & McGorry, P. D. (2015). Cognitive intervention in early psychosis: preserving abilities versus remediating deficits. *Current Opinion in Behavioral Sciences,* **4**, 63–72.

Paus, T., Keshavan, M., & Giedd, J. N. (2008). Why do many psychiatric disorders emerge during adolescence? *Nature Reviews Neuroscience,* **9**, 947–957.

Pinkham, A. E., Penn, D. L., Green, M. F., Buck, B., Healey, K., & Harvey, P. D. (2014). The Social Cognition Psychometric Evaluation Study: results of the expert survey and RAND panel. *Schizophrenia Bulletin,* **40**, 813–823.

Plana, I., Lavoie, M. A., Battaglia, M., & Achim, A. M. (2014). A meta-analysis and scoping review of social cognition performance in social phobia, posttraumatic stress disorder and other anxiety disorders. *Journal of Anxiety Disorders,* **28**(2), 169–177.

Polak, A. R., Witteveen, A. B., Reitsma, J. B., & Olff, M. (2012). The role of executive function in posttraumatic stress disorder: a systematic review. *Journal of Affective Disorders,* **141**(1), 11–21.

Pukrop, R., & Klosterkotter, J. (2010). Neurocognitive indicators of clinical high-risk states for psychosis: a critical review of the evidence. *Neurotoxicity Research,* **18**(3–4), 272–286.

Rajji, T. K., Ismail, Z., & Mulsant, B. H. (2009). Age at onset and cognition in schizophrenia: meta-analysis. *British Journal of Psychiatry,* **195**(4), 286–293.

Rajji, T. K., & Mulsant, B. H. (2008). Nature and course of cognitive function in late-life schizophrenia: a systematic review. *Schizophrenia Research,* **102**(1–3), 122–140.

Ratheesh, A., Lin, A., Nelson, B., Wood, S. J., Brewer, W., Betts, J., . . . Bechdolf, A. (2013). Neurocognitive functioning in the prodrome of mania: an exploratory study. *Journal of Affective Disorders,* **147**(1–3), 441–445.

Reichenberg, A., Caspi, A., Harrington, H., Houts, R., Keefe, R. S. E., Murray, R. M., . . . Moffitt, T. E. (2010). Static and dynamic cognitive deficits in childhood preceding adult schizophrenia: a 30-year study. *American Journal of Psychiatry,* **167**(2), 160–169.

Reichenberg, A., Harvey, P. D., Bowie, C. R., Mojtabai, R., Rabinowitz, J., Heaton, R. K., & Bromet, E. (2009). Neuropsychological function and dysfunction in schizophrenia and psychotic affective disorders. *Schizophrenia Bulletin,* **35**(5), 1022–1029.

Reichenberg, A., Weiser, M., Rabinowitz, J., Caspi, A., Schmeidler, J., Mark, M., . . . Davidson, M. (2002). A population-based cohort study of premorbid intellectual, language, and behavioral functioning in patients with schizophrenia, schizoaffective disorder, and nonpsychotic bipolar disorder. *American Journal of Psychiatry*, **159**(12), 2027–2035.

Reichenberg, A., Weiser, M., Rapp, M. A., Rabinowitz, J., Caspi, A., Schmeidler, J., . . . Davidson, M. (2005). Elaboration on premorbid intellectual performance in schizophrenia: premorbid intellectual decline and risk for schizophrenia. *Archives of General Psychiatry*, **62**(12), 1297–1304.

Reinares, M., Papachristou, E., Harvey, P., Mar Bonnin, C., Sanchez-Moreno, J., Torrent, C., . . . Frangou, S. (2013). Towards a clinical staging for bipolar disorder: defining patient subtypes based on functional outcome. *Journal of Affective Disorders*, **144**(1–2), 65–71.

Robinson, L. J., & Ferrier, I. N. (2006). Evolution of cognitive impairment in bipolar disorder: a systematic review of cross-sectional evidence. *Bipolar Disorders*, **8**(2), 103–116.

Robinson, L. J., Thompson, J. M., Gallagher, P., Goswami, U., Young, A. H., Ferrier, I. N., & Moore, P. B. (2006). A meta-analysis of cognitive deficits in euthymic patients with bipolar disorder. *Journal of Affective Disorders*, **93**, 105–115.

Rock, P. L., Roiser, J. P., Riedel, W. J., & Blackwell, A. D. (2014). Cognitive impairment in depression: a systematic review and meta-analysis. *Psychological Medicine*, **44**(10), 2029–2040.

Rosa, A. R., Magalhaes, P. V., Czepielewski, L., Sulzbach, M. V., Goi, P. D., Vieta, E., . . . Kapczinski, F. (2014). Clinical staging in bipolar disorder: focus on cognition and functioning. *Journal of Clinical Psychiatry*, **75**(5), e450–e456.

Samame, C., Martino, D. J., & Strejilevich, S. A. (2012). Social cognition in euthymic bipolar disorder: systematic review and meta-analytic approach. *Acta Psychiatrica Scandinavica*, **125**(4), 266–280.

Samame, C., Martino, D. J., & Strejilevich, S. A. (2013). A quantitative review of neurocognition in euthymic late-life bipolar disorder. *Bipolar Disorders*, **15**(6), 633–644.

Samame, C., Martino, D. J., & Strejilevich, S. A. (2014). Longitudinal course of cognitive deficits in bipolar disorder: a meta-analytic study. *Journal of Affective Disorders*, **164**, 130–138.

Sarapas, C., Shankman, S. A., Harrow, M., & Goldberg, J. F. (2012). Parsing trait and state effects of depression severity on neurocognition: evidence from a 26-year longitudinal study. *Journal of Abnormal Psychology*, **121**(4), 830–837.

Savla, G. N., Vella, L., Armstrong, C. C., Penn, D. L., & Twamley, E. W. (2013). Deficits in domains of social cognition in schizophrenia: a meta-analysis of the empirical evidence. *Schizophrenia Bulletin*, **39**(5), 979.

Schmid, M., & Hammar, A. (2013). A follow-up study of first episode major depressive disorder: impairment in inhibition and semantic fluency – potential predictors for relapse? *Frontiers in Psychology*, **4**, 633.

Scott, J. C., Matt, G. E., Wrocklage, K. M., Crnich, C., Jordan, J., Southwick, S. M., . . . Schweinsburg, B. C. (2015). A quantitative meta-analysis of neurocognitive functioning in posttraumatic stress disorder. *Psychological Bulletin*, **141**(1), 105–140.

Seaton, B. E., Goldstein, G., & Allen, D. N. (2001). Sources of heterogeneity in schizophrenia: the role of neuropsychological functioning. *Neuropsychology Review*, **11**(1), 45–67.

Shen, C., Popescu, F. C., Hahn, E., Ta, T. T., Dettling, M., & Neuhaus, A. H. (2014). Neurocognitive pattern analysis reveals classificatory hierarchy of attention deficits in schizophrenia. *Schizophrenia Bulletin*, **40**(4), 878–885.

Shin, N. Y., Lee, T. Y., Kim, E., & Kwon, J. S. (2014). Cognitive functioning in obsessive-compulsive disorder: a meta-analysis. *Psychological Medicine*, **44**(6), 1121–1130.

Simonsen, C., Sundet, K., Vaskinn, A., Birkenaes, A. B., Engh, J. A., Faerden, A. . . . & Andreassen, O. A. (2011). Neurocognitive dysfunction in bipolar and schizophrenia spectrum disorders depends on history of psychosis rather than diagnostic group. *Schizophrenia Bulletin*, **37**(1), 73–83.

Sitskoorn, M. M., Aleman, A., Ebisch, S. J. H., Appels, M. C. M., & Kahn, R. S. (2004). Cognitive deficits in relatives of patients with schizophrenia: a meta-analysis. *Schizophrenia Research,* **71**(2–3), 285–295.

Snitz, B. E., Macdonald, A. W., 3rd, & Carter, C. S. (2006). Cognitive deficits in unaffected first-degree relatives of schizophrenia patients: a meta-analytic review of putative endophenotypes. *Schizophrenia Bulletin,* **32**(1), 179–194.

Snyder, H. R. (2013). Major depressive disorder is associated with broad impairments on neuropsychological measures of executive function: a meta-analysis and review. *Psychological Bulletin,* **139**(1), 81–132.

Snyder, H. R., Kaiser, R. H., Warren, S. L., & Heller, W. (2015a). Obsessive-compulsive disorder is associated with broad impairments in executive function: a meta-analysis. *Clinical Psychological Science,* **3**(2), 301–330.

Snyder, H. R., Miyake, A., & Hankin, B. L. (2015b). Advancing understanding of executive function impairments and psychopathology: bridging the gap between clinical and cognitive approaches. *Frontiers in Psychology,* **6**, 24.

Sole, B., Martinez-Aran, A., Torrent, C., Bonnin, C. M., Reinares, M., Popovic, D., . . . Vieta, E. (2011). Are bipolar II patients cognitively impaired? A systematic review. *Psychological Medicine,* **41**(9), 1791–1803.

Sprong, M., Schothorst, P., Vos, E., Hox, J., & van Engeland, H. (2007). Theory of mind in schizophrenia. *British Journal of Psychiatry,* **191**, 5–13.

Stefanopoulou, E., Manoharan, A., Landau, S., Geddes, J. R., Goodwin, G., & Frangou, S. (2009). Cognitive functioning in patients with affective disorders and schizophrenia: a meta-analysis. *International Review of Psychiatry,* **21**(4), 336–356.

Strejilevich, S. A., Samame, C., & Martino, D. J. (2015). The trajectory of neuropsychological dysfunctions in bipolar disorders: a critical examination of a hypothesis. *Journal of Affective Disorders,* **175**, 396–402.

Sutterby, S. R., & Bedwell, J. S. (2012). Lack of neuropsychological deficits in generalized social phobia. *PLoS One,* **7**(8), e42675.

Svirskis, T., Korkeila, J., Heinimaa, M., Huttunen, J., Ilonen, T., Ristkari, T., . . .

Salokangas, R. K. R. (2005). Axis-I disorders and vulnerability to psychosis. *Schizophrenia Research,* **75**(2–3), 439–446.

Szoke, A., Trandafir, A., Dupont, M.-E., Meary, A., Schurhoff, F., & Leboyer, M. (2008). Longitudinal studies of cognition in schizophrenia: meta-analysis. *British Journal of Psychiatry,* **192**, 248–257.

Talarowska, M., Zajaczkowska, M., & Galecki, P. (2015). Cognitive functions in first-episode depression and recurrent depressive disorder. *Psychiatria Danubina,* **27**(1), 38–43.

Tempesta, D., Mazza, M., Serroni, N., Moschetta, F. S., Di Giannantonio, M., Ferrara, M., & De Berardis, D. (2013). Neuropsychological functioning in young subjects with generalized anxiety disorder with and without pharmacotherapy. *Progress in Neuro-Psychopharmacology and Biological Psychiatry,* **45**, 236–241.

Tiihonen, J., Haukka, J., Henriksson, M., Cannon, M., Kieseppa, T., Laaksonen, I., . . . Lonnqvist, J. (2005). Premorbid intellectual functioning in bipolar disorder and schizophrenia: results from a cohort study of male conscripts. *American Journal of Psychiatry,* **162**(10), 1904–1910.

Torres, I. J., Boudreau, V. G., & Yatham, L. N. (2007). Neuropsychological functioning in euthymic bipolar disorder: a meta-analysis. *Acta Psychiatrica Scandinavica,* **116**(Suppl. 434), 17–26.

Torres, I. J., Kozicky, J., Popuri, S., Bond, D. J., Honer, W. G., Lam, R. W., & Yatham, L. N. (2014). 12-month longitudinal cognitive functioning in patients recently diagnosed with bipolar disorder. *Bipolar Disorders,* **16**, 159–171.

Treasure, J., Stein, D., & Maguire, S. (2015). Has the time come for a staging model to map the course of eating disorders from high risk to severe enduring illness? An examination of the evidence. *Early Intervention in Psychiatry,* **9**(3), 173–184.

Trotta, A., Murray, R. M., & MacCabe, J. H. (2015). Do premorbid and post-onset cognitive functioning differ between schizophrenia and bipolar disorder? A systematic review and meta-analysis. *Psychological Medicine,* **45**, 381–394.

Uren, J., Cotton, S., Killackey, E., Saling, M., & Allott, K. (2017). Cognitive clusters in first-episode psychosis: overlap with healthy controls and relationship to concurrent and prospective symptoms and functioning. *Neuropsychology, 31*(7), 787–797.

Van den Eynde, F., Guillaume, S., Broadbent, H., Stahl, D., Campbell, I. C., Schmidt, U., & Tchanturia, K. (2011). Neurocognition in bulimic eating disorders: a systematic review. *Acta Psychiatrica Scandinavica, 124*(2), 120–140.

Viswanath, B., Janardhan Reddy, Y. C., Kumar, K. J., Kandavel, T., & Chandrashekar, C. R. (2009). Cognitive endophenotypes in OCD: a study of unaffected siblings of probands with familial OCD. *Progress in Neuro-Psychopharmacology and Biological Psychiatry, 33*(4), 610–615.

Vorstman, J. A., Breetvelt, E. J., Duijff, S. N., Eliez, S., Schneider, M., Jalbrzikowski, M., . . . Bassett, A. S. (2015). Cognitive decline preceding the onset of psychosis in patients with 22q11.2 deletion syndrome. *JAMA Psychiatry, 72*(4), 377–385.

Weiser, M., Reichenberg, A., Kravitz, E., Lubin, G., Shmushkevich, M., Glahn, D. C., . . . Davidson, M. (2008). Subtle cognitive dysfunction in nonaffected siblings of individuals affected by nonpsychotic disorders. *Biological Psychiatry, 63*(6), 602–608.

Weiser, M., Reichenberg, A., Rabinowitz, J., Knobler, H. Y., Lubin, G., Yazvitzky, R., . . . Davidson, M. (2004). Cognitive performance of male adolescents is lower than controls across psychiatric disorders: a population-based study. *Acta Psychiatrica Scandinavica, 110*(6), 471–475.

Whitney, J., Howe, M., Shoemaker, V., Li, S., Sanders, E. M., Dijamco, C., . . . Chang, K. (2013). Socio-emotional processing and functioning of youth at high risk for bipolar disorder. *Journal of Affective Disorders, 148*(1), 112–117.

Wood, S. J., Yung, A. R., McGorry, P. D., & Pantelis, C. (2011). Neuroimaging and treatment evidence for clinical staging in psychotic disorders: from the at-risk mental state to chronic schizophrenia. *Biological Psychiatry, 70*(7), 619–625.

Wood, S. J., Yung, A. R., & Pantelis, C. (2013). Cognitive precursors of severe mental disorders. *Cognitive Neuropsychiatry, 18*(1–2), 1–8.

Woodberry, K. A., Giuliano, A. J., & Seidman, L. J. (2008). Premorbid IQ in schizophrenia: a meta-analytic review. *American Journal of Psychiatry, 165*(5), 579–587.

Wu, M., Brockmeyer, T., Hartmann, M., Skunde, M., Herzog, W., & Friederich, H. C. (2014). Set-shifting ability across the spectrum of eating disorders and in overweight and obesity: a systematic review and meta-analysis. *Psychological Medicine, 44*(16), 3365–3385.

Zakzanis, K. K., Campbell, Z., & Polsinelli, A. (2010). Quantitative evidence for distinct cognitive impairment in anorexia nervosa and bulimia nervosa. *Journal of Neuropsychology, 4*(Pt 1), 89–106.

Zammit, S., Allebeck, P., David, A. S., Dalman, C., Hemmingsson, T., Lundberg, I., & Lewis, G. (2004). A longitudinal study of premorbid IQ score and risk of developing schizophrenia, bipolar disorder, severe depression, and other nonaffective psychoses. *Archives of General Psychiatry, 61*(4), 354–360.

Chapter

8

Neuroinflammation and Staging

Bernhard T. Baune

Introduction

As many areas of clinical medicine move towards the introduction of more personalised treatment selection, linked to the stage of illness at which one presents for care, we are still early in the process of evaluation of the relevance of clinical staging for the major psychiatric disorders (McGorry, 2007; McGorry et al., 2006; 2010). Clinical staging in psychiatry builds on strong epidemiological evidence indicating that what we regard as the major mental illnesses evolve over time and in terms of severity. The model aims to differentiate earlier and milder clinical phenomena from those that mark illness progression and extension, moving outside the traditional diagnostic boundaries to place strong emphasis on where a person sits within the evolution of the course of their illness. Advances in research, particularly in the area of early psychosis, have shown that treatment in the very early stages of illness can produce significantly better clinical and functional outcomes for patients (Bertelsen et al., 2008; Hegelstad et al., 2012; Larsen et al., 2011; McGorry et al., 2010; Norman et al., 2011). This research has opened the way for a paradigm shift in psychiatry: the movement towards a pre-emptive, rather than largely palliative psychiatry (Insel, 2007).

To date, the classification of the early stages of schizophrenia and other psychotic disorders is based on clinical characteristics, which is of limited predictive value, and there is a pressing need for further enhancement of predictive models (McGorry et al., 2014). The identification of biomarkers that provide accurate assessments of risk and illness progression is of crucial importance, with diagnostic and treatment implications. It was recently shown that a combination of clinical and biological markers can be employed to characterise the longitudinal course of first-episode psychosis at the onset of disease (Schubert et al., 2015) and to delineate groups of patients at high risk for transition to psychosis from those who do not develop the full clinical picture of psychosis (Clark et al., 2015). Such clinical and biological markers ideally should link to a relevant pathophysiology of the disease and enhance our understanding of the biological mechanisms that underlie the onset and progression of illness. Biomarkers in particular may be of value as predictors of treatment response.

Neuroinflammation in Psychosis and Schizophrenia

Among other theories on the aetiology and pathophysiology, more and more studies in recent years suggest a role of inflammation and specifically of cytokines in the pathophysiology and pathogenetics of schizophrenia (Figure 8.1). In summary, cytokines are

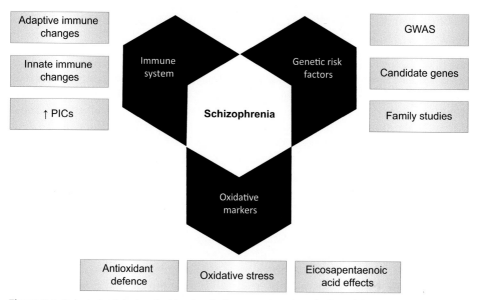

Figure 8.1 Biological aetiologies of schizophrenia. Among various classic biological theories involving genetic risk factors and monoamines as a cause of schizophrenia, new theories have emerged to suggest a role of the immune system, inflammation and oxidative stress in the aetiology of schizophrenia. PICs, pro-inflammatory cytokines; GWAS, genome-wide association studies.

humoral mediators and play an important role in cell development and survival of almost every tissue, including the brain; hence, cytokines likely are directly or indirectly involved in neurodevelopmental and neurodegenerative processes in schizophrenia. Robust findings obtained from peripheral blood indicate that IL-2, IL-6, TNF-α and IGFN cytokine systems are regulated differently in schizophrenia compared to controls. Although there is strong evidence that dopaminergic transmission is involved in schizophrenia, the exact mechanisms leading to dopaminergic dysfunction are still unclear. It has been postulated that a dysbalance in the immune response associated with a slight inflammatory process of the central nervous system (CNS) presents a mechanism as the basis for the 'mild encephalitis' concept. A dysfunction in the activation of the type-1 immune response appears to be associated with decreased activity of the key enzyme of the tryptophan/kynurenine metabolism, indoleamine 2,3-dioxygenase (IDO), which may interact with glutamatergic neurotransmission in schizophrenia (Muller et al., 2012). However, the role of inflammatory markers appears to be non-specific to schizophrenia as the dysregulation applies to other pathophysiological processes in the CNS as well. It is therefore important to enhance the understanding of the role of inflammation in people with schizophrenia and in individuals with attenuated psychotic manifestations at ultra-high risk (UHR) of psychosis. Although a clinical stage-specific approach using inflammatory markers to characterise clinical disease stages in schizophrenia has not been systematically undertaken, such a stage-specific characterisation of biomarkers and inflammation specifically is an important step to enhance diagnostic and therapeutic processes and accuracy in predicting the course of the illness in psychosis/schizophrenia.

Inflammation in Schizophrenia: An Elevated Inflammatory Response May Define a Subgroup of Individuals with Schizophrenia

Multiple lines of evidence point to increased inflammatory and immune processes in schizophrenia. Immune system-related genes, such as the major histocompatibility complex (Shi et al., 2009) and genes coding cytokines (Ripke et al., 2011; Xu & He, 2010) have been associated with schizophrenia. Elevated cytokines or cytokine receptor expression has been consistently identified in the peripheral blood of individuals with schizophrenia, with some cytokines (e.g. TNF-α) considered as trait markers and others (e.g. IL-1β, IL-6) as state markers specific to acute illness (Miller et al., 2011). Post-mortem studies have reported increased expression of inflammation-related genes in the prefrontal cortex (PFC) of individuals with schizophrenia (Arion et al., 2007; Saetre et al., 2007), although in genes not classically involved in chronic or acute inflammation. Also, adjunctive treatment with immunomodulatory drugs has some efficacy in treating active illness (Muller et al., 2002) and atypical antipsychotics have been shown to inhibit pro-inflammatory cytokines (Monji et al., 2009), suggesting anti-inflammatory actions may contribute to their therapeutic response.

Numerous studies have found that people with schizophrenia have increased blood concentrations of inflammatory cytokines (Miller et al., 2011). Two important themes emerge from these studies. First, inflammatory abnormalities are present in subjects with first-episode, drug-naïve psychosis (FEP) compared with healthy controls (HCs), suggesting an association that may be independent of the effects of antipsychotic medications. Second, the concentrations of some inflammatory molecules may vary with the clinical status of patients (see Figure 8.2): i.e. there appears to be separate groups for state and trait markers. The state-related markers include IL-1β, IL-6 and TGF-β. People with schizophrenia have higher concentrations of these cytokines than controls during an exacerbation of symptoms, but there is no difference during periods of clinical stability. IL-12, IFN-γ and TNF-α appear to be trait markers. Concentrations of these cytokines are higher in patients with FEP than in HCs. C-reactive protein (CRP), another pro-inflammatory molecule, also appears to be a state marker (Miller et al., 2014).

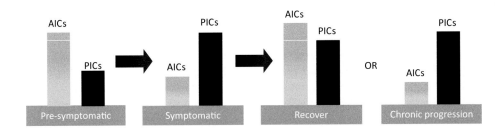

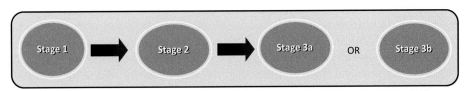

Figure 8.2 Pro- and anti-inflammatory phases during stages of psychosis and schizophrenia. Clinical stages of psychosis and schizophrenia may be reflected by the regulation of pro- and anti-inflammatory cytokines (AICs, PICs).

Inflammation in UHR Individuals: Inflammatory Markers May Predict Conversion to Psychosis

Most studies exploring the role of inflammatory markers in psychosis have been conducted on subjects with long durations of illness, and only a few studies suggest that inflammatory abnormalities are present in newly diagnosed antipsychotic-naïve patients (Borovcanin et al., 2012; Garcia-Rizo et al., 2012). Only one preliminary study compared 17 UHR individuals with individuals diagnosed with a psychotic disorder and HCs (Stojanovic et al., 2014). UHR subjects exhibited significantly higher IL-6 levels than did controls ($p = 0.019$). Six of the 17 UHR subjects (35 per cent) exhibited a transition to psychosis during the follow-up period of 26 months. UHR subjects who developed psychosis exhibited increased median IL-6 levels compared with those who did not transition (0.61 vs 0.35 pg/mL). However, this difference was not statistically significant, which could be explained by a lack of statistical power due to the small sample size. The authors concluded that IL-6 may be a biomarker for early psychotic symptoms; however, further studies in larger samples are needed to confirm this result.

Oxidative Stress in Schizophrenia

Oxidative stress refers to an imbalance of free radicals, such as reactive oxygen and nitrogen species, which are generated from both normal metabolism – including neurotransmitters associated with schizophrenia such as dopamine and glutamate – and from various environmental exposures. The failure of antioxidant defences to protect against free-radical generation damages cell membranes, with resulting dysfunction that might impact on neurotransmission and, ultimately, symptomatology in schizophrenia (Yao & Keshavan, 2011). Important free radicals in humans include hydrogen peroxide (H_2O_2), the hydroxyl radical (OH^-), nitric oxide (NO) and the superoxide radical (O_2^-). Superoxide dismutase (SOD) catalyses the conversion of superoxide radicals to hydrogen peroxide. Reduced glutathione (GSH) is oxidised by glutathione peroxidase to oxidised GSH (GSSG). Radicals promote apoptosis, DNA damage and lipid peroxidation. Thiobarbituric acid reactive substances and malondialdehyde (MDA) are important end products of lipid peroxidation (Flatow et al., 2013).

Alterations in Antioxidant Defence Systems in Schizophrenia

Abnormal oxidative stress parameters have been consistently reported in peripheral blood cells, cerebrospinal fluid, and/or post-mortem brain in patients with schizophrenia (Flatow et al., 2013). One study found decreased in vivo GSH levels in the medial prefrontal cortex of patients with schizophrenia (Keshavan et al., 1993). Other results suggest that eicosapentaenoic acid (an omega-3 polyunsaturated fatty acid (PUFA)) alters GSH availability and modulates the glutamine/glutamate cycle in early psychosis, with some of the metabolic brain changes being correlated with negative symptom improvement (Berger et al., 2008; Do et al., 2000).

Clinical trials also support an association between oxidative stress and schizophrenia (Libov et al., 2007; Shamir et al., 2001; Zhang et al., 2004). Furthermore, it has been found that adjunctive treatment with the antioxidant N-acetyl-cysteine, a precursor of GSH, significantly reduced psychopathology in schizophrenia (Berk et al., 2008). Together with the finding that supplementation with omega-3 PUFAs – which reduce oxidative stress (Kiecolt-Glaser et al., 2013) – significantly reduced the progression to FEP in subjects with prodromal symptoms (Amminger et al., 2010), these studies suggest that oxidative stress levels might be a biomarker of psychosis and predictor of response to antioxidant treatment.

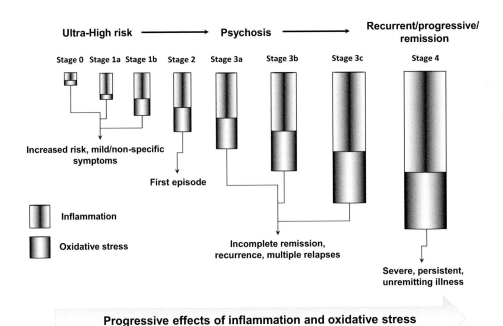

Figure 8.3 Inflammation and oxidative stress during conversion from ultra-high risk to psychosis. The figure suggests progressive effects of inflammation and oxidative stress during stages of psychosis.

Alterations in Antioxidant Defence Systems in UHR Individuals

Data from our lab recently for the first time indicated that lower levels of GSH at baseline predicted transition to psychosis at the longer-term follow-up (median = 6.6 years) in the participants of the Vienna UHR study (Lavoie et al., 2017), described in detail by Amminger et al. (2010). This is important evidence highlighting the crucial role of oxidative stress for illness progression of psychotic disorder (see Figure 8.3 for the progressive effects of inflammation and oxidative stress).

In summary, the current proposal will allow us for the first time to compare markers of inflammation and oxidative stress in patients with schizophrenia and UHR patients from large representative samples with healthy controls.

Neuroinflammation in Depression

Among biological theories of depression, factors of the immune system exerting effects on key processes such as neuroplasticity, neurotransmission, oxidative stress and neuroendocrinological functions are considered to be central to the development and chronic course of depression (Dantzer et al., 2008; Eyre & Baune, 2012; Haroon et al., 2012; McAfoose & Baune, 2009; Miller et al., 2009). Inflammation has been associated with the clinical presentation of depression and with anatomical, functional and biochemical disturbances relevant to depression (Baune, 2009; Mahar et al., 2014; Moylan et al., 2014; Slavich & Irwin, 2014). The most established immune-based model of depression is the inflammatory or cytokine model of depression (Dantzer et al., 2008; McAfoose & Baune, 2009; Miller et al., 2009). This model postulates that a pro-inflammatory state characterised by elevations in pro-inflammatory cytokines (PICs) and reductions in anti-inflammatory cytokines (AIC) is involved in the development of depression-like behaviour in animals and clinical depression in humans. The net pro-inflammatory state is found to impair hippocampal neuroplasticity (e.g. neurogenesis, synaptic plasticity, long-term potentiation (LTP)), induce glucocorticoid insensitivity of the hypothalamic–pituitary–adrenal (HPA) axis, increase oxidative stress in the hippocampus, reduce serotonin levels and create neurotoxic serotonergic metabolites (i.e. 3-hydroxy-kynurenine (3-HK) and quinolinic acid (QA)) (Dantzer et al., 2008; Eyre & Baune, 2012; Leonard & Maes, 2012; Miller et al., 2009; Moylan et al., 2013). Although this model suggests that anti-inflammatory treatments could alleviate symptoms of depression by reducing the net pro-inflammatory state in the brain, recent findings appear to be inconclusive on the clinical efficacy of anti-inflammatory treatments (Gallagher et al., 2012; Muller et al., 2006; 2011; Raison et al., 2012; Warner-Schmidt et al., 2011) and concerns of a blanket approach to anti-inflammatory treatments have been raised (Baune, 2015; Eyre & Baune, 2015; Eyre et al., 2014). This caution may also be due to the difference of immune alterations during various stages of depression, as discussed in the following.

In line with a pro-inflammatory state in the depressed brain is the neuroprogression model recently published by Moylan et al. (2013). This model suggests that a neuroprogressive process occurs in some patients with major depressive disorder (MDD), leading to poorer symptomatic, treatment and functional outcomes. In such patients, longer and more frequent episodes appear to increase vulnerability to develop further episodes (Kendler et al., 2001). The neuroprogressive nature of such a course of disease is believed to be associated with structural brain changes and changes in inflammatory, neurotransmission, oxidative and nitrosative stress pathways, neuroplasticity, HPA axis modulation and mitochondrial dysfunction (Maes et al., 2012; Moylan et al., 2013; Sheline et al., 2003; Videbech & Ravnkilde, 2004). However, this model of depression may only apply to a subgroup of patients diagnosed with depression.

Inflammation during Phases of Depression

Different phases of depression can be distinguished. A pre-clinical phase of depression is characterised by subthreshold symptoms and risk factors for the development of depression. In this phase, a proportion of people may not go on to develop a depressive episode, whereas some patients may develop a first or recurrent major depressive episode. When symptomatology is not self-limited and endures or reaches higher severity, an onset of a clinical phase of depression occurs during which the depressive symptoms may be mild, moderate or severe and may include melancholic, atypical, psychotic and non-melancholic symptomatology. This clinical phase can be a first episode for an individual; interestingly, studies suggest that 60–90 per cent of adolescents with depressive episode show remission within one year (Dunner et al., 2006; March et al., 2004). However, 50–70 per cent of remitted patients suffer one or more subsequent depressive episodes within five years (Lewinsohn et al., 2000). Importantly, only a few adults experience a full symptomatic and functional remission between depressive episodes with a high risk of long-term loss of function (Conradi et al., 2011; Fava et al., 2007). These data suggest that it is important to identify markers according to the phase or stage of the disease in order to predict the course of depression and to determine which patients may benefit from phase- and stage-specific interventions. The activity of innate and adaptive immune factors according to the phase and stage of depression is presented in Figures 8.4 and 8.5.

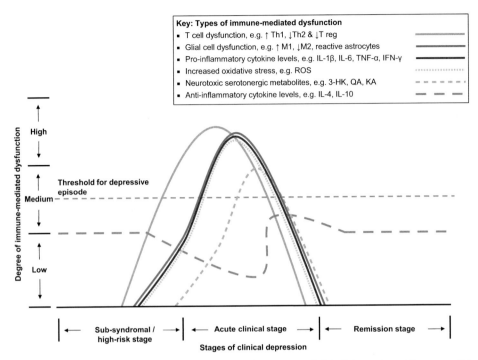

Figure 8.4 Dynamic changes of the immune response during stages of clinical depression until recovery. This figure represents an acute clinical depressive episode with full remission in the context of the three phases of the phase-specific neuroimmune model of clinical depression: sub-syndromal, acute clinical and remission stages as shown on the x-axis show the relevant phases; the y-axis shows the degree of immune-mediated dysfunction. The shaded lines represent the various types of immune-mediated dysfunction. The horizontal grey dashed line indicates an immune dysfunction threshold line whereby a clinically significant depressive episode is diagnosable. 3-HK, 3-hydroxykynurenine; IFN, interferon; IL, interleukin; KA, kynurenic acid; QA, quinolinic acid; ROS, reactive oxygen species; T reg, T regulatory cell; Th, T helper; TNF, tumour necrosis factor. *A black and white version of this figure will appear in some formats. For the colour version, please refer to the plate section.*

Neuroprotection and Neuroinflammation in Stages of Psychiatric Diseases

It is proposed that immune system-related pathophysiological changes in psychiatric disorders are due to impaired neuroprotective immune processes (Berger et al., 2003), as well as enhanced neuroinflammatory and possibly neurodegenerative (in some subgroups of patients) immune processes in various psychiatric disorders such as schizophrenia, depression and cognitive ageing.

In a multi-immune factor model involving cytokines, chemokines, glial cells and peripheral immune cells, it is suggested here that physiological, healthy adult conditions are associated with a positive balance of neuroprotective immune effects (see Figure 8.6). Physiological and healthy conditions are associated with increased IL-4, IL-10, neuroprotective functions of TNF-α (signalling via R2) and IL-6, increased levels of CNS- and Aβ-specific autoreactive CD4+ T cells, M2 microglia, quiescent astrocytes, increased CX3CL1, CD200 and insulin-like growth factor 1 (IGF-1). In addition, less neurodegenerative activity of TNF-α (signalling via R1), IL-1β, M1 microglia and reactive astrocytes is observed under physiological conditions.

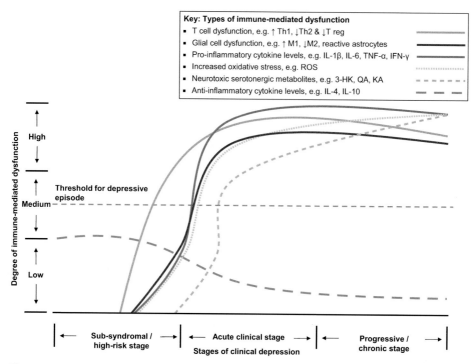

Figure 8.5 Progressive immune changes during a progressive course of clinical depression. This figure represents a chronic and progressive major depressive episode. The x-axis shows the relevant phases (sub-syndromal/ high-risk stage, acute clinical stage, progressive/chronic stage); the y-axis shows the degree of immune-mediated dysfunction. The shaded lines represent the various types of immune-mediated dysfunction. The horizontal grey dashed line indicates an immune dysfunction threshold line whereby a clinically significant depressive episode is diagnosable. 3-HK, 3-hydroxykynurenine; IFN, interferon; IL, interleukin; KA, kynurenic acid; QA, quinolinic acid; ROS, reactive oxygen species; T reg, T regulatory cell; Th, T helper; TNF, tumour necrosis factor. *A black and white version of this figure will appear in some formats. For the colour version, please refer to the plate section.*

On the other hand, during ageing conditions, cognitive decline appears to be associated with a predominantly neurodegenerative effect of immune factors. Age-related cognitive decline conditions are associated with increased CRP, TNF-α (via R1), IL-6, IL-1β, M1 microglia and reactive astrocytes, CCR2-deficiency monocytes and Th1 CD4+ T cells. There are lower levels of neuroprotective factors (listed above).

Based on the strong relationship between the neuroimmune system and other neuro-biological systems (i.e. neuroplasticity, neurotransmission, mitochondrial physiology, oxidative stress (Krstic & Knuesel, 2013; Liu et al., 2013; Monsonego et al., 2013; Naert & Rivest, 2013; Wyss-Coray & Rogers, 2012)), we believe age-related cognitive decline may exert immune-mediated detrimental effects on these systems. Age-related cognitive decline's neuroimmune effects are likely involved with reduced neuroplasticity, dysfunctional neurotransmission (i.e. increased glutamate), excessive Aβ and tau protein deposition, mitochondrial dysfunction and elevated oxidative stress, as reviewed above in detail.

The suggested model of balance/imbalance of neuroinflammation and neuroprotection during depression has several clinical and preventive implications. It is important to consider treatment and preventive strategies that may promote neuroprotective

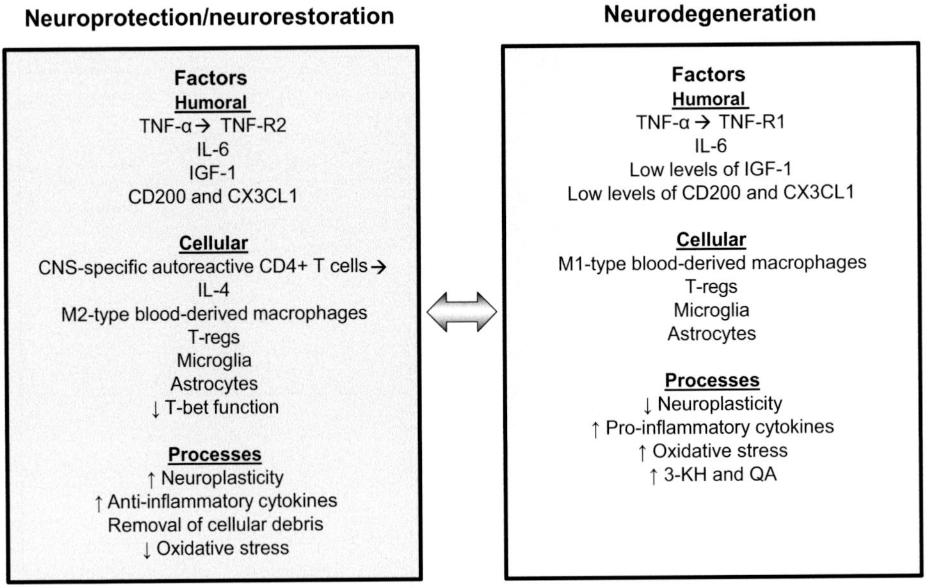

Neuroprotection/neurorestoration	Neurodegeneration
Factors	**Factors**
Humoral	**Humoral**
TNF-α → TNF-R2	TNF-α → TNF-R1
IL-6	IL-6
IGF-1	Low levels of IGF-1
CD200 and CX3CL1	Low levels of CD200 and CX3CL1
Cellular	**Cellular**
CNS-specific autoreactive CD4+ T cells →	M1-type blood-derived macrophages
IL-4	T-regs
M2-type blood-derived macrophages	Microglia
T-regs	Astrocytes
Microglia	
Astrocytes	**Processes**
↓ T-bet function	↓ Neuroplasticity
	↑ Pro-inflammatory cytokines
Processes	↑ Oxidative stress
↑ Neuroplasticity	↑ 3-KH and QA
↑ Anti-inflammatory cytokines	
Removal of cellular debris	
↓ Oxidative stress	

Figure 8.6 Mechanisms of neuroprotection and neurodegeneration. The figure presents that both humoral and cellular immune processes affect neurobiological, inflammatory and oxidative stress processes in specific ways either during neuroprotection or neurodegeneration. 3-KH, 3-hydroxykynurenine; CD200, OX-2 membrane glycoprotein, also named CD200 (cluster of differentiation 200); CD4+ T cells, T helper cells; CX3CL1, CXC3 chemokine receptor 1, also known as the fractalkine receptor or G-protein coupled receptor 13 (GPR13); IGF-1, insulin-like growth factor 1; IL-4, interleukin 4; IL-6, interleukin 6; QA, quinolinic acid; T-bet, a T cell-specific T-box transcription factor; T-regs, regulatory T cells; TNF-R1, tumor necrosis factor receptor 1; TNF-R2, tumor necrosis factor receptor 2; TNF-α, tumor necrosis factor alpha.

processes, and hence counterbalance neurodegenerative dysbalance. Physical activity (Erickson et al., 2013; Hamer et al., 2012), the Mediterranean diet (Lourida et al., 2013) and omega-3 PUFA supplementation (Loef & Walach, 2013) are treatment and preventive strategies that exert positive effects on the immune system. The Mediterranean diet (Barbaresko et al., 2013) and omega-3 PUFA supplementation (Calviello et al., 2013) have anti-inflammatory effects, as shown by a number of observational clinical studies. From an immunological perspective, physical activity (PA) has been shown to increase IL-10, IL-6 (acutely), MIF, CNS-specific autoreactive CD4+ T cells, M2 microglia, quiescent astrocytes, CX3CL1 and IGF-1 (Eyre et al., 2013). It is also shown to reduce Th1/Th2 balance, PICs, CRP, M1 microglia and reactive astrocytes (Eyre et al., 2013). A variety of other immune factors require further investigation. These include micro ribonucleic acid (miRNA) (Ponomarev et al., 2013), chemokines (Torres et al., 2012), CD200 (Blank & Prinz, 2013), IGF-1 (Park et al., 2011), glial cells (e.g. oligodendrocytes and astrocytes (Nagelhus et al., 2013)), peripheral immune cells (B cells, neutrophils) (Aguilar-Valles et al., 2014; Eyre & Baune, 2012) (Figure 8.7).

Anti-inflammatory Treatments According to Stages of Disease

Following on from the increasing and consistent evidence in support of an up-regulated pro-inflammatory environment in the above-mentioned conditions, the possible use of

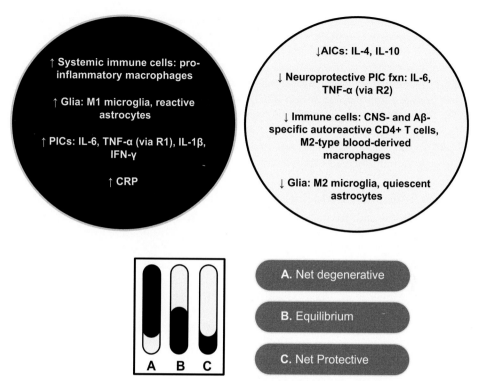

Figure 8.7 Balance and dysbalance of neuroprotective and neurodegenerative mechanisms. The figure indicates that depending on the degree and balance of neuroprotection and neurodegeneration, three stages can be distinguished: (1) net degenerative; (2) equilibrium; and (3) net protective.

anti-inflammatory drugs is gaining momentum in the scientific discussion and in clinical exploration as a treatment modality. However, anti-inflammatory treatments have so far been mainly explored in acute disease settings rather than throughout different disease stages. We will briefly review the main components of some of these interventions and make a suggestion where these interventions could possibly be useful. Moreover, the study base is very limited and inconclusive. Some possibilities will be discussed.

Omega-3 Polyunsaturated Fatty Acids

Omega-3 PUFAs are a potential prevention and treatment strategy; however, their mechanism of action is poorly understood (Freund-Levi et al., 2006; 2009; Orr et al., 2013). Omega-3 PUFAs exert beneficial effects on inflammation (Hjorth et al., 2013) through decreased expression of TNF-α, IL-6, IL-1β, reduced microglial activation and reduced astrocyte and monocyte PIC production (Gupta et al., 2012; Labrousse et al., 2012; Mizwicki et al., 2013). The effects on other humoral and cellular immune factors are poorly understood, but include improved Aβ phagocytosis, prevention of astrocyte dysfunction and senescence, and possibly microglial phagocytosis of Aβ (Hjorth et al., 2013; Latour et al., 2013; Mizwicki et al., 2013). Additionally, physical activity (Erickson et al., 2013; Hamer et al., 2012), the Mediterranean diet (Lourida et al., 2013) and omega-3 PUFA supplementation (Loef & Walach, 2013) are treatment and preventive strategies that exert positive effects on the immune system. The Mediterranean diet (Barbaresko et al., 2013) and omega-3 PUFA supplementation (Calviello et al., 2013) have anti-inflammatory effects, as shown by a number of observational clinical studies. It can therefore be speculated that these anti-inflammatory and neuroprotective effects may translate into clinical benefits. In support of such a translational notion is the finding that long-chain omega-3 PUFAs reduce the risk of progression to psychotic disorder and may offer a safe and efficacious strategy for indicated prevention in young people with subthreshold psychotic states (Amminger et al., 2010), and that decreased nervonic acid in erythrocyte membranes predicts psychosis in help-seeking ultra-high-risk individuals (Amminger et al., 2012).

Non-steroidal Anti-inflammatory Drugs (NSAIDs) Treatment

Given this clinical and mechanistic relationship between inflammation and depression, both selective cyclooxygenase (COX)-2 and non-selective COX inhibitor non-steroidal anti-inflammatory drugs (NSAIDs) have been investigated as possible adjuncts in the treatment of depression with antidepressants, yielding mixed results (Akhondzadeh et al., 2009; Almeida et al., 2010; 2012; Fields et al., 2012; Fond et al., 2014; Gallagher et al., 2012; Muller, 2013; Muller et al., 2006; Musil et al., 2011; Nery et al., 2008; Pasco et al., 2010; Shelton, 2012; Uher et al., 2012; Warner-Schmidt et al., 2011) and others have found detrimental effects suggesting NSAIDs may reduce the antidepressant effect of selective serotonin reuptake inhibitors (SSRIs) (Gallagher et al., 2012; Warner-Schmidt et al., 2011). These mixed results may be due to various reasons such as differing antidepressant utilisation and doses, the use of varying selective COX-2 and/or non-selective COX inhibitor NSAIDs, study design, age of study population, as well as study populations with varying degrees of depressive symptomatology and presence of general medication conditions.

In 2012, a Cochrane review evaluated the efficacy and side-effects of aspirin, steroidal and non-steroidal anti-inflammatory drugs in the treatment of Alzheimer's disease (AD), compared to placebo in 14 randomised controlled trials comprising 352, 138 and 1745 participants for aspirin, steroid and NSAIDs groups, respectively. The review showed no significant improvement in cognitive decline for aspirin, steroid, traditional NSAIDs and selective COX-2 inhibitors. Compared to controls, patients receiving aspirin experienced more bleeding while patients receiving steroid experienced more hyperglycaemia, abnormal lab results and face oedema. Patients receiving NSAIDs experienced nausea, vomiting, elevated creatinine, elevated LFT and hypertension. A trend towards higher death rates was observed among patients treated with NSAIDs compared with placebo and this was somewhat higher for selective COX-2 inhibitors than for traditional NSAIDs. Based on the comprehensive evaluation of these studies carried out so far, the authors concluded that the efficacy of aspirin, steroid and NSAIDs (traditional NSAIDs and COX-2 inhibitors) is not proven and cannot be recommended for the treatment of AD (Jaturapatporn et al., 2012).

Anti-inflammatory Interventions with Targeted Antagonists

A range of biological antagonists are available, such as infliximab and etanercept. Additionally anti-TNF therapy is being considered as an option in improving postoperative cognitive dysfunction (Terrando et al., 2010). Research into the effects of centrally and peripherally administered TNF-α blockade has shown clinical efficacy on cognition and depressive symptoms (Couch et al., 2013; Miller & Cole, 2012; Tobinick & Gross, 2008). In addition, a recently published trial in an animal model under peripheral lipopolysaccharide (LPS) stimulation showed that centrally administered etanercept reduced anxiety-like behaviours, but not spatial memory, and was associated with a decrease in hippocampal microglia numbers, being suggestive that etanercept recovers anxiety-like behaviour possibly mediated by a reduction of TNF-α-related central inflammation (Camara et al., 2015). However, there are two important problems limiting the clinical usefulness of these techniques. First, the blood–brain barrier prevents deep penetration into the CNS tissue; and second, basal levels of TNF-α are still required for normal functioning, and animal models have shown that the complete lack of TNF-α due to genetic modification results in cognitive impairment (Baune et al., 2008). This is possibly due to the influence that TNF-α exerts on nerve growth factor (NGF) and brain-derived neurotrophic factor (BDNF). Overall, this approach appears to be of limited use in early stages of psychiatric disorders, but may have a role in acute and progressive stages of the disease pending further studies (Figure 8.8).

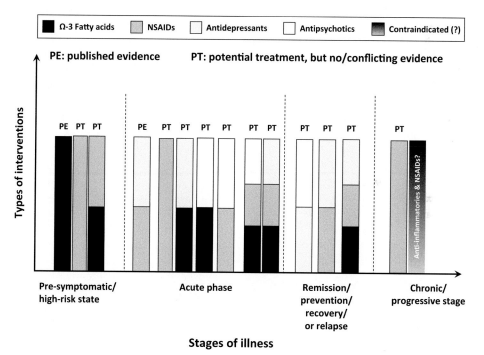

Figure 8.8 Anti-inflammatory interventions according to stages of mental illness. The figure shows various types of treatments with evidence-based or potential anti-inflammatory efficacy at various stages of psychiatric illnesses, such as psychosis and depressive/affective disorders. While evidence for omega-3 fatty acids has been published for prevention of transition to psychosis in high-risk states, their use during acute and post-acute stages lacks evidence. Likewise, NSAIDs, which are widely used during acute illness, could possibly also be used in combination with omega-3 fatty acids during pre-symptomatic/high-risk stages to prevent transition to full acute disease stages, as well as during remission and chronic stages for the prevention of relapse of illness and faster recovery. However, continuous use of NSAIDs for a longer period of time could potentially negatively affect the immune system and may enhance blood clotting; hence NSAIDs may be contraindicated for chronic use. Additionally, antidepressants and antipsychotics can be combined with NSAIDs and/or omega-3 fatty acids to control acute illness, and during remission/recovery and relapse prevention. Other possible treatments during a remission stage could be a combination of antidepressants and antipsychotics. An evidence-based treatment algorithm using the above interventions alone or in combination is still lacking and requires extensive future investigations and clinical trials.

Conclusions

The staging model of mental illness is developing beyond the clinical level, aiming to include biological processes and markers that may reflect the dynamic biological processes of stages of mental illness. The neurobiology of inflammation in mental illness has gained much attention in recent years. Since neuroinflammation has been shown to be an important possible feature of psychosis, schizophrenia and depression, it was attempted to map changes and dysregulation of the immune system and inflammation to the different clinical stages of severe mental illness. The literature suggests that an increased inflammatory response may define a subgroup of individuals in ultra-high-risk states, in acute disease episodes and in those with severe mental illness. In addition, the literature clearly points to the dynamic nature of the immune response in mental illness and shows an involvement of both the innate and adaptive immune system in mental illness. A focus on inflammation only might be shortsighted. While it has been shown that inflammation can be detrimental to the neurobiology of the brain, it has also been suggested that inflammation may lead to an increase in impaired neuroprotective mechanisms; hence the concept of enhancing the restoration of neuroprotection plus a reduction in inflammation may be an extended avenue for future interventions. While progress has been made in the understanding of the role of inflammation in mental illness, the dynamic nature of immune response during different stages of mental illness may require an indicated approach of interventions rather than a blanket 'anti-inflammatory' approach according to both the dynamic stages of the immune response and clinical stages of mental illness.

References

Aguliar-Valles, A., Kim, J., Jung, S., Woodside, B., & Luheshi, G. N. (2014). Role of brain transmigrating neutrophils in depression-like behavior during systemic infection. *Molecular Psychiatry,* **19**(5), 599–606.

Akhondzadeh, S., Jafari, S., Raisi, F., Nasehi, A. A., Ghoreishi, A., Salehi, B., . . . Kamalipour, A. (2009). Clinical trial of adjunctive celecoxib treatment in patients with major depression: a double blind and placebo controlled trial. *Depression and Anxiety,* **26**(7), 607–611.

Almeida, O. P., Alfonso, H., Jamrozik, K., Hankey, G. J., & Flicker, L. (2010). Aspirin use, depression, and cognitive impairment in later life: the health in men study. *Journal of the American Geriatrics Society,* **58**(5), 990–992.

Almeida, O. P., Flicker, L., Yeap, B. B., Alfonso, H., McCaul, K., & Hankey, G. J. (2012). Aspirin decreases the risk of depression in older men with high plasma homocysteine. *Translational Psychiatry,* **2**, e151.

Amminger, G. P., Schafer, M. R., Klier, C. M., Slavik, J. M., Holzer, I., Holub, M., . . . Berk, M. (2012). Decreased nervonic acid levels in erythrocyte membranes predict psychosis in help-seeking ultra-high-risk individuals. *Molecular Psychiatry,* **17**(12), 1150–1152.

Amminger, G. P., Schafer, M. R., Papageorgiou, K., Klier, C. M., Cotton, S. M., Harrigan, S. M., . . . Berger, G. E. (2010). Long-chain omega-3 fatty acids for indicated prevention of psychotic disorders: a randomized, placebo-controlled trial. *Archives of General Psychiatry,* **67**(2), 146–154.

Arion, D., Unger, T., Lewis, D. A., Levitt, P., & Mirnics, K. (2007). Molecular evidence for increased expression of genes related to immune and chaperone function in the prefrontal cortex in schizophrenia. *Biological Psychiatry,* **62**(7), 711–721.

Barbaresko, J., Koch, M., Schulze, M. B., & Nothlings, U. (2013). Dietary pattern analysis and biomarkers of low-grade inflammation: a systematic literature review. *Nutrition Reviews,* **71**(8), 511–527.

Baune, B. (2009). Conceptual challenges of a tentative model of stress-induced depression. *PLoS One,* **4**(1), e4266.

Baune, B. T. (2015). Inflammation and neurodegenerative disorders: is there still hope for therapeutic intervention? *Current Opinion in Psychiatry,* **28**(2), 148–154.

Baune, B. T., Wiede, F., Braun, A., Golledge, J., Arolt, V., & Koerner, H. (2008). Cognitive dysfunction in mice deficient for TNF- and its receptors. *American Journal of Medical Genetics Part B: Neuropsychiatric Genetics,* **147B**(7), 1056–1064.

Berger, G. E., Wood, S., & McGorry, P. (2003). Incipient neurovulnerability and neuroprotection in early psychosis. *Psychopharmacology Bulletin,* **37**(2), 79–101.

Berger, G. E., Wood, S. J., Wellard, R. M., Proffitt, T. M., McConchie, M., Amminger, G. P., . . . McGorry, P. D. (2008). Ethyl-eicosapentaenoic acid in first-episode psychosis: a 1H-MRS study. *Neuropsychopharmacology,* **33**(10), 2467–2473.

Berk, M., Copolov, D., Dean, O., Lu, K., Jeavons, S., Schapkaitz, I., . . . Bush, A. (2008). N-acetyl cysteine as a glutathione precursor for schizophrenia: a double-blind, randomized, placebo-controlled trial. *Biological Psychiatry,* **64**, 361–368.

Bertelsen, M., Jeppesen, P., Petersen, L., Thorup, A., Ohlenschlaeger, J., le Quach, P., . . . Nordentoft, M. (2008). Five-year follow-up of a randomized multicenter trial of intensive early intervention vs standard treatment for patients with a first episode of psychotic illness: the OPUS trial. *Archives of General Psychiatry,* **65**(7), 762–771.

Blank, T., & Prinz, M. (2013). Microglia as modulators of cognition and neuropsychiatric disorders. *Glia,* **61**(1), 62–70.

Borovcanin, M., Jovanovic, I., Radosavljevic, G., Djukic Dejanovic, S., Bankovic, D., Arsenijevic, N., & Lukic, M. L. (2012). Elevated serum level of type-2 cytokine and low IL-17 in first episode psychosis and schizophrenia in relapse. *Journal of Psychiatric Research,* **46**(11), 1421–1426.

Calviello, G., Su, H. M., Weylandt, K. H., Fasano, E., Serini, S., & Cittadini, A. (2013). Experimental evidence of omega-3 polyunsaturated fatty acid modulation of inflammatory cytokines and bioactive lipid mediators: their potential role in inflammatory, neurodegenerative, and neoplastic diseases. *BioMed Research International,* **2013**, 743171.

Camara, M. L., Corrigan, F., Jaehne, E. J., Jawahar, M. C., Anscomb, H., & Baune, B. T. (2015). Effects of centrally administered etanercept on behavior, microglia, and astrocytes in mice following a peripheral immune challenge. *Neuropsychopharmacology,* **40**(2), 502–512.

Clark, S. R., Schubert, K. O., & Baune, B. T. (2015). Towards indicated prevention of psychosis: using probabilistic assessments of transition risk in psychosis prodrome. *Journal of Neural Transmission,* **122**(1), 155–169.

Conradi, H. J., Ormel, J., & De Jonge, P. (2011). Presence of individual (residual) symptoms during depressive episodes and periods of remission: a 3-year prospective study. *Psychological Medicine,* **41**(6), 1165–1174.

Couch, Y., Anthony, D. C., Dolgov, O., Revischin, A., Festoff, B., Santos, A. I., . . . Strekalova, T. (2013). Microglial activation, increased TNF and SERT expression in the prefrontal cortex define stress-altered behaviour in mice susceptible to anhedonia. *Brain, Behavior, and Immunity,* **29**, 136–146.

Dantzer, R., O'Connor, J. C., Freund, G. G., Johnson, R. W., & Kelley, K. W. (2008). From inflammation to sickness and depression: when the immune system subjugates the brain. *Nature Reviews Neuroscience,* **9**(1), 46–56.

Do, K. Q., Trabesinger, A. H., Kirsten-Krüger, M., Lauer, C. J., Dydak, U., Hell, D., . . . Cuénod, M. (2000). Schizophrenia: glutathione deficit in cerebrospinal fluid and prefrontal cortex in vivo. *European Journal of Neuroscience,* **12**, 3721–3728.

Dunner, D. L., Rush, A. J., Russell, J. M., Burke, M., Woodard, S., Wingard, P., & Allen, J. (2006). Prospective, long-term, multicenter study of the naturalistic outcomes of patients with treatment-resistant depression. *Journal of Clinical Psychiatry, 67*(5), 688–695.

Erickson, K. I., Gildengers, A. G., & Butters, M. A. (2013). Physical activity and brain plasticity in late adulthood. *Dialogues in Clinical Neuroscience, 15*(1), 99–108.

Eyre, H. A., Air, T., Proctor, S., Rositano, S., & Baune, B. T. (2014). A critical review of the efficacy of non-steroidal anti-inflammatory drugs in depression. *Progress in Neuro-Psychopharmacology and Biological Psychiatry, 57C*, 11–16.

Eyre, H., & Baune, B. T. (2012). Neuroplastic changes in depression: a role for the immune system. *Psychoneuroendocrinology, 37*(9), 1397–1416.

Eyre, H. A., & Baune, B. T. (2015). Anti-inflammatory intervention in depression. *JAMA Psychiatry, 72*(5), 511.

Eyre, H., Papps, E., & Baune, B. T. (2013). Treating depression and depression-like behaviour with physical activity: an immune perspective. *Frontiers in Psychiatry, 4*, 3.

Fava, G. A., Ruini, C., & Belaise, C. (2007). The concept of recovery in major depression. *Psychological Medicine, 37*(3), 307–317.

Fields, C., Drye, L., Vaidya, V., & Lyketsos, C. (2012). Celecoxib or naproxen treatment does not benefit depressive symptoms in persons age 70 and older: findings from a randomized controlled trial. *American Journal of Geriatric Psychiatry, 20*(6), 505–513.

Flatow, J., Buckley, P., & Miller, B. J. (2013). Meta-analysis of oxidative stress in schizophrenia. *Biological Psychiatry, 74*, 400–409.

Fond, G., Hamdani, N., Kapczinski, F., Boukouaci, W., Drancourt, N., Dargel, A., . . . Leboyer, M. (2014). Effectiveness and tolerance of anti-inflammatory drugs' add-on therapy in major mental disorders: a systematic qualitative review. *Acta Psychiatrica Scandinavica, 129*(3), 163–179.

Freund-Levi, Y., Eriksdotter-Jonhagen, M., Cederholm, T., Basun, H., Faxen-Irving, G., Garlind, A., . . . Palmblad, J. (2006). Omega-3 fatty acid treatment in 174 patients with mild to moderate Alzheimer disease: OmegAD study – a randomized double-blind trial. *Archives of Neurology, 63*(10), 1402–1408.

Freund-Levi, Y., Hjorth, E., Lindberg, C., Cederholm, T., Faxen-Irving, G., Vedin, I., . . . Eriksdotter Jonhagen, M. (2009). Effects of omega-3 fatty acids on inflammatory markers in cerebrospinal fluid and plasma in Alzheimer's disease: the OmegAD study. *Dementia and Geriatric Cognitive Disorders, 27*(5), 481–490.

Gallagher, P. J., Castro, V., Fava, M., Weilburg, J. B., Murphy, S. N., Gainer, V. S., . . . Perlis, R. H. (2012). Antidepressant response in patients with major depression exposed to NSAIDs: a pharmacovigilance study. *American Journal of Psychiatry, 169*(10), 1065–1072.

Garcia-Rizo, C., Fernandez-Egea, E., Oliveira, C., Justicia, A., Bernardo, M., & Kirkpatrick, B. (2012). Inflammatory markers in antipsychotic-naïve patients with nonaffective psychosis and deficit vs. nondeficit features. *Psychiatry Research, 198*(2), 212–215.

Gupta, S., Knight, A. G., Keller, J. N., & Bruce-Keller, A. J. (2012). Saturated long-chain fatty acids activate inflammatory signaling in astrocytes. *Journal of Neurochemistry, 120*(6), 1060–1071.

Hamer, M., Sabia, S., Batty, G. D., Shipley, M. J., Tabak, A. G., Singh-Manoux, A., & Kivimaki, M. (2012). Physical activity and inflammatory markers over 10 years: follow-up in men and women from the Whitehall II cohort study. *Circulation, 126*(8), 928–933.

Haroon, E., Raison, C. L., & Miller, A. H. (2012). Psychoneuroimmunology meets neuropsychopharmacology: translational implications of the impact of inflammation on behavior. *Neuropsychopharmacology, 37*(1), 137–162.

Hegelstad, W. T., Larsen, T. K., Auestad, B., Evensen, J., Haahr, U., Joa, I., . . . McGlashan, T. (2012). Long-term follow-up of the TIPS early detection in psychosis study: effects on 10-year outcome. *American Journal of Psychiatry, 169*(4), 374–380.

Hjorth, E., Zhu, M., Toro, V. C., Vedin, I., Palmblad, J., Cederholm, T., . . . Schultzberg, M. (2013). Omega-3 fatty acids enhance phagocytosis of Alzheimer's disease-related amyloid-beta42 by human microglia and decrease inflammatory markers. *Journal of Alzheimer's Disease,* **35**(4), 697–713.

Insel, T. (2007). The arrival of preemptive psychiatry. *Early Intervention in Psychiatry,* **1**, 5–6.

Jaturapatporn, D., Isaac, M. G., McCleery, J., & Tabet, N. (2012). Aspirin, steroidal and non-steroidal anti-inflammatory drugs for the treatment of Alzheimer's disease. *Cochrane Database of Systematic Reviews,* **2**, CD006378.

Kendler, K. S., Thornton, L. M., & Gardner, C. O. (2001). Genetic risk, number of previous depressive episodes, and stressful life events in predicting onset of major depression. *American Journal of Psychiatry,* **158**(4), 582–586.

Keshavan, M. S., Sanders, R. D., Pettegrew, J. W., Dombrowsky, S. M., & Panchalingam, K. (1993). Frontal lobe metabolism and cerebral morphology in schizophrenia: 31P MRS and MRI studies. *Schizophrenia Research,* **10**, 241–246.

Kiecolt-Glaser, J. K., Epel, E. S., Belury, M. A., Andridge, R., Lin, J., Glaser, R., ... Blackburn, E. (2013). Omega-3 fatty acids, oxidative stress, and leukocyte telomere length: a randomized controlled trial. *Brain, Behavior, and Immunity,* **28**, 16–24.

Krstic, D., & Knuesel, I. (2013). Deciphering the mechanism underlying late-onset Alzheimer disease. *Nature Reviews: Neurology,* **9**(1), 25–34.

Labrousse, V. F., Nadjar, A., Joffre, C., Costes, L., Aubert, A., Gregoire, S., ... Laye, S. (2012). Short-term long chain omega3 diet protects from neuroinflammatory processes and memory impairment in aged mice. *PLoS One,* **7**(5), e36861.

Larsen, T. K., Melle, I., Auestad, B., Haahr, U., Joa, I., Johannessen, J. O., ... McGlashan, T. (2011). Early detection of psychosis: positive effects on 5-year outcome. *Psychological Medicine,* **41**(7), 1461–1469.

Latour, A., Grintal, B., Champeil-Potokar, G., Hennebelle, M., Lavialle, M., Dutar, P., ... Denis, I. (2013). Omega-3 fatty acids

deficiency aggravates glutamatergic synapse and astroglial aging in the rat hippocampal CA1. *Aging Cell,* **12**(1), 76–84.

Lavoie, S., Berger, M., Schlögelhofer, M., Schäfer, M. R., Rice, S., Kim, S. W., ... Amminger, G. P. (2017). Erythrocyte glutathione levels as long-term predictor of transition to psychosis. *Translational Psychiatry,* **7**(3), e1064.

Leonard, B., & Maes, M. (2012). Mechanistic explanations how cell-mediated immune activation, inflammation and oxidative and nitrosative stress pathways and their sequels and concomitants play a role in the pathophysiology of unipolar depression. *Neuroscience and Biobehavioral Reviews,* **36**(2), 764–785.

Lewinsohn, P. M., Rohde, P., Seeley, J. R., Klein, D. N., & Gotlib, I. H. (2000). Natural course of adolescent major depressive disorder in a community sample: predictors of recurrence in young adults. *American Journal of Psychiatry,* **157**(10), 1584–1591.

Libov, I., Miodownik, C., Bersudsky, Y., Dwolatzky T., Lerner, V. (2007). Efficacy of piracetam in the treatment of tardive dyskinesia in schizophrenic patients: a randomized, double-blind, placebo-controlled crossover study. *Journal of Clinical Psychiatry,* **68**, 1031–1037.

Liu, Y. H., Zeng, F., Wang, Y. R., Zhou, H. D., Giunta, B., Tan, J., & Wang, Y. J. (2013). Immunity and Alzheimer's disease: immunological perspectives on the development of novel therapies. *Drug Discovery Today,* **18**(23–24), 1212–1220.

Loef, M., & Walach, H. (2013). The omega-6/omega-3 ratio and dementia or cognitive decline: a systematic review on human studies and biological evidence. *Journal of Nutrition in Gerontology and Geriatrics,* **32**(1), 1–23.

Lourida, I., Soni, M., Thompson-Coon, J., Purandare, N., Lang, I. A., Ukoumunne, O. C., & Llewellyn, D. J. (2013). Mediterranean diet, cognitive function, and dementia: a systematic review. *Epidemiology,* **24**(4), 479–489.

Maes, M., Mihaylova, I., Kubera, M., & Ringel, K. (2012). Activation of cell-mediated immunity in depression: association with inflammation, melancholia, clinical staging and the fatigue and somatic symptom cluster of depression. *Progress in Neuro-Psychopharmacology and Biological Psychiatry, 36*(1), 169–175.

Mahar, I., Bambico, F. R., Mechawar, N., & Nobrega, J. N. (2014). Stress, serotonin, and hippocampal neurogenesis in relation to depression and antidepressant effects. *Neuroscience and Biobehavioral Reviews, 38,* 173–192.

March, J., Silva, S., Petrycki, S., Curry, J., Wells, K., Fairbank, J., . . . Treatment for Adolescents with Depression Study Team. (2004). Fluoxetine, cognitive-behavioral therapy, and their combination for adolescents with depression: treatment for Adolescents with Depression Study (TADS) randomized controlled trial. *JAMA, 292*(7), 807–820.

McAfoose, J., & Baune, B. T. (2009). Evidence for a cytokine model of cognitive function. *Neuroscience and Biobehavioral Reviews, 33* (3), 355–366.

McGorry, P. D. (2007). Issues for DSM-V: clinical staging – a heuristic pathway to valid nosology and safer, more effective treatment in psychiatry. *American Journal of Psychiatry, 164*(6), 859–860.

McGorry, P. D., Hickie, I. B., Yung, A. R., Pantelis, C., & Jackson, H. J. (2006). Clinical staging of psychiatric disorders: a heuristic framework for choosing earlier, safer and more effective interventions. *Australian and New Zealand Journal of Psychiatry, 40*(8), 616–622.

McGorry, P., Keshavan, M., Goldstone, S., Amminger, P., Allott, K., Berk, M., . . . Hickie, I. (2014). Biomarkers and clinical staging in psychiatry. *World Psychiatry, 13* (3), 211–223.

McGorry, P. D., Nelson, B., Goldstone, S., & Yung, A. R. (2010). Clinical staging: a heuristic and practical strategy for new research and better health and social outcomes for psychotic and related mood disorders. *Canadian Journal of Psychiatry, 55* (8), 486–497.

Miller, A. H., Maletic, V., & Raison, C. L. (2009). Inflammation and its discontents: the role of cytokines in the pathophysiology of major depression. *Biological Psychiatry, 65*(9), 732–741.

Miller, B. J., Buckley, P., Seabolt, W., Mellor, A., & Kirkpatrick, B. (2011). Meta-analysis of cytokine alterations in schizophrenia: clinical status and antipsychotic effects. *Biological Psychiatry, 70*(7), 663–671.

Miller, B. J., Culpepper, N., & Rapaport, M. H. (2014). C-reactive protein levels in schizophrenia. *Clinical Schizophrenia & Related Psychoses, 7,* 223–230.

Miller, G. E., & Cole, S. W. (2012). Clustering of depression and inflammation in adolescents previously exposed to childhood adversity. *Biological Psychiatry, 72*(1), 34–40.

Mizwicki, M. T., Liu, G., Fiala, M., Magpantay, L., Sayre, J., Siani, A., . . . Teplow, D. B. (2013). 1alpha,25-dihydroxyvitamin D3 and resolvin D1 retune the balance between amyloid-beta phagocytosis and inflammation in Alzheimer's disease patients. *Journal of Alzheimer's Disease, 34*(1), 155–170.

Monji, A., Kato, T., & Kanba, S. (2009). Cytokines and schizophrenia: microglia hypothesis of schizophrenia. *Psychiatry and Clinical Neurosciences, 63*(3), 257–265.

Monsonego, A., Nemirovsky, A., & Harpaz, I. (2013). CD4 T cells in immunity and immunotherapy of Alzheimer's disease. *Immunology, 139*(4), 438–446.

Moylan, S., Berk, M., Dean, O. M., Samuni, Y., Williams, L. J., O'Neil, A., . . . Maes, M. (2014). Oxidative & nitrosative stress in depression: why so much stress? *Neuroscience and Biobehavioral Reviews, 45C,* 46–62.

Moylan, S., Maes, M., Wray, N. R., & Berk, M. (2013). The neuroprogressive nature of major depressive disorder: pathways to disease evolution and resistance, and therapeutic implications. *Molecular Psychiatry, 18*(5), 595–606.

Muller, N. (2013). The role of anti-inflammatory treatment in psychiatric disorders. *Psychiatria Danubina, 25*(3), 292–298.

Muller, N., Myint, A. M., & Schwarz, M. J. (2011). Inflammatory biomarkers and depression. *Neurotoxicity Research, 19*(2), 308–318.

Muller, N., Myint, A. M., & Schwarz, M. J. (2012). Inflammation in schizophrenia. *Advances in Protein Chemistry and Structural Biology, 88*, 49–68.

Muller, N., Riedel, M., Scheppach, C., Brandstatter, B., Sokullu, S., Krampe, K., . . . Schwarz, M. J. (2002). Beneficial antipsychotic effects of celecoxib add-on therapy compared to risperidone alone in schizophrenia. *American Journal of Psychiatry, 159*(6), 1029–1034.

Muller, N., Schwarz, M. J., Dehning, S., Douhe, A., Cerovecki, A., Goldstein-Muller, B., . . . Riedel, M. (2006). The cyclooxygenase-2 inhibitor celecoxib has therapeutic effects in major depression: results of a double-blind, randomized, placebo controlled, add-on pilot study to reboxetine. *Molecular Psychiatry, 11* (7), 680–684.

Musil, R., Schwarz, M. J., Riedel, M., Dehning, S., Cerovecki, A., Spellmann, I., . . . Muller, N. (2011). Elevated macrophage migration inhibitory factor and decreased transforming growth factor-beta levels in major depression: no influence of celecoxib treatment. *Journal of Affective Disorders, 134* (1–3), 217–225.

Naert, G., & Rivest, S. (2013). A deficiency in CCR2+ monocytes: the hidden side of Alzheimer's disease. *Journal of Molecular Cell Biology, 5*(5), 284–293.

Nagelhus, E. A., Amiry-Moghaddam, M., Bergersen, L. H., Bjaalie, J. G., Eriksson, J., Gundersen, V., . . . Tonjum, T. (2013). The glia doctrine: addressing the role of glial cells in healthy brain ageing. *Mechanisms of Ageing and Development, 134*(10), 449–459.

Nery, F. G., Monkul, E. S., Hatch, J. P., Fonseca, M., Zunta-Soares, G. B., Frey, B. N., . . . Soares, J. C. (2008). Celecoxib as an adjunct in the treatment of depressive or mixed episodes of bipolar disorder: a double-blind, randomized, placebo-controlled study. *Human Psychopharmacology, 23*(2), 87–94.

Norman, R. M., Manchanda, R., Malla, A. K., Windell, D., Harricharan, R., & Northcott, S. (2011). Symptom and functional outcomes for a 5 year early intervention program for psychoses. *Schizophrenia Research, 129*(2–3), 111–115.

Orr, S. K., Trepanier, M. O., & Bazinet, R. P. (2013). n-3 polyunsaturated fatty acids in animal models with neuroinflammation. *Prostaglandins, Leukotrienes and Essential Fatty Acids, 88*(1), 97–103.

Park, S. E., Dantzer, R., Kelley, K. W., & McCusker, R. H. (2011). Central administration of insulin-like growth factor-I decreases depressive-like behavior and brain cytokine expression in mice. *Journal of Neuroinflammation, 8*, 12.

Pasco, J. A., Jacka, F. N., Williams, L. J., Henry, M. J., Nicholson, G. C., Kotowicz, M. A., & Berk, M. (2010). Clinical implications of the cytokine hypothesis of depression: the association between use of statins and aspirin and the risk of major depression. *Psychotherapy and Psychosomatics, 79*(5), 323–325.

Ponomarev, E. D., Veremeyko, T., & Weiner, H. L. (2013). MicroRNAs are universal regulators of differentiation, activation, and polarization of microglia and macrophages in normal and diseased CNS. *Glia, 61*(1), 91–103.

Raison, C. L., Rutherford, R. E., Woolwine, B. J., Shuo, C., Schettler, P., Drake, D. F., . . . Miller, A. H. (2012). A randomized controlled trial of the tumor necrosis factor antagonist infliximab for treatment-resistant depression: the role of baseline inflammatory biomarkers. *Archives of General Psychiatry, 70*, 31–41.

Ripke, S., Sanders, A. R., Kendler, K. S., Levinson, D. F., Sklar, P., Holmans, P. A., . . . Cichon, S. (2011). Genome-wide association study identifies five new schizophrenia loci. *Nature Genetics, 43*(10), 969–976.

Saetre, P., Emilsson, L., Axelsson, E., Kreuger, J., Lindholm, E., & Jazin, E. (2007). Inflammation-related genes up-regulated in schizophrenia brains. *BMC Psychiatry, 7*, 46.

Schubert, K. O., Clark, S. R., & Baune, B. T. (2015). The use of clinical and biological characteristics to predict outcome following first episode psychosis. *Australian and New Zealand Journal of Psychiatry, 49* (1), 24–35.

Shamir, E., Barak, Y., Shalman, I., Laudon, M., Zisapel, N., Tarrasch, R., . . . Weizman, R. (2001). Melatonin treatment for tardive dyskinesia: a double-blind, placebo-controlled, crossover study. *Archives of General Psychiatry, 58,* 1049–1052.

Sheline, Y. I., Gado, M. H., & Kraemer, H. C. (2003). Untreated depression and hippocampal volume loss. *American Journal of Psychiatry,* **160**(8), 1516–1518.

Shelton, R. C. (2012). Does concomitant use of NSAIDs reduce the effectiveness of antidepressants? *American Journal of Psychiatry,* **169**(10), 1012–1015.

Shi, J., Levinson, D. F., Duan, J., Sanders, A. R., Zheng, Y., Pe'er, I., ... Gejman, P. V. (2009). Common variants on chromosome 6p22.1 are associated with schizophrenia. *Nature,* **460**, 753–757.

Slavich, G. M., & Irwin, M. R. (2014). From stress to inflammation and major depressive disorder: a social signal transduction theory of depression. *Psychological Bulletin,* **140**(3), 774–815.

Stojanovic, A., Martorell, L., Montalvo, I., Ortega, L., Monseny, R., Vilella, E., & Labad, J. (2014). Increased serum interleukin-6 levels in early stages of psychosis: associations with at-risk mental states and the severity of psychotic symptoms. *Psychoneuroendocrinology,* **41**, 23–32.

Terrando, N., Monaco, C., Ma, D., Foxwell, B. M., Feldmann, M., & Maze, M. (2010). Tumor necrosis factor-alpha triggers a cytokine cascade yielding postoperative cognitive decline. *Proceedings of the National Academy of Sciences of the United States of America,* **107**(47), 20518–20522.

Tobinick, E. L., & Gross, H. (2008). Rapid cognitive improvement in Alzheimer's disease following perispinal etanercept administration. *Journal of Neuroinflammation,* **5**, 2.

Torres, K. C., Santos, R. R., de Lima, G. S., Ferreira, R. O., Mapa, F. C., Pereira, P. A., ... Romano-Silva, M. A. (2012). Decreased expression of CCL3 in monocytes and CCR5

in lymphocytes from frontotemporal dementia as compared with Alzheimer's disease patients. *Journal of Neuropsychiatry and Clinical Neurosciences,* **24**(3), E11–E12.

Uher, R., Carver, S., Power, R. A., Mors, O., Maier, W., Rietschel, M., ... McGuffin, P. (2012). Non-steroidal anti-inflammatory drugs and efficacy of antidepressants in major depressive disorder. *Psychological Medicine,* **42**(10), 2027–2035.

Videbech, P., & Ravnkilde, B. (2004). Hippocampal volume and depression: a meta-analysis of MRI studies. *American Journal of Psychiatry,* **161**(11), 1957–1966.

Warner-Schmidt, J. L., Vanover, K. E., Chen, E. Y., Marshall, J. J., & Greengard, P. (2011). Antidepressant effects of selective serotonin reuptake inhibitors (SSRIs) are attenuated by antiinflammatory drugs in mice and humans. *Proceedings of the National Academy of Sciences of the United States of America,* **108**(22), 9262–9267.

Wyss-Coray, T., & Rogers, J. (2012). Inflammation in Alzheimer disease: a brief review of the basic science and clinical literature. *Cold Spring Harbor Perspectives in Medicine,* **2**(1), a006346.

Xu, M., & He, L. (2010). Convergent evidence shows a positive association of interleukin-1 gene complex locus with susceptibility to schizophrenia in the Caucasian population. *Schizophrenia Research,* **120**(1–3), 131–142.

Yao, J. K., & Keshavan, M. S. (2011). Antioxidants, redox signaling, and pathophysiology in schizophrenia: an integrative view. *Antioxidants & Redox Signaling,* **15**, 2011–2035.

Zhang, X. Y., Zhou, D. F., Cao, L. Y., Xu, C. Q., Chen, D. C., & Wu, G. Y. (2004). The effect of vitamin E treatment on tardive dyskinesia and blood superoxide dismutase: a double-blind placebo-controlled trial. *Journal of Clinical Psychopharmacology,* **24**, 83–86.

Chapter

9

Bioactive and Inflammatory Markers in Emerging Psychotic Disorders

Gregor E. Berger

Introduction

The quest for biological markers in psychiatry has been disappointing (Keshavan et al., 2005). Despite over a century of intensive research, no single biological marker has successfully translated into daily clinical practice. One of the key challenges in psychiatric research is that traditional diagnostic categories represent phenomenological constructs that do not necessarily circumscribe a biological homogeneous entity, but encompass a whole range of disorders presenting with similar phenotypes. This was highlighted in 1911 by Eugen Bleuler, who reported in his seminal book, *Dementia Praecox or the Group of Schizophrenias* (German: *Dementia praecox oder die Gruppe der Schizophrenien*), that schizophrenia is not a single disease entity, but a group of disorders with different courses and different presentations (Bleuler, 1950). The quest to find biological markers to better characterise heterogeneous entities such as schizophrenia-spectrum disorders has resulted in several thousand papers (Schmitt et al., 2017), trying to overcome the limitations of purely psychopathological-based approaches. A range of markers have been explored, including rapid eye movement, electro-dermal activity, electrophysiological markers such as event-related brain potentials, cognitive markers such as attention or memory deficits, brain imaging markers ranging from structural, functional to metabolic imaging, as well as metabolic and genetic markers. Despite these attempts, all approaches have failed to identify a single diagnostic biological marker for any psychiatric disorder.

The recent Research Domain Criteria (RDoC) initiative (Carcone & Ruocco, 2017) tries to address some of these conceptual limitations of current diagnostic categories in psychiatry by establishing a research framework for new ways of studying and understanding mental disorders. The RDoC tries to integrate many levels of information (from genomics to psychopathology) to better understand basic dimensions of functioning underlying the full range of human behaviours from normal to abnormal. To a certain extent, the RDoC approach abandons the categorical diagnostic approach that has been applied over more than a century and attempts to better understand common underlying pathological processes that may lead to the identification of novel neurobiological targets that are of prognostic and therapeutic relevance.

What Can We Learn from Oncology?

A more clinically focused framework complementary to the RDoC approach is to investigate the different stages of mental disorders from a developmental perspective using a staging model (Nelson et al., 2017). This approach is well established in other areas of medicine such as oncology. In cancer, staging is a routine component of daily clinical practice that is informed by biological markers, providing the basis for prognosis and therapeutic options across different stages of particular tumour types and stages. A key example of a clinically relevant biomarker is the prostate-specific antigen (PSA) in pT3N0M0 prostate cancer survivors. The PSA level informs affected patients and doctors after radical prostatectomy about a biochemical relapse, providing two potential treatment pathways. In the first option, patients can start radiation therapy (RT) directly after radical prostatectomy, called adjuvant radiotherapy, the current recommended standard treatment of a T3N0M0 stage prostate cancer. The second option is a more experimental approach called early salvage radiotherapy, which starts RT as soon as the PSA level starts to rise. In stark contrast, psychiatry is far away from such differentiated approaches to screening for disease, to stage the illness more accurately, to define subgroups for personalised treatment or to detect relapse or progression of the illness. Given the high burden of disease associated with emerging and potentially chronic mental disorders and the devastating consequences of relapses and disability, we are in urgent need of such marker-driven approaches that are linked to various stages of mental illness. The potential benefits are enormous, with biological markers informing clinicians and patients about prognosis and treatment choices. However, at this stage we lack such markers, which will inevitably span existing diagnostic categories.

Implications for Early Intervention in Psychiatry

In oncology, in later stages of disease in particular, patients are agreeable to performing very invasive treatments such as operations, chemotherapy or radiotherapy, even if the beneficial effect in terms of overall survival rate is often limited (Hamdy et al., 2016; Wilt et al., 2017). Psychiatry faces the opposite problem. Although some of our treatments (e.g. stimulants for ADHD, or mood stabilisers for bipolar affective disorders, or antidepressants in relapse prevention of recurrent depression) have excellent evidence-based efficacy as well as relatively better safety profiles, patients seem to weigh this evidence-based knowledge differently compared to cancer treatments (even if these treatments are usually more invasive and often less efficacious in terms of reducing the burden of disease) (Gore et al., 2011). Even when symptoms are present and already disabling, such as in the subthreshold ultra-high-risk (UHR) state or first-episode psychosis, there is a reluctance to accept the need for indicated or secondary preventive interventions (such as antipsychotic or antidepressant medication) to prevent progression to full-blown and persistent disorders. Biomarkers would potentially strengthen our field (Fusar-Poli et al., 2015; Tadokoro et al., 2011) to make informed decisions in relation to selecting appropriate and effective interventions at particular stages of mental disorders.

At the current state of knowledge, it is quite difficult for psychiatric parents and their relatives to make an informed decision on whether one should treat early stages of mental disorders or not. While effective psychosocial interventions certainly exist for first-line use and may be acceptable, if these are not effective in an individual case, parents may ask themselves if they should accept a prescription of an antipsychotic for their 15-year old son who presents with attenuated psychotic symptoms, in view of the fact that only 1–2 out of 10 individuals with attenuated psychotic symptoms will ever progress towards a first psychotic episode within the next 1–2 years, with only about half of those progressing towards chronic schizophrenia (Yung, 2017). On the risk side of the equation, there is the issue of side-effects. Such a young man may gain 20 kg in weight and get bullied at school because of his obesity, and further be at risk for diabetes and metabolic syndrome.

Currently published intervention studies in individuals at UHR for psychosis have mainly focused on transition rates (Nelson et al., 2018); some recent UHR studies have also started to better characterise those UHR subjects that do not progress towards psychosis but are still help-seeking (Michel et al., 2018). However, our knowledge regarding how to deal with such early stages of a disorder (Stage 1) is limited. There are no biological markers to guide whether a UHR patient will solely benefit from psychosocial support, specific psychological therapies (Bechdolf et al., 2005), antidepressants (beside treating the often occurring depression in UHR, selective serotonin reuptake inhibitors (SSRIs) may have neurotrophic and neuroprotective effects counteracting the progression towards full-blown psychosis) (Amminger et al., 2010; McGorry et al., 2016), low-dose lithium (Berger et al., 2012), omega-3 PUFAs (Amminger et al., 2010; 2015b) or antipsychotic medication (McGorry et al., 2002). In contrast to the plethora of markers that have been investigated in the context of the 'diagnosis schizophrenia' (Schmitt et al., 2017), relatively few studies have attempted to identify predictors of response in UHR states and none have really succeeded yet (Amminger et al., 2015a).

Once again, perhaps we can learn from oncology and their use of genetic or metabolic markers in daily clinical practice? The use of PSA as a screening parameter in the general population is heavily debated, with a significant proportion of false-positive elevated PSA levels potentially resulting in overdiagnosis and overtreatment of low-grade prostate cancer. However, enrichment of the sample overcomes this issue. In subjects with a strong family history of prostate cancer, the use of PSA screening is recommended, as the likelihood of an early onset and poor course of prostate cancer is higher and early intervention is likely to save lives. Also, the use of PSA monitoring in secondary prevention is widely accepted (see above). Another noteworthy example of a successful biological marker in oncology is the discovery of breast cancer risk gene variants (*BRCA1* and *BRCA2*) that have contributed to the identification of a rare but relevant subgroup of early-onset breast cancer cases that affect about 5 per cent of breast cancer patients. However, the usefulness of *BRCA* gene variants is limited to women who have a family history of breast cancer in a first-degree relative occurring prior to the age of 50. The likelihood of being affected by breast cancer rises dramatically to 85 per cent or more in women who meet this criterion and are carriers of the *BRCA* gene variants. While such examples of biological markers are limited to certain circumstances, they have had a critical impact on clinical practice and point the way to a more complete form of personalised medicine. In psychiatry, progression has been slower and the application of similar research approaches to identify biological markers in such a differentiated way remains elusive. The genetics of psychiatric disorders is much more complex. A factor potentially contributing to this is the continuing search for diagnostic markers specific to century-old syndromal concepts of uncertain validity, rather than stage-dependent markers relevant for prognosis or certain subgroups of patients (e.g. those with a strong family history of psychotic or other disorders). The latter approach may be more likely to be successful and contribute to more personalised early intervention approaches (McGorry et al., 2014).

However, as yet this is largely an aspirational goal in psychiatry, despite significant advances in our understanding of the biochemical, genetic and neurobiological processes underlying major mental disorders. Bringing together a clinical staging model for severe mental disorders with biological markers that have already undergone some systematic evaluation could be the basis of a new framework for a stage-dependent detection approach, as well as stage-dependent interventions. The advantage of such a new framework is that it not only uses the evolution of psychopathology during the development of a mental illness, but also integrates the underlying neurobiology of progression of illness, and more importantly how personalised interventions that target individual modifiable risk and protective factors that potentially can alter the disease trajectory. The specific goals of such tailored therapeutic interventions are therefore broadened to include the prevention of illness onset or the prevention of progression towards a chronic end-stage phenomenon based on biological markers, and is hopefully able to minimise the risk of harm associated with more complex treatment regimens. The integration of biological, social and environmental factors in a stage-dependent manner for emerging mental disorders would be a major step forward in the development of a truly pre-emptive psychiatry (Berger et al., 2003; McGorry et al., 2014).

Limitations of Biological Markers in Psychiatry

The limitations of our current categorical diagnostic approach become even more prominent in child and adolescent psychiatry, where diagnostic stability is even less clear compared to adult psychiatry. ICD-10 child and adolescent criteria (F9) are usually less specific than their adult counterparts. Many psychiatric-like features are present across a range of child and adolescent diagnostic categories and are often of limited prognostic or therapeutic relevance. For example, psychotic-like features such as hallucinations are not uncommon in late childhood or early adolescence, but only a minority of those affected minors will ever progress towards a full-blown psychotic disorder such as schizophrenia. Further, many children display aberrant behaviour during certain developmental phases, but a large proportion of these children will transition into healthy, independent and fully functional adults. The importance of the developmental perspective in child, adolescent and youth mental health may be one of the key differences compared to traditional adult psychiatry, where most presentations are in middle-aged and older adults and characterised by phenomenologically more stable syndromes that are often deemed as an 'end-stage phenomenon' requiring long-term and often palliative treatment approaches (e.g. chronic schizophrenia or recurrent depression).

Most research investigating genetic or metabolic markers is carried out in adult psychiatric samples, where established and often chronic illness is the rule. At this stage, it may be too late to investigate the underlying neurobiology relevant for the emergence of a particular mental disorder. An end-stage phenotype may not be suitable to understand the underlying pathology associated with the emergence of a particular disorder. Put another way, the neurobiology of different stages may be very different and evolving over time. However, as more than 80 per cent of all psychiatric conditions emerge in adolescence, it may be important to identify markers that are particularly relevant to the peri-onset phase of disorders (Haggerty & Mrazek, 1994). A pertinent example to illustrate this dilemma is 'heart failure' (Tamargo et al., 2017). It is generally accepted that heart failure is a heterogeneous group of disorders with many different aetiopathologies, such as (multiple) myocardial infarctions, myocarditis or a valve defect, but also rare genetic disorders. Therefore, quite diverse disease entities may result in the same end-stage phenomena of 'heart failure'. In internal medicine, no serious researcher would try to understand acute myocardial infarction or a valve defect by solely studying patients with heart failure. However, in the case of many mental disorders, that has been the standard approach to both research and treatment, until recently when early intervention has gained ground. The clinical staging model shifts our focus to search for markers relevant to particular stages of mental disorders and provides a useful framework to differentiate overlapping and heterogeneous syndromes, e.g. by differentiating age of onset or familial subtypes. The identification of such 'stage'-dependent markers may be more meaningful and of greater prognostic and therapeutic value than our quest for categorical disease markers.

Bioactive Lipids, Neuroinflammation and Brain Development

As already outlined in Chapter 8, the balance between pro-inflammatory and anti-inflammatory markers is important to regulate normal brain development and brain plasticity. Animal studies have demonstrated that an excessive pro-inflammatory hit in early development can have detrimental effects on later brain development (Meyer & Feldon, 2009), potentially raising the susceptibility for future mental disorders. Neuroinflammation has been associated with psychiatric disorders for a long time (Horrobin, 1977; Stevens, 1982). In the early 1980s, Janice R. Stevens (1982) discovered periventricular signs of gliosis in schizophrenia and suggested that schizophrenia may be associated with a low-grade inflammation. Neuroinflammation in the central nervous system (CNS) plays a different role compared to the rest of the body. Neuroinflammatory mediators modulate various physiological cellular processes in the living human brain important for normal brain development and functioning, such as neurogenesis, gliagenesis, cell differentiation, cell migration, synaptic plasticity, as well as synaptic pruning (Deverman & Patterson, 2009; Rao et al., 2012).

Key cells important for the regulation of inflammatory processes are microglia cells that have a comparable role to macrophages in the periphery. Microglia cells account for approximately 15 per cent of the total cellular compartments of the brain. Beside the immunological role, microglia cells are involved in various neural and synaptic activities. If microglia cells are not in a resting state, they usually exert neurotrophic activities important for synaptogenesis and neurogenesis via a physiological release of cytokines (Domenici et al., 2010). During conditions in which the brain is injured and the homeostasis of the micro-environment is disturbed, microglia cells can become excessively active and produce large amounts of pro-inflammatory cytokines and reactive oxidants (Lehnardt, 2010). The brain attempts to defend or restore neural integrity. However, under certain circumstances an uncontrolled and/or sustained inflammatory reaction can have detrimental effects and contribute to a vulnerability to or onset of future mental disorders (Beumer et al., 2012b).

Already the Feinberg Hypothesis suggests that the onset of psychosis is the result of an excessive elimination of synapses in adolescence (Berger et al., 2003; Feinberg, 1982). This hypothesis has gained momentum in the last couple of years, as molecular genetic approaches have been able to identify key molecules responsible for synaptic elimination with schizophrenia-spectrum disorders that involves variation in the major histocompatibility complex (MHC) locus that is associated, at least in part, with many structurally diverse alleles of the complement component 4 (*C4*) genes. These alleles generated widely varying levels of C4A and C4B expression in the brain, with each common *C4* allele associating with schizophrenia in proportion to its tendency to generate greater expression of C4A. Human C4 protein is localised to neuronal synapses, dendrites, axons and cell bodies. In mice, C4 mediated synapse elimination during postnatal development. These results implicate excessive complement activity in the development of schizophrenia, potentially explaining the reduced number of synapses in the brains of individuals with schizophrenia. Excessive synaptic pruning is likely to be associated with the excessive release of pro-inflammatory mediators, as well as the production of radicals (Stevens et al., 2007). An excess of pro-inflammatory markers and radicals has been observed at the onset of psychotic disorders (Berger et al., 2003; Lasic et al., 2014). First-episode schizophrenia patients demonstrate an increase in pro-inflammatory, alongside a decrease in anti-inflammatory, mediators. Based on the increasing literature of altered neuroinflammatory markers in schizophrenia (Bergink et al., 2014; Miller et al., 2011), several authors suggest that increased activity of pro-inflammatory pathways along with decreased activity of anti-inflammatory pathways may increase the vulnerability to the emergence and/or progression of mental disorders, in particular schizophrenia (García-Bueno et al., 2015; Leza et al., 2015; Schmitt et al., 2017). Related systems such as homocysteine plasma levels together with nitric oxide synthase and cyclooxygenase activity have also been suggested as reliable risk markers in first-episode schizophrenia (García-Bueno et al., 2013). The latter raises the potential to modulate inflammatory processes as new therapeutic targets, in particular in the early course of disorders. However, not all patients have signs of neuroinflammation, but those patients who have may benefit from neuroprotective and/or anti-inflammatory agents (Muller et al., 2013). The use of biological markers of neuroinflammation may enhance the likelihood of identifying subgroups within the schizophrenia-spectrum that may benefit from neuroinflammatory mediators, as outlined in Chapter 8. Neuroinflammatory markers are very diverse and have different roles in regulating important processes in brain homeostasis. Preclinical data suggest that some markers are mainly state-dependent (e.g. interleukin (IL) IL-1β, IL-2, IL-6 of transforming growth factor (TGF)-β), whereas others behave more like trait markers (e.g. IL-12, interferon-γ and TNF-α) (Bergink et al., 2014; Drexhage et al., 2010; Kirkpatrick & Miller, 2013). The in vivo investigation and characterisation of such neuroinflammatory markers in humans is a challenge as psychiatric medication modulates such markers (Kim et al., 2001; Kim et al., 2009; Na et al., 2014). These processes have been studied across current phenotypic syndromes and are likely to be transdiagnostic.

Bioactive Lipids and Immune Markers in Psychiatry

Major depressive disorders (Jeon & Kim, 2016), schizophrenia (Na et al., 2014), but also neurological conditions such as Alzheimer's disease (Shaftel et al., 2008) and Parkinson's disease (More et al., 2013) have all been associated with elevated pro-inflammatory cytokines and chronic neuroinflammation (Hong et al., 2016). However, at this stage it is not known if the pro-inflammatory state is causal for the pathogenesis of these disorders, or just an epiphenomenon. Inflammatory markers such as cytokines are closely linked to bioactive lipids. Pro-inflammatory mediators induce COX-2, a key enzyme for the production of bioactive lipids such as prostaglandins from arachidonic acid (AA), a long-chain omega-6 fatty acid (Knorr et al., 2010; Kruger et al., 2016). Prostaglandin 15d-PGJ2 is linked to sustained attention and has been suggested as a potential marker for schizophrenia (Cabrera et al., 2016). The kynurenine pathway has been suggested to play a role in the pathophysiology of schizophrenia (Muller et al., 2015), as schizophrenia is often associated with excessive kynurenic acid levels, in particular in relation to cognitive deficits (Muller et al., 2013). Furthermore, elevated cerebrospinal fluid levels of the glia-derived N-methyl-D-aspartic acid receptor antagonist kynurenic acid could be linked to a common variant within 1p21.3 (SNX7), to positive psychotic symptoms and executive function deficits in bipolar disorder, supporting the notion that biomarkers may lead to novel drug targets (Sellgren et al., 2016).

Bioactive Lipids as Potential Response Predictors

For major depression, there is some evidence that omega-3 fatty acids may be particularly beneficial (Grosso et al., 2014) in those patients with an increased inflammatory index (Rapaport et al., 2016) or an altered omega-3 fatty acid profile (e.g. an omega-3 index <3); however, for the latter, more clinical data are warranted. At this stage, currently published omega-3 fatty acid randomised controlled trials (RCTs) in schizophrenia and related disorders have not taken omega-3 fatty acid levels or an inflammatory index as a potential marker to predict omega-3 fatty acid response. Future studies should investigate if first-episode psychosis patients with a pronounced deficit of omega-3 fatty acids (e.g. an omega-3 index <3) (Parletta et al., 2016) or an associated increase in omega-9 fatty acid may benefit from omega-3 supplementation.

Niacin sensitivity is another biological marker of interest closely linked to neuroin-flammation and bioactive lipids, in particular prostaglandins. A body of evidence has identified impaired niacin sensitivity in schizophrenia (Nadalin et al., 2010; Smesny et al., 2007). Interestingly, a recently published study in adolescents with at-risk mental state (Berger et al., 2016) demonstrated that those UHR subjects that progress towards a frank psychotic episode show higher niacin sensitivity than those who do not or normal controls. The latter finding was unexpected and counter-intuitive. As niacin is closely linked to the production of prostaglandin D2, an inflammatory marker and metabolite of AA, one can speculate that the period prior to the conversion to a frank psychotic episode is associated with a pro-inflammatory state. These changes according to stage support the validity of the clinical staging model, in particular for Stage 1b according to the Melbourne staging model (Nelson et al., 2018).

At this stage it is not clear whether dysfunctional neuroinflammatory systems are associated with the pathophysiology of the underlying neurobiology of disease or reflect an epiphenomenon, e.g. due to lifestyle factors such as smoking, obesity, medication or a consequence of chronic stress (Beumer et al., 2012a). Most psychiatric medications such as antidepressant or antipsychotic treatments have immune-modulating properties (Miller et al., 2011). However, family studies of non-affected relatives of schizophrenia patients are suggestive that neuroinflammatory processes contribute to the vulnerability of schizophrenia and related disorders (Martinez-Gras et al., 2012).

Phospholipase A2 Family as a Modulator of Brain Immune Homeostasis

Not only enzymes downstream of the pro-inflammatory arachidonic acid–eicosanoid pathway have been associated with schizophrenia and related disorders, but also the key upstream enzymes, the superfamily of phospholipase A2 (PLA2) that play major roles in membrane phospholipid homeostasis, but also in glial and neuronal progenitor cell func-tioning, myelination, synaptic functioning, and brain immune responses, which finally influence brain development, function and behaviour (Law et al., 2006). PLA2 catalyses the hydrolysis of the sn-2 position of membrane phospholipids, triggering the release of polyunsaturated fatty acids (PUFAs) from membrane phospholipids, in particular the pro-inflammatory AA, and the lysophospholipids. AA is then converted into pro-inflammatory lipid mediators, such as prostaglandins, leukotrienes and thromboxanes (Berger et al., 2006). Increased PLA2 activity was detected in serum, plasma and platelets of unmedicated and medicated patients with schizophrenia, as well as in *post-mortem* brain tissue (for further reading, see Berger et al. (2006) and Smesny et al. (2005)). Antipsychotic medication inhibits PLA2 activity (Gattaz et al., 1987; Schmitt et al., 2001). Also, in vivo 31P-magnetic spectroscopy (31P-MRS) studies suggest an acceleration of phospholipid metabolism in the frontal and parietal lobes of schizophrenia patients, suggesting a decrease in the membrane precursors phosphomonoesters (PMEs) and an increase of membrane breakdown products phosphodiesters (PDEs) (for references, see Berger et al. (2002)). Our group interpreted these findings as a possible attempt of the brain to maintain a structural and functional integrity, potentially as a compensatory process after a developmental deficit and/or a neurotoxic effect of an acute psychotic state (Berger et al., 2006). The dynamic remodelling includes both synthesis and breakdown of phospholipid bilayers. A link between morphometric abnormalities in schizophrenia and PLA2 activity supports the hypothesis that PLA2 activity is associated with certain regional brain structural changes in schizophrenia, in particular in the early phase of illness (Smesny et al., 2010). Once again this supports the staging approach in that the biology seems to change over time.

Bioactive Lipids as Potential Biomarkers of Interest for Individualised Psychiatric Interventions

Emerging data from the last two to three decades point towards the importance of lipid biology for mental disorders and its close link with neuroimmunological processes and its potential role in better understanding the underlying pathogenesis of these complex disorders. Key processes proposed to be involved in these disorders, such as brain development, synaptogenesis, neurogenesis, myelination, pruning, as well as ion channel and receptor functioning, highlight the importance of lipid biology for mental disorders. Targeted and non-targeted lipidomics and proteomics have shown that there is an interplay between bioactive lipids and their associated enzymes with a range of mental disorders, in particular schizophrenia and major depressive disorders. We are now in a position to investigate a range of pro- and anti-inflammatory lipid markers in the context of these disorders across different stages of emerging mental disorders, in particular schizophrenia and major depression.

Several groups have investigated neuroprotective strategies in a range of mental disorders across different stages of disorders. The use of eicosapentaenoic acid-enriched omega-3 fatty acids in emerging psychotic disorders is promising. Such benign strategies are probably not effective once the first psychotic episode has passed, but even in this group omega-3 fatty acids, probably through the antioxidant mechanism of action, were able to increase tolerability of antipsychotic treatments. More promising might be the pre-emptive use of neuroprotective strategies in UHR samples. However, definitive proof is lacking so far as the initial study by Amminger et al. (2010) could not be replicated in a multi-centre study (McGorry et al., 2017). Several reasons might have accounted for this failure, such as the effective background psychosocial treatment in the placebo group resulting in a very low transition rate, as well as the very low compliance rate, with less than 50 per cent of patients being even partially compliant until the first follow-up assessment (Berger, 2016). Two follow-up trials are underway to address the question of whether bioactive lipid markers and immunomarkers may be able to identify those UHR patients that may benefit from omega-3 fatty acid supplementation. N-acetyl-cysteine (NAC) is another interesting neuroprotective agent that may have particular importance as a pre-emptive treatment approach in combination with a biological marker of increased oxidation (Skvarc et al., 2017).

Future research should therefore investigate whether there are lipid and/or immune-endophenotypes of these disorders that may respond to more benign immunomodulatory interventions, such as COX-2-inhibitors, omega-3 fatty acids, NAC or other neuroprotective substances, in particular in the early stages of these disorders. Such research would pave the way for an individualised treatment regime that can be applied in conjunction with biological markers that are linked to their associated mechanism of action, such as the omega-3 index, or an inflammatory index. Phospholipids, polyunsaturated fatty acids, and their bioactive lipids (e.g. prostaglandins, leukotrienes, resolvins, maresins) and lysophospholipids may all represent such potential biomarkers for investigation in future research as response predictors for such interventions at different stages and spanning the boundaries of our current psychiatric diagnostic categories.

References

Amminger, G. P., Mechelli, A., Rice, S., Kim, S. W., Klier, C. M., McNamara, R. K., . . . Schafer, M. R. (2015a). Predictors of treatment response in young people at ultra-high risk for psychosis who received long-chain omega-3 fatty acids. *Translational Psychiatry, 5,* e495.

Amminger, G. P., Schafer, M. R., Papageorgiou, K., Klier, C. M., Cotton, S. M., Harrigan, S. M., . . . Berger, G. E. (2010). Long-chain omega-3 fatty acids for indicated prevention of psychotic disorders: a randomized, placebo-controlled trial. *Archives of General Psychiatry, 67*(2), 146–154.

Amminger, G. P., Schafer, M. R., Schlogelhofer, M., Klier, C. M., & McGorry, P. D. (2015b). Longer-term outcome in the prevention of psychotic disorders by the Vienna omega-3 study. *Nature Communications, 6,* 7934.

Bechdolf, A., Veith, V., Schwarzer, D., Schormann, M., Stamm, E., Janssen, B., . . . Klosterkötter, J. (2005). Cognitive-behavioral therapy in the pre-psychotic phase: an exploratory study. *Psychiatry Research, 136*(2), 251–255.

Berger, G. (2016). Comments on Bozzatello et al. Supplementation with omega-3 fatty acids in psychiatric disorders: a review of literature data. J. Clin. Med. 2016, 5, 67. *Journal of Clinical Medicine, 5*(8), 69.

Berger, G. E., Smesny, S., & Amminger, G. P. (2006). Bioactive lipids in schizophrenia.

International Review of Psychiatry, 18(2), 85–98.

Berger, G. E., Smesny, S., Schafer, M. R., Milleit, B., Langbein, K., Hipler, U. C., . . . Amminger, G. P. (2016). Niacin skin sensitivity is increased in adolescents at ultra-high risk for psychosis. *PLoS One, 11*(2), e0148429.

Berger, G. E., Wood, S., & McGorry, P. D. (2003). Incipient neurovulnerability and neuroprotection in early psychosis. *Psychopharmacology Bulletin, 37*(2), 79–101.

Berger, G. E., Wood, S. J., Pantelis, C., Velakoulis, D., Wellard, R. M., & McGorry, P. D. (2002). Implications of lipid biology for the pathogenesis of schizophrenia. *Australian and New Zealand Journal of Psychiatry, 36*(3), 355–366.

Berger, G. E., Wood, S. J., Ross, M., Hamer, C. A., Wellard, R. M., Pell, G., . . . McGorry, P. D. (2012). Neuroprotective effects of low-dose lithium in individuals at ultra-high risk for psychosis: a longitudinal MRI/MRS study. *Current Pharmaceutical Design, 18*(4), 570–575.

Bergink, V., Gibney, S. M., & Drexhage, H. A. (2014). Autoimmunity, inflammation, and psychosis: a search for peripheral markers. *Biological Psychiatry, 75*(4), 324–331.

Beumer, W., Drexhage, R. C., De Wit, H., Versnel, M. A., Drexhage, H. A., & Cohen, D. (2012a). Increased level of serum cytokines, chemokines and adipokines in patients with schizophrenia is associated with disease and metabolic syndrome. *Psychoneuroendocrinology, 37*(12), 1901–1911.

Beumer, W., Gibney, S. M., Drexhage, R. C., Pont-Lezica, L., Doorduin, J., Klein, H. C., . . . Drexhage, H. A. (2012b). The immune theory of psychiatric diseases: a key role for activated microglia and circulating monocytes. *Journal of Leukocyte Biology, 92*(5), 959–975.

Bleuler, E. (1950). *Dementia praecox or the group of schizophrenias* (German edition published in 1911). New York: International Universities Press.

Cabrera, B., Bioque, M., Penades, R., Gonzalez-Pinto, A., Parellada, M., Bobes, J., . . . Bernardo, M. (2016). Cognition and psychopathology in first-episode psychosis: are they related to inflammation? *Psychological Medicine, 46*(10), 2133–2144.

Carcone, D., & Ruocco, A. C. (2017). Six years of research on the National Institute of Mental Health's Research Domain Criteria (RDoC) Initiative: a systematic review. *Frontiers in Cellular Neuroscience, 11*, 46.

Deverman, B. E., & Patterson, P. H. (2009). Cytokines and CNS development. *Neuron, 64*(1), 61–78.

Domenici, E., Willé, D. R., Tozzi, F., Prokopenko, I., Miller, S., McKeown, A., . . . Turck, C. W. (2010). Plasma protein biomarkers for depression and schizophrenia by multi analyte profiling of case-control collections. *PLoS One, 5*(2), e9166.

Drexhage, R. C., Knijff, E. M., Padmos, R. C., Heul-Nieuwenhuijzen, L., Beumer, W., Versnel, M. A., & Drexhage, H. A. (2010). The mononuclear phagocyte system and its cytokine inflammatory networks in schizophrenia and bipolar disorder. *Expert Review of Neurotherapeutics, 10*(1), 59–76.

Feinberg, I. (1982). Schizophrenia: caused by a fault in programmed synaptic elimination during adolescence? *Journal of Psychiatric Research, 17*(4), 319–334.

Fusar-Poli, P., Frascarelli, M., Valmaggia, L., Byrne, M., Stahl, D., Rocchetti, M., . . . McGuire, P. (2015). Antidepressant, antipsychotic and psychological interventions in subjects at high clinical risk for psychosis:

OASIS 6-year naturalistic study. *Psychological Medicine, 45*(6), 1327–1339.

García-Bueno, B., Bioque, M., Mac-Dowell, K. S., Barcones, M. F., Martínez-Cengotitabengoa, M., Pina-Camacho, L., . . . Lafuente, A. (2013). Pro-/anti-inflammatory dysregulation in patients with first episode of psychosis: toward an integrative inflammatory hypothesis of schizophrenia. *Schizophrenia Bulletin, 40*(2), 376–387.

García-Bueno, B., Bioque, M., MacDowell, K. S., Santabárbara, J., Martínez-Cengotitabengoa, M., Moreno, C., . . . Barcones, M. F. (2015). Pro-/anti-inflammatory dysregulation in early psychosis: results from a longitudinal, case-control study. *International Journal of Neuropsychopharmacology, 18*(2), pyu037.

Gattaz, W. F., Kollisch, M., Thuren, T., Virtanen, J. A., & Kinnunen, P. K. (1987). Increased plasma phospholipase-A2 activity in schizophrenic patients: reduction after neuroleptic therapy. *Biological Psychiatry, 22*(4), 421–426.

Gore, F. M., Bloem, P. J., Patton, G. C., Ferguson, J., Joseph, V., Coffey, C., . . . Mathers, C. D. (2011). Global burden of disease in young people aged 10–24 years: a systematic analysis. *Lancet, 377*(9783), 2093–2102.

Grosso, G., Galvano, F., Marventano, S., Malaguarnera, M., Bucolo, C., Drago, F., & Caraci, F. (2014). Omega-3 fatty acids and depression: scientific evidence and biological mechanisms. *Oxidative Medicine and Cellular Longevity, 2014*, 313570.

Haggerty, R. J., & Mrazek, P. J. (1994). Can we prevent mental illness? *Bulletin of the New York Academy of Medicine, 71*(2), 300–306.

Hamdy, F. C., Donovan, J. L., Lane, J. A., Mason, M., Metcalfe, C., Holding, P., . . . Neal, D. E. (2016). 10-year outcomes after monitoring, surgery, or radiotherapy for localized prostate cancer. *New England Journal of Medicine, 375*(15), 1415–1424.

Hong, H., Kim, B. S., & Im, H. I. (2016). Pathophysiological role of neuroinflammation in neurodegenerative diseases and psychiatric disorders. *International Neurourology Journal, 20* (Suppl. 1), S2–S7.

Horrobin, D. F. (1977). Schizophrenia as a prostaglandin deficiency disease. *Lancet,* 1(8018), 936–937.

Jeon, S. W., & Kim, Y. K. (2016). Neuroinflammation and cytokine abnormality in major depression: cause or consequence in that illness? *World Journal of Psychiatry,* 6(3), 283–293.

Keshavan, M. S., Berger, G., Zipursky, R. B., Wood, S. J., & Pantelis, C. (2005). Neurobiology of early psychosis. *British Journal of Psychiatry Supplement,* 48, s8–s18.

Kim, D. J., Kim, W., Yoon, S. J., Go, H. J., Choi, B. M., Jun, T. Y., & Kim, Y. K. (2001). Effect of risperidone on serum cytokines. *International Journal of Neuroscience,* 111(1–2), 11–19.

Kim, Y. K., Myint, A. M., Verkerk, R., Scharpe, S., Steinbusch, H., & Leonard, B. (2009). Cytokine changes and tryptophan metabolites in medication-naive and medication-free schizophrenic patients. *Neuropsychobiology,* 59(2), 123–129.

Kirkpatrick, B., & Miller, B. J. (2013). Inflammation and schizophrenia. *Schizophrenia Bulletin,* 39(6), 1174–1179.

Knorr, C., Marks, D., Gerstberger, R., Muhlradt, P. F., Roth, J., & Rummel, C. (2010). Peripheral and central cyclooxygenase (COX) products may contribute to the manifestation of brain-controlled sickness responses during localized inflammation induced by macrophage-activating lipopeptide-2 (MALP-2). *Neuroscience Letters,* 479(2), 107–111.

Kruger, K., Bredehoft, J., Mooren, F. C., & Rummel, C. (2016). Different effects of strength and endurance exercise training on COX-2 and mPGES expression in mouse brain are independent of peripheral inflammation. *Journal of Applied Physiology,* 121(1), 248–254.

Lasic, D., Bevanda, M., Bosnjak, N., Uglesic, B., Glavina, T., & Franic, T. (2014). Metabolic syndrome and inflammation markers in patients with schizophrenia and recurrent depressive disorder. *Psychiatria Danubina,* 26(3), 214–219.

Law, M. H., Cotton, R. G., & Berger, G. E. (2006). The role of phospholipases A2 in schizophrenia. *Molecular Psychiatry,* 11(6), 547–556.

Lehnardt, S. (2010). Innate immunity and neuroinflammation in the CNS: the role of microglia in Toll-like receptor-mediated neuronal injury. *Glia,* 58(3), 253–263.

Leza, J. C., García-Bueno, B., Bioque, M., Arango, C., Parellada, M., Do, K., . . . Bernardo, M. (2015). Inflammation in schizophrenia: a question of balance. *Neuroscience and Biobehavioral Reviews,* 55, 612–626.

Martinez-Gras, I., Garcia-Sanchez, F., Guaza, C., Rodriguez-Jimenez, R., Andres-Esteban, E., Palomo, T., . . . Borrell, J. (2012). Altered immune function in unaffected first-degree biological relatives of schizophrenia patients. *Psychiatry Research,* 200(2–3), 1022–1025.

McGorry, P. D., Goldstone, S., Berger, G. E., Chen, E., de Haan, L., Hickie, I., . . . Amminger, G. P. (2016). The neurapro-e study: a multicentre RCT of omega-3 fatty acids and cognitive-behavioral case management for patients at ultra-high risk of psychosis. Paper presented at the 5th Biennial Schizophrenia International Research Society Conference, Florence, Italy.

McGorry, P., Keshavan, M., Goldstone, S., Amminger, P., Allott, K., Berk, M., . . . Hickie, I. (2014). Biomarkers and clinical staging in psychiatry. *World Psychiatry,* 13(3), 211–223.

McGorry, P. D., Nelson, B., Markulev, C., Yuen, H. P., Schafer, M. R., Mossaheb, N., . . . Amminger, G. P. (2017). Effect of omega-3 polyunsaturated fatty acids in young people at ultrahigh risk for psychotic disorders: the NEURAPRO randomized clinical trial. *JAMA Psychiatry,* 74(1), 19–27.

McGorry, P. D., Yung, A. R., Phillips, L. J., Yuen, H. P., Francey, S., Cosgrave, E. M., . . . Blair, A. (2002). Randomized controlled trial of interventions designed to reduce the risk of progression to first-episode psychosis in a clinical sample with subthreshold symptoms. *Archives of General Psychiatry,* 59(10), 921–928.

Meyer, U., & Feldon, J. (2009). Neural basis of psychosis-related behaviour in the infection model of schizophrenia. *Behavioural Brain Research,* 204(2), 322–334.

Michel, C., Ruhrmann, S., Schimmelmann, B. G., Klosterkötter, J., & Schultze-Lutter, F. (2018). Course of clinical high-risk states for psychosis beyond conversion. *European Archives of Psychiatry and Clinical Neuroscience,* **268**(1), 39–48.

Miller, B. J., Buckley, P., Seabolt, W., Mellor, A., & Kirkpatrick, B. (2011). Meta-analysis of cytokine alterations in schizophrenia: clinical status and antipsychotic effects. *Biological Psychiatry,* **70**(7), 663–671.

More, S. V., Kumar, H., Kim, I. S., Song, S. Y., & Choi, D. K. (2013). Cellular and molecular mediators of neuroinflammation in the pathogenesis of Parkinson's disease. *Mediators of Inflammation,* **2013**, 952375.

Muller, N., Myint, A. M., Krause, D., Weidinger, E., & Schwarz, M. J. (2013). Anti-inflammatory treatment in schizophrenia. *Progress in Neuro-Psychopharmacology and Biological Psychiatry,* **42**, 146–153.

Muller, N., Weidinger, E., Leitner, B., & Schwarz, M. J. (2015). The role of inflammation in schizophrenia. *Frontiers in Neuroscience,* **9**, 372.

Na, K. S., Jung, H. Y., & Kim, Y. K. (2014). The role of pro-inflammatory cytokines in the neuroinflammation and neurogenesis of schizophrenia. *Progress in Neuro-Psychopharmacology and Biological Psychiatry,* **48**, 277–286.

Nadalin, S., Buretic-Tomljanovic, A., Rubesa, G., Tomljanovic, D., & Gudelj, L. (2010). Niacin skin flush test: a research tool for studying schizophrenia. *Psychiatria Danubina,* **22**(1), 14–27.

Nelson, B., Amminger, G. P., Yuen, H. P., Wallis, N. J. Kerr, M., Dixon, L., . . . Shumway, M. (2018). Staged treatment in early psychosis: a sequential multiple assignment randomised trial of interventions for ultra high risk of psychosis patients. *Early Intervention in Psychiatry,* **12**(3), 292–306.

Nelson, B., McGorry, P. D., Wichers, M., Wigman, J. T., & Hartmann, J. A. (2017). Moving from static to dynamic models of the onset of mental disorder: a review. *JAMA Psychiatry,* **74**(5), 528–534.

Parletta, N., Zarnowiecki, D., Cho, J., Wilson, A., Procter, N., Gordon, A., . . . Meyer, B. J. (2016). People with schizophrenia and

depression have a low omega-3 index. *Prostaglandins, Leukotrienes and Essential Fatty Acids,* **110**, 42–47.

Rao, J. S., Kellom, M., Kim, H. W., Rapoport, S. I., & Reese, E. A. (2012). Neuroinflammation and synaptic loss. *Neurochemical Research,* **37**(5), 903–910.

Rapaport, M. H., Nierenberg, A. A., Schettler, P. J., Kinkead, B., Cardoos, A., Walker, R., & Mischoulon, D. (2016). Inflammation as a predictive biomarker for response to omega-3 fatty acids in major depressive disorder: a proof-of-concept study. *Molecular Psychiatry,* **21**(1), 71–79.

Schmitt, A., Maras, A., Petroianu, G., Braus, D. F., Scheuer, L., & Gattaz, W. F. (2001). Effects of antipsychotic treatment on membrane phospholipid metabolism in schizophrenia. *Journal of Neural Transmission,* **108**(8–9), 1081–1091.

Schmitt, A., Martins-de-Souza, D., Akbarian, S., Cassoli, J. S., Ehrenreich, H., Fischer, A., . . . Gerlach, M. (2017). Consensus paper of the WFSBP Task Force on Biological Markers: criteria for biomarkers and endophenotypes of schizophrenia, part III – molecular mechanisms. *World Journal of Biological Psychiatry,* **18**(5), 330–356.

Sellgren, C. M., Kegel, M. E., Bergen, S. E., Ekman, C. J., Olsson, S., Larsson, M., . . . Landen, M. (2016). A genome-wide association study of kynurenic acid in cerebrospinal fluid: implications for psychosis and cognitive impairment in bipolar disorder. *Molecular Psychiatry,* **21**(10), 1342–1350.

Shaftel, S. S., Griffin, W. S., & O'Banion, M. K. (2008). The role of interleukin-1 in neuroinflammation and Alzheimer disease: an evolving perspective. *Journal of Neuroinflammation,* **5**, 7.

Skvarc, D. R., Dean, O. M., Byrne, L. K., Gray, L., Lane, S., Lewis, M., . . . Marriott, A. (2017). The effect of N-acetylcysteine (NAC) on human cognition: a systematic review. *Neuroscience and Biobehavioral Reviews,* **78**, 44–56.

Smesny, S., Kinder, D., Willhardt, I., Rosburg, T., Lasch, J., Berger, G., & Sauer, H. (2005). Increased calcium-independent phospholipase A2 activity in first but not in multiepisode chronic schizophrenia. *Biological Psychiatry, 57*(4), 399–405.

Smesny, S., Klemm, S., Stockebrand, M., Grunwald, S., Gerhard, U.-J., Rosburg, T., . . . Blanz, B. (2007). Endophenotype properties of niacin sensitivity as marker of impaired prostaglandin signalling in schizophrenia. *Prostaglandins, Leukotrienes and Essential Fatty Acids, 77*(2), 79–85.

Smesny, S., Milleit, B., Nenadic, I., Preul, C., Kinder, D., Lasch, J., . . . Gaser, C. (2010). Phospholipase A2 activity is associated with structural brain changes in schizophrenia. *NeuroImage, 52*(4), 1314–1327.

Stevens, B., Allen, N. J., Vazquez, L. E., Howell, G. R., Christopherson, K. S., Nouri, N., . . . Stafford, B. (2007). The classical complement cascade mediates CNS synapse elimination. *Cell, 131*(6), 1164–1178.

Stevens, J. R. (1982). Neuropathology of schizophrenia. *Archives of General Psychiatry, 39*(10), 1131–1139.

Tadokoro, S., Kanahara, N., Kikuchi, S., Hashimoto, K., & Masaomi, I. (2011). Fluvoxamine may prevent onset of psychosis: a case report of a patient at ultra-high risk of psychotic disorder. *Annals of General Psychiatry, 10*, 26.

Tamargo, J., Rosano, G. M., Delpon, E., Ruilope, L., & Lopez-Sendon, J. (2017). Pharmacological reasons that may explain why randomized clinical trials have failed in acute heart failure syndromes. *International Journal of Cardiology, 233*, 1–11.

Wilt, T. J., Jones, K. M., Barry, M. J., Andriole, G. L., Culkin, D., Wheeler, T., . . . Brawer, M. K. (2017). Follow-up of prostatectomy versus observation for early prostate cancer. *New England Journal of Medicine, 377*(2), 132–142.

Yung, A. R. (2017). Treatment of people at ultra-high risk for psychosis. *World Psychiatry, 16*(2), 207–208.

Chapter

10

Electroencephalography and Staging

Suzie Lavoie

Introduction

This chapter will cover the development (from Stages 0 to 4) of the most important brain functioning impairments, as measured with electroencephalography (EEG) in the psychosis spectrum and in severe mood disorders.

EEG measures voltage fluctuations resulting from ionic current flows within the neurons of the brain. Electrodes are used to record the summation of electrical dipoles along the scalp. EEG has been used to measure the activity of the resting brain during sleep and wakefulness, as well as the brain's response to stimuli. At rest, scalp EEG activity shows oscillations at a variety of frequencies. Several of these oscillations have characteristic frequency ranges and spatial distributions, and are associated with different states of brain functioning. Following the presentation of stimuli, averaging the EEG activity time-locked to the onset of the presentation leads to a stereotyped electrophysiological response called an event-related potential (ERP). ERP waveforms consist of a series of positive and negative voltage deflections, and the amplitude of these waves depends on the strength of the underlying generators. Abnormalities in both resting state EEG and ERPs have been observed in schizophrenia, major depressive disorders (MDDs) and bipolar disorder (BD).

Resting EEG

For the measurement of resting brain activity, participants are instructed to sit quietly and comfortably for a few minutes with their eyes open, then a few minutes with their eyes closed. The raw EEG data recorded are subsequently Fourier-decomposed into a voltage (power) by frequency spectral graphing. Each defined frequency band, i.e. delta (< 4 Hz), theta (4–7 Hz), alpha (8–15 Hz), beta (16–31 Hz) and gamma (> 32 Hz), is associated with a variety of physiological functions, and the power calculated for each of these frequency bands is compared between studied groups in research settings.

No single pattern of quantitative resting EEG abnormalities has been identified in schizophrenia. The most consistent observation obtained from spectral analysis in both medicated and unmedicated patients suffering from schizophrenia is the increased activity in the slow wave bands (delta and theta), mainly in the frontal area (see meta-analyses: Boutros et al., 2008; Galderisi et al., 2009), consistent with the decrease in the frontal brain activity observed in schizophrenia. Activity in the delta and theta bands is associated with slow wave sleep (Stages 3 and 4) and is potentially pathological in the waking state. It may therefore indicate some brain pathology in schizophrenia (Chen et al., 2016). Chronicity has a significant effect on both the delta and theta bands, with the effect size of the difference between patients and controls being much higher in chronic than in first-episode psychosis (FEP) patients and intermediate in mixed samples (Galderisi et al., 2009). EEG spectral power analyses performed in individuals at ultra-high risk (UHR) of psychosis showed no difference when compared to a control population and did not predict transition to psychosis (Lavoie et al., 2012; Ranlund et al., 2014; Zimmermann et al., 2010). The increase in slow wave activity has been associated with more severe negative symptoms in schizophrenia (Gattaz et al., 1992; Gerez & Tello, 1995; Gross et al., 2006; Sponheim et al., 2000; Venables et al., 2009), in FEP (Gschwandtner et al., 2009) and in UHR (Lavoie et al., 2012; Zimmermann et al., 2010), making this observation a fairly robust marker of the illness.

Studies have reported large decreases in alpha activity in drug-free BD euthymic patients (Basar et al., 2012; Kano et al., 1992; Ozerdem et al., 2008) compared to healthy controls, whereas in schizophrenia, spontaneous alpha activity is only slightly reduced (Basar et al., 2016). In BP patients with acute hypomania or depression, alpha activity was rather increased (Moeini et al., 2015) and the authors concluded that the increased alpha power, which corresponds to a decrease in the thalamic metabolism leading to diminished attention, is consistent with BD presentation. Another group demonstrated increased alpha activity in BD patients; however, the current state of the patient at the time of EEG recording was not specified (Narayanan et al., 2014). In this study, all PD patients presented with psychotic features, and their EEG profiles (increased delta, theta and alpha) matched those of the schizophrenia group. It could therefore be hypothesised that resting EEG activity is a reflection of the psychotic symptoms rather than a specific marker of psychiatric illness. Indeed, in a heterogeneous BD group with only 9 out of 30 patients showing psychotic symptoms, no resting EEG impairment was observed (Venables et al., 2009). In first-episode BP patients with psychotic features, increased low-frequency and alpha power were observed (Clementz et al., 1994), while only the increase in alpha band was reported in first-episode BP patients in acute hypomania or depressive state (Moeini et al., 2015). However, in light of the results available, it could be that the increased slow activity is specific to psychotic symptoms rather than schizophrenia itself.

In patients with MDD, higher alpha power with the eyes closed and greater alpha suppression with the eyes open were observed when compared to healthy controls (for reviews, see Olbrich & Arns, 2013; Pollock & Schneider, 1990). An increase in alpha power is thought to reflect a relative decrease in the proportion of local cortical neurons engaged in a particular task performance. It has been suggested that impaired alpha activity can be considered an endophenotype for MDD, mediating the pathway between the brain-derived neurotrophic factor BDNF Val66Met polymorphism and depressed mood (Gatt et al., 2008; Zoon et al., 2013). However, the most reproducible resting EEG observation in MDD is the increased frontal alpha asymmetry (see review by Thibodeau et al., 2006). Indeed, this meta-analytic review demonstrates that studies on resting EEG in depression show relative right-sided resting frontal alpha asymmetry among adults with MDD, but also in infants of afflicted mothers. While there are conflicting findings, it appears that alpha asymmetry may be a marker for developing a depressive disorder. Indeed, alpha asymmetry indicative of relatively less right than left parieto-temporal activity has been observed in second-generation (Bruder et al., 2005) and third-generation (Bruder et al., 2007) offspring of parents and/or grandparents suffering from depression. These results, including data collected in children without a lifetime history of depression, support the hypothesis that right parieto-temporal hypoactivation is an endophenotypic marker of vulnerability to the disease.

Gamma Phase Synchrony

The synchronous activity of neurons, mediated by oscillations in the gamma-band (30–100 Hz) of the EEG, has been proposed to play an important role in the linking of neurons into cell assemblies that code information in the brain. This synchronisation (phase-locking) has been proposed as a mechanism for the integration, or binding, of activity in distributed neural networks (Uhlhaas & Singer, 2006). Research using EEG in both animals and humans have shown that gamma-band synchronisation contributes to a variety of cognitive functions including attention and memory (for a review, see Rieder et al., 2011). Reduced gamma activity and a lack of lateralisation in response to various stimuli have been repeatedly observed in patients suffering from schizophrenia (for reviews, see Lee et al., 2003; Uhlhaas & Singer, 2010). Decreased gamma phase synchrony relative to a pre-stimulus baseline has also been demonstrated in FEP (Slewa-Younan et al., 2004; Spencer et al., 2008; Symond et al., 2005). In another study with FEP patients, it was shown that the absolute magnitude of gamma synchrony is enhanced, markedly in the left centro-temporal region, when the reference to this baseline period is removed (Flynn et al., 2008). The authors suggested that diminished neural synchronisation to stimuli, regardless of their task relevance, is occurring in an environment of generally excessive synchrony. Tada et al. (2014) investigated the time-course of the auditory gamma-band response in an FEP group and a UHR group and they showed a reduction of early-latency (0–100 ms) gamma-band in the FEP group and a reduction of late-latency (300–500 ms) gamma-band in both UHR and FEP groups. These findings suggest that the early gamma-band response may be reduced after the onset of psychosis in accordance with the staging model, whereas the late gamma-band response may be impaired before the onset of psychosis and considered an endophenotype. However, these results are not supported by the other gamma-band investigations conducted in UHR individuals to date (Leicht et al., 2016; Perez et al., 2013). In those studies, impairment of early-latency gamma-band was observed in UHR individuals, leading the authors to suggest that the reduced activation of this type of network is likely to reflect the clinical risk for transition to psychosis.

Although the study of gamma-band oscillations in BD has received less attention than in schizophrenia, the same reduced gamma power in response to auditory stimuli has been observed repeatedly (for a review, see Onitsuka et al., 2013). Therefore, reduced gamma-band activity may not represent an efficient diagnostic tool, although it has been suggested that the mechanisms underpinning this impairment in schizophrenia involves the cortical inhibition by GABA inter-neurons, while this is not the case in BD (Farzan et al., 2010).

In contrast with schizophrenia and BD, MDD individuals displayed an increased gamma-band power sustained during eight seconds following presentation of negative versus neutral words, compared to control participants and to individuals with schizophrenia (Siegle et al., 2010). Similarly, in individuals with a first episode of depression, the gamma-band showed increased cortical activity both at rest and during the performance of an arithmetic counting task and a spatial imagination task (Strelets et al., 2002).

Event-Related Potentials

P50

During an auditory dual-click paradigm, a positive polarity on the EEG trace occurs approximately 50 ms post-stimulus; this is the so-called P50. The relative decrease of the

P50 wave to the second click compared with the first is thought to reflect a sensory gating mechanism, aiming to protect against information overload. The abnormal auditory gating observed in schizophrenia, i.e. a decreased attenuation in the amplitude of the second P50, has been suggested to be a candidate endophenotype of the illness (see meta-analyses by Bramon et al., 2004 and Patterson et al., 2008). Indeed, a reduced P50 suppression has been linked to several gene loci and was found in healthy relatives of schizophrenia patients (for a review, see Turetsky et al., 2007). A central hypothesis proposed to account for perception and attention deficits in schizophrenia is that these patients cannot inhibit, or 'gate', irrelevant sensory input, leading to an overload of information reaching the brain. Impaired sensory gating has been demonstrated in FEP patients (Devrim-Ucok et al., 2008a; Hong et al., 2009), but not by all (de Wilde et al., 2007; Morales-Munoz et al., 2016). In UHR, the results are also inconsistent, with some studies showing impaired P50 (Brockhaus-Dumke et al., 2008; Myles-Worsley et al., 2004), while others did not (Cadenhead et al., 2005; Hsieh et al., 2012; van Tricht et al., 2015). While P50 reflects pre-attentional gating mechanisms, recent studies have extended the evaluation of sensory gating to later stages, namely N1 and P2, for which deficits have also been observed in UHR, FEP and schizophrenia (Brockhaus-Dumke et al., 2008; Morales-Munoz et al., 2016). Van Tricht et al. (2015) found a reduced suppression of N100 (N1) in UHR individuals who later transitioned to psychosis compared to UHR individuals who did not and to controls, and the N1 difference score contributed modestly to the prediction of FEP. Hsieh et al. (2012) suggest that both P50 and N1 are potential predictors of psychosis and Morales-Munoz et al. (2016) extended this suggestion to the P2 component.

A recent meta-analysis has shown that sensory gating impairment, as indexed by the decrease in P50 suppression, is present in BP patients and it is likely to worsen with a history of psychosis (Cheng et al., 2016). BP is associated with the decrease in P50 suppression with a high genetic component (Hall et al., 2007a; Sanchez-Morla et al., 2008), and therefore P50 suppression impairment is a good candidate for an endophenotype of this mental disease. To our knowledge, only two studies have looked at the P50 in MDD and they have both demonstrated sensory gating impairment (Kuang et al., 2016; Wang et al., 2009b). Interestingly, impaired P50 sensory gating measured in 40-month-old infants was predictive of attention problems and anxious/depressed symptoms three years later (Hutchison et al., 2017), indicative of the neurophysiological dysfunction being present long before the behaviour or symptoms manifest.

Mismatch Negativity

Mismatch negativity (MMN) is a change in the activity of the brain induced by the occurrence of novel stimuli, leading to a switch of attention in the subject (for a review, see Naatanen et al., 2011). MMN is thought to reflect the functioning of NMDA receptors (Javitt et al., 1995; Umbricht et al., 2002). A meta-analysis of 32 studies reports that a decrease in the amplitude of MMN has been consistently replicated in schizophrenia (Umbricht & Krljes, 2005). This MMN deficit is a remarkably robust finding, and is one of the most replicable findings in schizophrenia (for a review, see Naatanen et al., 2015). Impaired MMN has been associated with poor social cognition (Wynn et al., 2010) and poor global functioning (Kawakubo & Kasai, 2006; Light et al., 2005a, 2005b; Rasser et al., 2011). Kiang et al. (2007) suggested that auditory memory encoding deficits in schizophrenia patients could lead to a reduced capacity for short-term storage of verbal information.

This impairment could in turn interfere not only with abstract thinking, but also with everyday tasks. During a classic auditory oddball paradigm (AOP), MMN is induced by the occurrence of a deviant sound in an otherwise contiguous stream of events. The most widely used deviant stimuli in schizophrenia research are sounds differing in their duration or pitch frequency.

Frequency MMN (fMMN) illustrates the theoretical concept of the staging model. Indeed, the Umbricht and Krljes (2005) meta-analysis showed that the effect sizes of fMMN were significantly correlated with the duration of illness, indicating that the fMMN amplitude attenuation could reflect disease progression. While this impairment is well established in chronic schizophrenia, and it may be present in FEP (Bodatsch et al., 2011; Oades et al., 2006), most FEP studies show that the fMMN is intact in these patients (Devrim-Ucok et al., 2008b; Magno et al., 2008; Mondragon-Maya et al., 2013; Salisbury et al., 2002; 2007; Todd et al., 2007; Umbricht et al., 2006; Valkonen-Korhonen et al., 2003). However, a significant decrease in the fMMN amplitude was observed in the same participants in the post-acute phase (Devrim-Ucok et al., 2008b) or one year after their first psychotic episode (Salisbury et al., 2007). Worsening of the MMN generation has been correlated with grey matter volume reduction in the primary auditory cortex, a correlation that was also observed in chronic schizophrenia (Rasser et al., 2011). Very few studies have measured fMMN in young individuals presenting with an at-risk mental state, although the amplitude was shown to be intact compared to that seen in controls in three studies (Bodatsch et al., 2011; Brockhaus-Dumke et al., 2005; Mondragon-Maya et al., 2013), while it was decreased in another study (Perez et al., 2014). Finally, the generation of fMMN was shown to be intact in first-degree relatives (Magno et al., 2008) and in twins of affected patients (Ahveninen et al., 2006), making it a poor contender as a biomarker for the illness. Altogether, the literature suggests that fMMN impairment worsens with deterioration of illness, and this hypothesis has been recently investigated using longitudinal study designs. One study supported the hypothesis, showing a significant decline in fMMN following transition (Lavoie et al., 2018), while the other did not (Atkinson et al., 2017).

For the amplitude of the MMN in response to a change in the duration of the sound (dMMN), it is equally attenuated in schizophrenia and FEP patients (Atkinson et al., 2012; Bodatsch et al., 2011; Hermens et al., 2010; Kaur et al., 2011; Oades et al., 2006; Solis-Vivanco et al., 2014), although this was not reported in all studies (Magno et al., 2008; Umbricht et al., 2006). Almost all studies conducted in UHR individuals showed a decrease in the dMMN amplitude in these individuals compared to controls (Atkinson et al., 2012; Bodatsch et al., 2011; Higuchi et al., 2014; Jahshan et al., 2012a; Perez et al., 2014; Shaikh et al., 2012; Shin et al., 2009; Solis-Vivanco et al., 2014), apart from two studies (Higuchi et al., 2013; Mondragon-Maya et al., 2013). Most interestingly, studies in which UHR individuals who transitioned to psychosis were compared to UHR individuals who did not transition have revealed that the decrease in dMMN amplitude was significant only in those who transitioned (Atkinson et al., 2012; Bodatsch et al., 2011; Higuchi et al., 2013; 2014; Perez et al., 2014; Shaikh et al., 2012), and it was suggested that this impairment could be used as a predictor of the illness.

dMMN deficit seems to be related to the genetic disposition of the patient. Indeed, a modest but significant genetic correlation between the amplitude of dMMN and schizophrenia has been observed, suggesting that it is a potentially valid endophenotype for this disease (Hall et al., 2007b). On the other hand, it was shown that fMMN can be improved by the administration of N-acetyl-cysteine in schizophrenia patients (Lavoie et al., 2007), reinforcing its status as a state rather than a trait marker.

MMN has not been extensively studied in either BD or MDD, and most of the studies on this topic have been conducted in Stages 3 or 4 of the illnesses. A meta-analysis including seven studies looking at MMN in BD compared to controls showed that BD patients display a significantly reduced frontal MMN of moderate effect size (Chitty et al., 2013). However, close examination of the results obtained from each study included in the meta-analysis reveals highly inconsistent results. Indeed, only three studies showed a significant decrease in MMN amplitude in BD patients compared to controls (Andersson et al., 2008; Jahshan et al., 2012b; Kaur et al., 2012), while it was not significantly decreased in the other four studies (Catts et al., 1995; Hall et al., 2009; Salisbury et al., 2007; Umbricht et al., 2003). A recent comprehensive review of the literature on MMN in BD also demonstrates that MMN appears to be perturbed in BD but to a lesser degree than that observed in schizophrenia (Hermens et al., 2018). The heterogeneity, not only of the BD population, but also of the methodology followed by the various studies, can possibly explain these discrepancies. For example, while a great majority of the studies present results from a mix of bipolar I and bipolar II, regardless of the phase they are in, i.e. manic, depressive or euthymic, other studies only state that they have recruited patients with BP. To our knowledge, the MMN impairment in BD has not been rigorously studied in the early stages of the illness.

Similar to BD patients, no real consensus can be reached regarding MMN impairment in MDD patients. In schizophrenia research, the paradigm used to elicit the MMN and the methods used to measure the induced brain activity have become relatively standardised over the years. However, in MDD populations various methodologies have been used, such as visual paradigms instead of auditory paradigms, magnetoencephalography (MEG) instead of EEG, midline electrodes instead of temporal or frontocentral ones, etc. It appears that dMMN is decreased in MDD when compared to controls (Chen et al., 2014; Naismith et al., 2012; Qiao et al., 2013; Takei et al., 2009), while the amplitude of the fMMN remains the same (Umbricht et al., 2003) or even increases in some MDD patients (He et al., 2010; Kahkonen et al., 2007). At first sight, nothing striking can differentiate the participants in the various studies and it seems like the MNN amplitude is not related to depressive symptoms (He et al., 2010; Takei et al., 2009).

Until recent years, the MMN impairment was thought to be specific to schizophrenia. However, studies conducted in BD and MDD over the last decade or so have been contradicting this hypothesis, therefore threatening the use of the MMN impairment as a diagnostic tool for schizophrenia.

P300

The P300 (P3) waveform has been conceptualised as an index of endogenous cognitive processes appearing on EEG traces as a large positive component peaking around 300 ms post-stimulus. The preferred paradigm to elicit the P3 is an active button-press oddball paradigm. A meta-analysis including 46 studies (Bramon et al., 2004) and another including 104 studies (Jeon & Polich, 2003) showed large pooled effect sizes of 0.85 and 0.89 for P3 amplitude differences between schizophrenia patients and controls at midline electrodes, and the P3 latency was also significantly delayed. Abnormalities in P3 may reflect a failure to allocate attention resources to a stimulus and/or deficits in information processing and cognitive updating. P3 impairments are also consistently observed in neuroleptic-naïve FEP patients (Brown et al., 2002; de Wilde et al., 2008; Demiralp et al., 2002; Hermens et al., 2010; Hirayasu et al., 1998; Kaur et al., 2011; McCarley et al., 2002; Ozgurdal et al., 2008; Renoult et al., 2007; van der Stelt et al., 2005; Wang et al., 2009a; Xiong et al., 2010) and in individuals at clinical high risk for psychosis (Bramon et al., 2008; Frommann et al., 2008; Nieman et al., 2014; Ozgurdal et al., 2008; van der Stelt et al., 2005). Interestingly, it was shown that P300 peak amplitude significantly predicted later improvement in negative and general symptoms in high-risk individuals who did not transition to psychosis within two years of EEG recording (Kim et al., 2015). A meta-analysis including 11 studies on P3 amplitudes in unaffected relatives of schizophrenia patients showed that these healthy relatives have reduced P3 amplitudes and increased latency compared to controls (Bramon et al., 2005). Its high heritability and stability makes it a candidate of choice in the research of an endophenotype (for a review, see Turetsky et al., 2007). P3 amplitude is indeed a strong contender as a biomarker for psychosis, as demonstrated by a study that used Cox regression analysis to estimate the best predictors for transition to psychosis (Nieman et al., 2014). In their Cox model, poor social–personal adjustment and reduced P3 parietal amplitude at midline site predicted transition to a first psychotic episode with a sensitivity of 88.9 per cent and a specificity 82.5 per cent.

In light of these results, it appears that the P3 impairment, although present before the onset of psychosis, worsens with the establishment of the illness, showing better established localisation of the damaged source and slower processes. A study showing a decrease in P3 amplitude in at-risk, FEP and schizophrenia patients compared to controls revealed a progressive course from prodromal to chronic schizophrenia in terms of P3 amplitude impairment (Ozgurdal et al., 2008). A relationship with illness duration has been established for the P3 latency increase (Mathalon et al., 2000; O'Donnell et al., 1995). However, it is important to note that impaired P3 is not specific to schizophrenia, being impaired in other mental or brain disorders, but with less consistency (for a review, see Duncan et al., 2009).

P3 is delayed and its amplitude is reduced in BD (Hall et al., 2009; O'Donnell et al., 2004; Salisbury et al., 1999; Schulze et al., 2008). Unaffected relatives of BD patients also present with the same P3 impairments (Hall et al., 2009; Pierson et al., 2000; Schulze et al., 2008). Similar to P50 suppression, impairments in the generation of the P3 should be considered as a potential biological marker of BD.

Findings of deviant P3 are less consistent in depression than in schizophrenia and BD, and they may be related to patient subtypes or to the severity of the disease (for a review, see Duncan et al., 2009). For example, the increase in P3 latency seems to be associated with the presence of melancholic symptoms (Bruder et al., 1991; Kemp et al., 2010; Schlegel et al., 1991) or with cognitive impairments (Vandoolaeghe et al., 1998). Kemp et al. (2010) suggested that melancholia is not only associated with an increased P300 latency, but also with an exaggerated P200. Vandoolaeghe et al. (1998), who observed the same profile of impairments, associated the latter to non-responders to antidepressant therapy. Another proposition is that P3 is normal in depressed individuals, although in families with multiple members with schizophrenia, relatives who suffer from MDD may show the same P3 abnormalities as their relatives with schizophrenia (Blackwood et al., 1991). However, when the amplitude of P3 was measured in the offspring of parents suffering from depression, a decrease was observed when compared to the P3 amplitude of control subjects without a family history of psychiatric disorders (Zhang et al., 2007). These inconsistent results regarding ERPs in major depression do not allow us to draw any conclusion. A given impairment might be genetically linked to the disease and/or related to a given symptom or abnormality observed in major depression.

Conclusion

This review attempted to present some of the EEG impairment observed in the major psychiatric illnesses in relation to the stage of the illness. Our first observation is that although these impairments have been extensively studied in all stages of schizophrenia, the results remain highly inconsistent in chronic BD and MDD, and almost non-existent for the early stages of these disorders. The clinical stages of MDD and BD have been defined (Berk et al., 2007; Hetrick et al., 2008) and EEG studies in the early stages of these illnesses are needed in order to obtain a better understanding of the course of the observed impairments. This review of the literature clearly demonstrates how inconsistent the results are from one study to another. Possible reasons for these inconsistencies are small sample sizes, variable sample compositions, variable paradigm settings, medication and post-hoc grouping of patients, to name a few.

At the time of publication of this review, it is not possible to draw any conclusion with regard to the state or trait character of any of the EEG impairments in both MDD and BD. In schizophrenia, the most promising markers of the stage of the illness are fMMN and P3 amplitudes, as these components seem to deteriorate with the increasing severity of illness. Longitudinal studies will be necessary to follow the course of these impairments in at-risk individuals who, after experiencing an FEP, are later diagnosed with schizophrenia. Furthermore, and most importantly, if these markers are going to be used as diagnostic tools in the establishment of the stage of a psychotic disorder, a quantifying parameter will need to be identified as well as normal and pathological ranges. However, given the complexity of major psychiatric disorders, and that not a single impairment can be observed in all patients, future research should most likely consider combinations of markers in the quest for a better identification of the stages of psychiatric illnesses.

References

Ahveninen, J., Jaaskelainen, I. P., Osipova, D., Huttunen, M. O., Ilmoniemi, R. J., Kaprio, J., ... Cannon, T. D. (2006). Inherited auditory-cortical dysfunction in twin pairs discordant for schizophrenia. *Biological Psychiatry*, **60**(6), 612–620.

Andersson, S., Barder, H. E., Hellvin, T., Løvdahl, H., & Malt, U. F. (2008). Neuropsychological and electrophysiological indices of neurocognitive dysfunction in bipolar II disorder. *Bipolar Disorders*, **10**, 888–899.

Atkinson, R. J., Fulham, W. R., Michie, P. T., Ward, P. B., Todd, J., Stain, H., ... Schall, U. (2017). Electrophysiological, cognitive and clinical profiles of at-risk mental state: the longitudinal Minds in Transition (MinT) study. *PLoS One*, **12**(2), e0171657.

Atkinson, R. J., Michie, P. T., & Schall, U. (2012). Duration mismatch negativity and P3a in first-episode psychosis and individuals at ultra-high risk of psychosis. *Biological Psychiatry*, **71**(2), 98–104.

Basar, E., Guntekin, B., Atagun, I., Turp Golbasi, B., Tulay, E., & Ozerdem, A. (2012). Brain's alpha activity is highly reduced in euthymic bipolar disorder patients. *Cognitive Neurodynamics*, **6**(1), 11–20.

Basar, E., Schmiedt-Fehr, C., Mathes, B., Femir, B., Emek-Savas, D. D., Tulay, E., ... Basar-Eroglu, C. (2016). What does the broken brain say to the neuroscientist? Oscillations and connectivity in schizophrenia, Alzheimer's disease, and bipolar disorder. *International Journal of Psychophysiology,* **103**, 135–148.

Berk, M., Conus, P., Lucas, N., Hallam, K., Malhi, G. S., Dodd, S., ... McGorry, P. (2007). Setting the stage: from prodrome to treatment resistance in bipolar disorder. *Bipolar Disorders,* **9**(7), 671–678.

Blackwood, D. H., St Clair, D. M., Muir, W. J., & Duffy, J. C. (1991). Auditory P300 and eye tracking dysfunction in schizophrenic pedigrees. *Archives of General Psychiatry,* **48**(10), 899–909.

Bodatsch, M., Ruhrmann, S., Wagner, M., Muller, R., Schultze-Lutter, F., Frommann, I., ... Brockhaus-Dumke, A. (2011). Prediction of psychosis by mismatch negativity. *Biological Psychiatry,* **69**(10), 959–966.

Boutros, N. N., Arfken, C., Galderisi, S., Warrick, J., Pratt, G., & Iacono, W. (2008). The status of spectral EEG abnormality as a diagnostic test for schizophrenia. *Schizophrenia Research,* **99**(1–3), 225–237.

Bramon, E., McDonald, C., Croft, R. J., Landau, S., Filbey, F., Gruzelier, J. H., ... Murray, R. M. (2005). Is the P300 wave an endophenotype for schizophrenia? A meta-analysis and a family study. *NeuroImage,* **27**(4), 960–968.

Bramon, E., Rabe-Hesketh, S., Sham, P., Murray, R. M., & Frangou, S. (2004). Meta-analysis of the P300 and P50 waveforms in schizophrenia. *Schizophrenia Research,* **70**(2–3), 315–329.

Bramon, E., Shaikh, M., Broome, M., Lappin, J., Berge, D., Day, F., ... McGuire, P. (2008). Abnormal P300 in people with high risk of developing psychosis. *NeuroImage,* **41**(2), 553–560.

Brockhaus-Dumke, A., Schultze-Lutter, F., Mueller, R., Tendolkar, I., Bechdolf, A., Pukrop, R., ... Ruhrmann, S. (2008). Sensory gating in schizophrenia: P50 and N100 gating in antipsychotic-free subjects at risk, first-episode, and chronic patients. *Biological Psychiatry,* **64**(5), 376–384.

Brockhaus-Dumke, A., Tendolkar, I., Pukrop, R., Schultze-Lutter, F., Klosterkotter, J., & Ruhrmann, S. (2005). Impaired mismatch negativity generation in prodromal subjects and patients with schizophrenia. *Schizophrenia Research,* **73**(2–3), 297–310.

Brown, K. J., Gonsalvez, C. J., Harris, A. W. F., Williams, L. M., & Gordon, E. (2002). Target and non-target ERP disturbances in first episode vs. chronic schizophrenia. *Clinical Neurophysiology,* **113**(11), 1754–1763.

Bruder, G. E., Tenke, C. E., Warner, V., Nomura, Y., Grillon, C., Hille, J., ... Weissman, M. M. (2005). Electroencephalographic measures of regional hemispheric activity in offspring at risk for depressive disorders. *Biological Psychiatry,* **57**(4), 328–335.

Bruder, G. E., Tenke, C. E., Warner, V., & Weissman, M. M. (2007). Grandchildren at high and low risk for depression differ in EEG measures of regional brain asymmetry. *Biological Psychiatry,* **62**(11), 1317–1323.

Bruder, G. E., Towey, J. P., Stewart, J. W., Friedman, D., Tenke, C., & Quitkin, F. M. (1991). Event-related potentials in depression: influence of task, stimulus hemifield and clinical features on P3 latency. *Biological Psychiatry,* **30**(3), 233–246.

Cadenhead, K. S., Light, G. A., Shafer, K. M., & Braff, D. L. (2005). P50 suppression in individuals at risk for schizophrenia: the convergence of clinical, familial, and vulnerability marker risk assessment. *Biological Psychiatry,* **57**(12), 1504–1509.

Catts, S. V., Shelley, A. M., Ward, P. B., Liebert, B., McConaghy, N., Andrews, S., & Michie, P. T. (1995). Brain potential evidence for an auditory sensory memory deficit in schizophrenia. *American Journal of Psychiatry,* **152**(2), 213–219.

Chen, J., Zhang, Y., Wei, D., Wu, X., Fu, Q., Xu, F., ... Zhang, Z. (2014). Neurophysiological handover from MMN to P3a in first-episode and recurrent major depression. *Journal of Affective Disorders,* **174C**, 173–179.

Chen, Y. H., Stone-Howell, B., Edgar, J. C., Huang, M., Wootton, C., Hunter, M. A., ... Canive, J. M. (2016). Frontal slow-wave activity as a predictor of negative symptoms, cognition and functional capacity in schizophrenia. *British Journal of Psychiatry,* **208**(2), 160–167.

Cheng, C. H., Chan, P. Y., Liu, C. Y., & Hsu, S. C. (2016). Auditory sensory gating in patients with bipolar disorders: a meta-analysis. *Journal of Affective Disorders,* **203**, 199–203.

Chitty, K. M., Lagopoulos, J., Lee, R. S., Hickie, I. B., & Hermens, D. F. (2013). A systematic review and meta-analysis of proton magnetic resonance spectroscopy and mismatch negativity in bipolar disorder. *European Neuropsychopharmacology,* **23**(11), 1348–1363.

Clementz, B. A., Sponheim, S. R., Iacono, W. G., & Beiser, M. (1994). Resting EEG in first-episode schizophrenia patients, bipolar psychosis patients, and their first-degree relatives. *Psychophysiology,* **31**(5), 486–494.

de Wilde, O. M., Bour, L. J., Dingemans, P. M., Koelman, J. H., Boeree, T., & Linszen, D. H. (2008). P300 deficits are present in young first-episode patients with schizophrenia and not in their healthy young siblings. *Clinical Neurophysiology,* **119**(12), 2721–2726.

de Wilde, O. M., Bour, L. J., Dingemans, P. M., Koelman, J. H., & Linszen, D. H. (2007). Failure to find P50 suppression deficits in young first-episode patients with schizophrenia and clinically unaffected siblings. *Schizophrenia Bulletin,* **33**(6), 1319–1323.

Demiralp, T., Ucok, A., Devrim, M., Isoglu-Alkac, U., Tecer, A., & Polich, J. (2002). N2 and P3 components of event-related potential in first-episode schizophrenic patients: scalp topography, medication, and latency effects. *Psychiatry Research,* **111**(2–3), 167–179.

Devrim-Ucok, M., Keskin-Ergen, H. Y., & Ucok, A. (2008a). P50 gating at acute and post-acute phases of first-episode schizophrenia. *Progress in Neuro-Psychopharmacology and Biological Psychiatry,* **32**(8), 1952–1956.

Devrim-Ucok, M., Keskin-Ergen, H. Y., & Ucok, A. (2008b). Mismatch negativity at acute and post-acute phases of first-episode schizophrenia. *European Archives of Psychiatry and Clinical Neuroscience,* **258**(3), 179–185.

Duncan, C. C., Barry, R. J., Connolly, J. F., Fischer, C., Michie, P. T., Naatanen, R., ... Van Petten, C. (2009). Event-related potentials in clinical research: guidelines for eliciting, recording, and quantifying mismatch negativity, P300, and N400. *Clinical Neurophysiology,* **120**(11), 1883–1908.

Farzan, F., Barr, M. S., Levinson, A. J., Chen, R., Wong, W., Fitzgerald, P. B., & Daskalakis, Z. J. (2010). Evidence for gamma inhibition deficits in the dorsolateral prefrontal cortex of patients with schizophrenia. *Brain,* **133**(Pt 5), 1505–1514.

Flynn, G., Alexander, D., Harris, A., Whitford, T., Wong, W., Galletly, C., ... Williams, L. M. (2008). Increased absolute magnitude of gamma synchrony in first-episode psychosis. *Schizophrenia Research,* **105**(1–3), 262–271.

Frommann, I., Brinkmeyer, J., Ruhrmann, S., Hack, E., Brockhaus-Dumke, A., Bechdolf, A., ... Wagner, M. (2008). Auditory P300 in individuals clinically at risk for psychosis. *International Journal of Psychophysiology,* **70**(3), 192–205.

Galderisi, S., Mucci, A., Volpe, U., & Boutros, N. (2009). Evidence-based medicine and electrophysiology in schizophrenia. *Clinical EEG and Neuroscience,* **40**(2), 62–77.

Gatt, J. M., Kuan, S. A., Dobson-Stone, C., Paul, R. H., Joffe, R. T., Kemp, A. H., ... Williams, L. M. (2008). Association between BDNF Val66Met polymorphism and trait depression is mediated via resting EEG alpha band activity. *Biological Psychology,* **79**(2), 275–284.

Gattaz, W. F., Mayer, S., Ziegler, P., Platz, M., & Gasser, T. (1992). Hypofrontality on topographic EEG in schizophrenia: correlations with neuropsychological and psychopathological parameters. *European Archives of Psychiatry and Clinical Neuroscience,* **241**(6), 328–332.

Gerez, M., & Tello, A. (1995). Selected quantitative EEG (QEEG) and event-related potential (ERP) variables as discriminators for positive and negative schizophrenia. *Biological Psychiatry,* **38**(1), 34–49.

Gross, A., Joutsiniemi, S. L., Rimon, R., & Appelberg, B. (2006). Correlation of symptom clusters of schizophrenia with absolute powers of main frequency bands in quantitative EEG. *Behavioral and Brain Functions, 2*, 23.

Gschwandtner, U., Zimmermann, R., Pflueger, M. O., Riecher-Rossler, A., & Fuhr, P. (2009). Negative symptoms in neuroleptic-naive patients with first-episode psychosis correlate with QEEG parameters. *Schizophrenia Research, 115*(2–3), 231–236.

Hall, M. H., Rijsdijk, F., Kalidindi, S., Schulze, K., Kravariti, E., Kane, F., ... Murray, R. M. (2007a). Genetic overlap between bipolar illness and event-related potentials. *Psychological Medicine, 37*(5), 667–678.

Hall, M. H., Rijsdijk, F., Picchioni, M., Schulze, K., Ettinger, U., Toulopoulou, T., ... Sham, P. (2007b). Substantial shared genetic influences on schizophrenia and event-related potentials. *American Journal of Psychiatry, 164*(5), 804–812.

Hall, M. H., Schulze, K., Rijsdijk, F., Kalidindi, S., McDonald, C., Bramon, E., ... Sham, P. (2009). Are auditory P300 and duration MMN heritable and putative endophenotypes of psychotic bipolar disorder? A Maudsley Bipolar Twin and Family Study. *Psychological Medicine, 39*(8), 1277–1287.

He, W., Chai, H., Zheng, L., Yu, W., Chen, W., Li, J., & Wang, W. (2010). Mismatch negativity in treatment-resistant depression and borderline personality disorder. *Progress in Neuro-Psychopharmacology and Biological Psychiatry, 34*(2), 366–371.

Hermens, D. F., Chitty, K. M., & Kaur, M. (2018). Mismatch negativity in bipolar disorder: a neurophysiological biomarker of intermediate effect? *Schizophrenia Research, 191*, 132–139.

Hermens, D. F., Ward, P. B., Hodge, M. A., Kaur, M., Naismith, S. L., & Hickie, I. B. (2010). Impaired MMN/P3a complex in first-episode psychosis: cognitive and psychosocial associations. *Progress in Neuro-Psychopharmacology and Biological Psychiatry, 34*(6), 822–829.

Hetrick, S. E., Parker, A. G., Hickie, I. B., Purcell, R., Yung, A. R., & McGorry, P. D. (2008). Early identification and intervention in depressive disorders: towards a clinical staging model. *Psychotherapy and Psychosomatics, 77*(5), 263–270.

Higuchi, Y., Seo, T., Miyanishi, T., Kawasaki, Y., Suzuki, M., & Sumiyoshi, T. (2014). Mismatch negativity and p3a/reorienting complex in subjects with schizophrenia or at-risk mental state. *Frontiers in Behavioral Neuroscience, 8*, 172.

Higuchi, Y., Sumiyoshi, T., Seo, T., Miyanishi, T., Kawasaki, Y., & Suzuki, M. (2013). Mismatch negativity and cognitive performance for the prediction of psychosis in subjects with at-risk mental state. *PLoS One, 8*(1), e54080.

Hirayasu, Y., Asato, N., Ohta, H., Hokama, H., Arakaki, H., & Ogura, C. (1998). Abnormalities of auditory event-related potentials in schizophrenia prior to treatment. *Biological Psychiatry, 43*, 244–253.

Hong, X., Chan, R. C., Zhuang, X., Jiang, T., Wan, X., Wang, J., ... Weng, B. (2009). Neuroleptic effects on P50 sensory gating in patients with first-episode never-medicated schizophrenia. *Schizophrenia Research, 108*(1–3), 151–157.

Hsieh, M. H., Shan, J. C., Huang, W. L., Cheng, W. C., Chiu, M. J., Jaw, F. S., ... Liu, C. C. (2012). Auditory event-related potential of subjects with suspected pre-psychotic state and first-episode psychosis. *Schizophrenia Research, 140*(1–3), 243–249.

Hutchison, A. K., Hunter, S. K., Wagner, B. D., Calvin, E. A., Zerbe, G. O., & Ross, R. G. (2017). Diminished infant P50 sensory gating predicts increased 40-month-old attention, anxiety/depression, and externalizing symptoms. *Journal of Attention Disorders, 21*(3), 209–218.

Jahshan, C., Cadenhead, K. S., Rissling, A. J., Kirihara, K., Braff, D. L., & Light, G. A. (2012a). Automatic sensory information processing abnormalities across the illness course of schizophrenia. *Psychological Medicine, 42*(1), 85–97.

Jahshan, C., Wynn, J. K., Mathis, K. I., Altshuler, L. L., Glahn, D. C., & Green, M. F. (2012b). Cross-diagnostic comparison of duration mismatch negativity and P3a in bipolar disorder and schizophrenia. *Bipolar Disorders,* **14**(3), 239–248.

Javitt, D. C., Schroeder, C. E., Steinschneider, M., Arezzo, J. C., Ritter, W., & Vaughan, H. G., Jr. (1995). Cognitive event-related potentials in human and non-human primates: implications for the PCP/NMDA model of schizophrenia. *Electroencephalography and Clinical Neurophysiology Supplement,* **44**, 161–175.

Jeon, Y. W., & Polich, J. (2003). Meta-analysis of P300 and schizophrenia: patients, paradigms, and practical implications. *Psychophysiology,* **40**(5), 684–701.

Kahkonen, S., Yamashita, H., Rytsala, H., Suominen, K., Ahveninen, J., & Isometsa, E. (2007). Dysfunction in early auditory processing in major depressive disorder revealed by combined MEG and EEG. *Journal of Psychiatry and Neuroscience,* **32**(5), 316–322.

Kano, K., Nakamura, M., Matsuoka, T., Iida, H., & Nakajima, T. (1992). The topographical features of EEGs in patients with affective disorders. *Electroencephalography and Clinical Neurophysiology,* **83**(2), 124–129.

Kaur, M., Battisti, R. A., Lagopoulos, J., Ward, P. B., Hickie, I. B., & Hermens, D. F. (2012). Neurophysiological biomarkers support bipolar-spectrum disorders within psychosis cluster. *Journal of Psychiatry and Neuroscience,* **37**(5), 313–321.

Kaur, M., Battisti, R. A., Ward, P. B., Ahmed, A., Hickie, I. B., & Hermens, D. F. (2011). MMN/P3a deficits in first episode psychosis: comparing schizophrenia-spectrum and affective-spectrum subgroups. *Schizophrenia Research,* **130**(1–3), 203–209.

Kawakubo, Y., & Kasai, K. (2006). Support for an association between mismatch negativity and social functioning in schizophrenia. *Progress in Neuro-Psychopharmacology and Biological Psychiatry,* **30**(7), 1367–1368.

Kemp, A. H., Pe Benito, L., Quintana, D. S., Clark, C. R., McFarlane, A., Mayur, P., . . . Williams, L. M. (2010). Impact of depression heterogeneity on attention: an auditory oddball event related potential study. *Journal of Affective Disorders,* **123**(1–3), 202–207.

Kiang, M., Light, G. A., Prugh, J., Coulson, S., Braff, D. L., & Kutas, M. (2007). Cognitive, neurophysiological, and functional correlates of proverb interpretation abnormalities in schizophrenia. *Journal of the International Neuropsychological Society,* **13**(4), 653–663.

Kim, M., Lee, T. Y., Lee, S., Kim, S. N., & Kwon, J. S. (2015). Auditory P300 as a predictor of short-term prognosis in subjects at clinical high risk for psychosis. *Schizophrenia Research,* **165**(2–3), 138–144.

Kuang, W., Tian, L., Yue, L., & Li, J. (2016). Effects of escitalopram with a Chinese traditional compound Jiuweizhenxin-keli on mismatch negativity and P50 in patients with major depressive disorders. *Neuropsychiatric Disease and Treatment,* **12**, 1935–1941.

Lavoie, S., Jack, B. N., Griffiths, O., Ando, A., Amminger, P., Couroupis, A., . . . Whitford, T. J. (2018). Impaired mismatch negativity to frequency deviants in individuals at ultra-high risk for psychosis, and preliminary evidence for further impairment with transition to psychosis. *Schizophrenia Research,* **191**, 95–100.

Lavoie, S., Murray, M. M., Deppen, P., Knyazeva, M. G., Berk, M., Boulat, O., . . . Do, K. Q. (2007). Glutathione precursor, N-acetyl-cysteine, improves mismatch negativity in schizophrenia patients. *Neuropsychopharmacology,* **33**, 2187–2199.

Lavoie, S., Schafer, M. R., Whitford, T. J., Benninger, F., Feucht, M., Klier, C. M., . . . Amminger, G. P. (2012). Frontal delta power associated with negative symptoms in ultra-high risk individuals who transitioned to psychosis. *Schizophrenia Research,* **138**, 206–211.

Lee, K. H., Williams, L. M., Breakspear, M., & Gordon, E. (2003). Synchronous gamma activity: a review and contribution to an integrative neuroscience model of schizophrenia. *Brain Research Reviews,* **41**(1), 57–78.

Leicht, G., Vauth, S., Polomac, N., Andreou, C., Rauh, J., Mussmann, M., . . . Mulert, C. (2016). EEG-informed fMRI reveals a disturbed gamma-band-specific network in subjects at high risk for psychosis. *Schizophrenia Bulletin,* **42**(1), 239–249.

Light, G. A., & Braff, D. L. (2005a). Mismatch negativity deficits are associated with poor functioning in schizophrenia patients. *Archives of General Psychiatry, 62*(2), 127–136.

Light, G. A., & Braff, D. L. (2005b). Stability of mismatch negativity deficits and their relationship to functional impairments in chronic schizophrenia. *American Journal of Psychiatry, 162*(9), 1741–1743.

Magno, E., Yeap, S., Thakore, J. H., Garavan, H., De Sanctis, P., & Foxe, J. J. (2008). Are auditory-evoked frequency and duration mismatch negativity deficits endophenotypic for schizophrenia? High-density electrical mapping in clinically unaffected first-degree relatives and first-episode and chronic schizophrenia. *Biological Psychiatry, 64*(5), 385–391.

Mathalon, D. H., Ford, J. M., Rosenbloom, M., & Pfefferbaum, A. (2000). P300 reduction and prolongation with illness duration in schizophrenia. *Biological Psychiatry, 47*, 413–427.

McCarley, R. W., Salisbury, D. F., Hirayasu, Y., Yurgelun-Todd, D. A., Tohen, M., Zarate, C., . . . Shenton, M. E. (2002). Association between smaller left posterior superior temporal gyrus volume on magnetic resonance imaging and smaller left temporal P300 amplitude in first-episode schizophrenia. *Archives of General Psychiatry, 59*(4), 321–331.

Moeini, M., Khaleghi, A., & Mohammadi, M. R. (2015). Characteristics of alpha band frequency in adolescents with bipolar II disorder: a resting-state QEEG study. *Iranian Journal of Psychiatry, 10*(1), 8–12.

Mondragon-Maya, A., Solis-Vivanco, R., Leon-Ortiz, P., Rodriguez-Agudelo, Y., Yanez-Tellez, G., Bernal-Hernandez, J., . . . de la Fuente-Sandoval, C. (2013). Reduced P3a amplitudes in antipsychotic naive first-episode psychosis patients and individuals at clinical high-risk for psychosis. *Journal of Psychiatric Research, 47*(6), 755–761.

Morales-Munoz, I., Jurado-Barba, R., Fernandez-Guinea, S., Rodriguez-Jimenez, R., Jimenez-Arriero, M. A., Criado, J. R., & Rubio, G. (2016). Sensory gating deficits in first-episode psychosis: evidence from neurophysiology, psychophysiology, and neuropsychology. *Journal of Nervous and Mental Disease, 204*(12), 877–884.

Myles-Worsley, M., Ord, L., Blailes, F., Ngiralmau, H., & Freedman, R. (2004). P50 sensory gating in adolescents from a Pacific Island isolate with elevated risk for schizophrenia. *Biological Psychiatry, 55*(7), 663–667.

Naatanen, R., Kujala, T., & Winkler, I. (2011). Auditory processing that leads to conscious perception: a unique window to central auditory processing opened by the mismatch negativity and related responses. *Psychophysiology, 48*(1), 4–22.

Naatanen, R., Shiga, T., Asano, S., & Yabe, H. (2015). Mismatch negativity (MMN) deficiency: a break-through biomarker in predicting psychosis onset. *International Journal of Psychophysiology, 95*(3), 338–344.

Naismith, S. L., Mowszowski, L., Ward, P. B., Diamond, K., Paradise, M., Kaur, M., . . . Hermens, D. F. (2012). Reduced temporal mismatch negativity in late-life depression: an event-related potential index of cognitive deficit and functional disability? *Journal of Affective Disorders, 138*(1–2), 71–78.

Narayanan, B., O'Neil, K., Berwise, C., Stevens, M. C., Calhoun, V. D., Clementz, B. A., . . . Pearlson, G. D. (2014). Resting state electroencephalogram oscillatory abnormalities in schizophrenia and psychotic bipolar patients and their relatives from the bipolar and schizophrenia network on intermediate phenotypes study. *Biological Psychiatry, 76*(6), 456–465.

Nieman, D. H., Ruhrmann, S., Dragt, S., Soen, F., van Tricht, M. J., Koelman, J. H., . . . de Haan, L. (2014). Psychosis prediction: stratification of risk estimation with information-processing and premorbid functioning variables. *Schizophrenia Bulletin, 40*(6), 1482–1490.

O'Donnell, B. F., Faux, S. F., McCarley, R. W., Kimble, M. O., Salisbury, D. F., Nestor, P. G., . . . Shenton, M. E. (1995). Increased rate of P300 latency prolongation with age in schizophrenia: electrophysiological evidence for a neurodegenerative process. *Archives of General Psychiatry, 52*(7), 544–549.

O'Donnell, B. F., Vohs, J. L., Hetrick, W. P., Carroll, C. A., & Shekhar, A. (2004). Auditory event-related potential abnormalities in bipolar disorder and schizophrenia. *International Journal of Psychophysiology, 53*(1), 45–55.

Oades, R. D., Wild-Wall, N., Juran, S. A., Sachsse, J., Oknina, L. B., & Ropcke, B. (2006). Auditory change detection in schizophrenia: sources of activity, related neuropsychological function and symptoms in patients with a first episode in adolescence, and patients 14 years after an adolescent illness-onset. *BMC Psychiatry, 6*, 7.

Olbrich, S., & Arns, M. (2013). EEG biomarkers in major depressive disorder: discriminative power and prediction of treatment response. *International Review of Psychiatry, 25*(5), 604–618.

Onitsuka, T., Oribe, N., & Kanba, S. (2013). Neurophysiological findings in patients with bipolar disorder. *Supplements to Clinical Neurophysiology, 62*, 197–206.

Ozerdem, A., Guntekin, B., Tunca, Z., & Basar, E. (2008). Brain oscillatory responses in patients with bipolar disorder manic episode before and after valproate treatment. *Brain Research, 1235*, 98–108.

Ozgurdal, S., Gudlowski, Y., Witthaus, H., Kawohl, W., Uhl, I., Hauser, M., . . . Juckel, G. (2008). Reduction of auditory event-related P300 amplitude in subjects with at-risk mental state for schizophrenia. *Schizophrenia Research, 105*(1–3), 272–278.

Patterson, J. V., Hetrick, W. P., Boutros, N. N., Jin, Y., Sandman, C., Stern, H., . . . Bunney, W. E., Jr. (2008). P50 sensory gating ratios in schizophrenics and controls: a review and data analysis. *Psychiatry Research, 158*(2), 226–247.

Perez, V. B., Roach, B. J., Woods, S. W., Srihari, V. H., McGlashan, T. H., Ford, J. M., & Mathalon, D. H. (2013). Early auditory gamma-band responses in patients at clinical high risk for schizophrenia. *Supplements to Clinical Neurophysiology, 62*, 147–162.

Perez, V. B., Woods, S. W., Roach, B. J., Ford, J. M., McGlashan, T. H., Srihari, V. H., & Mathalon, D. H. (2014). Automatic auditory processing deficits in schizophrenia and clinical high-risk patients: forecasting psychosis risk with mismatch negativity. *Biological Psychiatry, 75*(6), 459–469.

Pierson, A., Jouvent, R., Quintin, P., Perez-Diaz, F., & Leboyer, M. (2000). Information processing deficits in relatives of manic depressive patients. *Psychological Medicine, 30*(3), 545–555.

Pollock, V. E., & Schneider, L. S. (1990). Quantitative, waking EEG research on depression. *Biological Psychiatry, 27*(7), 757–780.

Qiao, Z., Yu, Y., Wang, L., Yang, X., Qiu, X., Zhang, C., . . . Yang, Y. (2013). Impaired pre-attentive change detection in major depressive disorder patients revealed by auditory mismatch negativity. *Psychiatry Research, 211*(1), 78–84.

Ranlund, S., Nottage, J., Shaikh, M., Dutt, A., Constante, M., Walshe, M., . . . Bramon, E. (2014). Resting EEG in psychosis and at-risk populations: a possible endophenotype? *Schizophrenia Research, 153*(1–3), 96–102.

Rasser, P. E., Schall, U., Todd, J., Michie, P. T., Ward, P. B., Johnston, P., . . . Thompson, P. M. (2011). Gray matter deficits, mismatch negativity, and outcomes in schizophrenia. *Schizophrenia Bulletin, 37*(1), 131–140.

Renoult, L., Prevost, M., Brodeur, M., Lionnet, C., Joober, R., Malla, A., & Debruille, J. B. (2007). P300 asymmetry and positive symptom severity: a study in the early stage of a first episode of psychosis. *Schizophrenia Research, 93*(1–3), 366–373.

Rieder, M. K., Rahm, B., Williams, J. D., & Kaiser, J. (2011). Human gamma-band activity and behavior. *International Journal of Psychophysiology, 79*(1), 39–48.

Salisbury, D. F., Kuroki, N., Kasai, K., Shenton, M. E., & McCarley, R. W. (2007). Progressive and interrelated functional and structural evidence of post-onset brain reduction in schizophrenia. *Archives of General Psychiatry, 64*(5), 521–529.

Salisbury, D. F., Shenton, M. E., Griggs, C. B., Bonner-Jackson, A., & McCarley, R. W. (2002). Mismatch negativity in chronic schizophrenia and first-episode schizophrenia. *Archives of General Psychiatry, 59*(8), 686–694.

Salisbury, D. F., Shenton, M. E., & McCarley, R. W. (1999). P300 topography differs in schizophrenia and manic psychosis. *Biological Psychiatry, 45*(1), 98–106.

Sanchez-Morla, E. M., Garcia-Jimenez, M. A., Barabash, A., Martinez-Vizcaino, V., Mena, J., Cabranes-Diaz, J. A., . . . Santos, J. L. (2008). P50 sensory gating deficit is a common marker of vulnerability to bipolar disorder and schizophrenia. *Acta Psychiatrica Scandinavica, 117*(4), 313–318.

Schlegel, S., Nieber, D., Herrmann, C., & Bakauski, E. (1991). Latencies of the P300 component of the auditory event-related potential in depression are related to the Bech–Rafaelsen Melancholia Scale but not to the Hamilton Rating Scale for Depression. *Acta Psychiatrica Scandinavica, 83*(6), 438–440.

Schulze, K. K., Hall, M. H., McDonald, C., Marshall, N., Walshe, M., Murray, R. M., & Bramon, E. (2008). Auditory P300 in patients with bipolar disorder and their unaffected relatives. *Bipolar Disorders, 10*(3), 377–386.

Shaikh, M., Valmaggia, L., Broome, M. R., Dutt, A., Lappin, J., Day, F., . . . Bramon, E. (2012). Reduced mismatch negativity predates the onset of psychosis. *Schizophrenia Research, 134*(1), 42–48.

Shin, K. S., Kim, J. S., Kang, D. H., Koh, Y., Choi, J. S., O'Donnell, B. F., . . . Kwon, J. S. (2009). Pre-attentive auditory processing in ultra-high-risk for schizophrenia with magnetoencephalography. *Biological Psychiatry, 65*(12), 1071–1078.

Siegle, G. J., Condray, R., Thase, M. E., Keshavan, M., & Steinhauer, S. R. (2010). Sustained gamma-band EEG following negative words in depression and schizophrenia. *International Journal of Psychophysiology, 75*(2), 107–118.

Slewa-Younan, S., Gordon, E., Harris, A. W., Haig, A. R., Brown, K. J., Flor-Henry, P., & Williams, L. M. (2004). Sex differences in functional connectivity in first-episode and chronic schizophrenia patients. *American Journal of Psychiatry, 161*(9), 1595–1602.

Solis-Vivanco, R., Mondragon-Maya, A., Leon-Ortiz, P., Rodriguez-Agudelo, Y., Cadenhead, K. S., & de la Fuente-Sandoval, C. (2014). Mismatch negativity reduction in the left cortical regions in first-episode psychosis and in individuals at ultra high-risk for psychosis. *Schizophrenia Research, 158*(1–3), 58–63.

Spencer, K. M., Salisbury, D. F., Shenton, M. E., & McCarley, R. W. (2008). Gamma-band auditory steady-state responses are impaired in first episode psychosis. *Biological Psychiatry, 64*(5), 369–375.

Sponheim, S. R., Clementz, B. A., Iacono, W. G., & Beiser, M. (2000). Clinical and biological concomitants of resting state EEG power abnormalities in schizophrenia. *Biological Psychiatry, 48*(11), 1088–1097.

Strelets, V. B., Novototsky-Vlasov, V. Y., & Golikova, J. V. (2002). Cortical connectivity in high frequency beta-rhythm in schizophrenics with positive and negative symptoms. *International Journal of Psychophysiology, 44*, 101–115.

Symond, M. P., Harris, A. W., Gordon, E., & Williams, L. M. (2005). 'Gamma synchrony' in first-episode schizophrenia: a disorder of temporal connectivity? *American Journal of Psychiatry, 162*(3), 459–465.

Tada, M., Nagai, T., Kirihara, K., Koike, S., Suga, M., Araki, T., . . . Kasai, K. (2014). Differential alterations of auditory gamma oscillatory responses between pre-onset high-risk individuals and first-episode schizophrenia. *Cerebral Cortex, 26*(3), 1027–1035.

Takei, Y., Kumano, S., Hattori, S., Uehara, T., Kawakubo, Y., Kasai, K., . . . Mikuni, M. (2009). Preattentive dysfunction in major depression: a magnetoencephalography study using auditory mismatch negativity. *Psychophysiology, 46*(1), 52–61.

Thibodeau, R., Jorgensen, R. S., & Kim, S. (2006). Depression, anxiety, and resting frontal EEG asymmetry: a meta-analytic review. *Journal of Abnormal Psychology, 115*(4), 715–729.

Todd, J., Michie, P. T., Schall, U., Karayanidis, F., Yabe, H., & Naatanen, R. (2007). Deviant matters: duration, frequency, and intensity deviants reveal different patterns of mismatch negativity reduction in early and late schizophrenia. *Biological Psychiatry,* 63(1), 58–64.

Turetsky, B. I., Calkins, M. E., Light, G. A., Olincy, A., Radant, A. D., & Swerdlow, N. R. (2007). Neurophysiological endophenotypes of schizophrenia: the viability of selected candidate measures. *Schizophrenia Bulletin,* 33(1), 69–94.

Uhlhaas, P. J., & Singer, W. (2006). Neural synchrony in brain disorders: relevance for cognitive dysfunctions and pathophysiology. *Neuron,* 52(1), 155–168.

Uhlhaas, P. J., & Singer, W. (2010). Abnormal neural oscillations and synchrony in schizophrenia. *Nature Reviews Neuroscience,* 11(2), 100–113.

Umbricht, D. S., Bates, J. A., Lieberman, J. A., Kane, J. M., & Javitt, D. C. (2006). Electrophysiological indices of automatic and controlled auditory information processing in first-episode, recent-onset and chronic schizophrenia. *Biological Psychiatry,* 59(8), 762–772.

Umbricht, D., Koller, R., Schmid, L., Skrabo, A., Grubel, C., Huber, T., & Stassen, H. (2003). How specific are deficits in mismatch negativity generation to schizophrenia? *Biological Psychiatry,* 53(12), 1120–1131.

Umbricht, D., Koller, R., Vollenweider, F. X., & Schmid, L. (2002). Mismatch negativity predicts psychotic experiences induced by NMDA receptor antagonist in healthy volunteers. *Biological Psychiatry,* 51(5), 400–406.

Umbricht, D., & Krljes, S. (2005). Mismatch negativity in schizophrenia: a meta-analysis. *Schizophrenia Bulletin,* 76(1), 1–23.

Valkonen-Korhonen, M., Purhonen, M., Tarkka, I. M., Sipila, P., Partanen, J., Karhu, J., & Lehtonen, J. (2003). Altered auditory processing in acutely psychotic never-medicated first-episode patients. *Cognitive Brain Research,* 17(3), 747–758.

van der Stelt, O., Lieberman, J. A., & Belger, A. (2005). Auditory P300 in high-risk, recent-onset and chronic schizophrenia. *Schizophrenia Research,* 77(2–3), 309–320.

van Tricht, M. J., Nieman, D. H., Koelman, J. T., Mensink, A. J., Bour, L. J., van der Meer, J. N., . . . de Haan, L. (2015). Sensory gating in subjects at ultra high risk for developing a psychosis before and after a first psychotic episode. *World Journal of Biological Psychiatry,* 16(1), 12–21.

Vandoolaeghe, E., van Hunsel, F., Nuyten, D., & Maes, M. (1998). Auditory event related potentials in major depression: prolonged P300 latency and increased P200 amplitude. *Journal of Affective Disorders,* 48(2–3), 105–113.

Venables, N. C., Bernat, E. M., & Sponheim, S. R. (2009). Genetic and disorder-specific aspects of resting state EEG abnormalities in schizophrenia. *Schizophrenia Bulletin,* 35(4), 826–839.

Wang, J., Tang, Y., Li, C., Mecklinger, A., Xiao, Z., Zhang, M., . . . Li, H. (2009a). Decreased P300 current source density in drug-naive first episode schizophrenics revealed by high density recording. *International Journal of Psychophysiology,* 75(3), 249–257.

Wang, Y., Fang, Y. R., Chen, X. S., Chen, J., Wu, Z. G., Yuan, C. M., . . . Cao, L. (2009b). A follow-up study on features of sensory gating P50 in treatment-resistant depression patients. *Chinese Medical Journal,* 122(24), 2956–2960.

Wynn, J. K., Sugar, C., Horan, W. P., Kern, R., & Green, M. F. (2010). Mismatch negativity, social cognition, and functioning in schizophrenia patients. *Biological Psychiatry,* 67(10), 940–947.

Xiong, P., Zeng, Y., Zhu, Z., Tan, D., Xu, F., Lu, J., . . . Ma, M. (2010). Reduced NGF serum levels and abnormal P300 event-related potential in first episode schizophrenia. *Schizophrenia Research,* 119(1–3), 34–39.

Zhang, Y., Hauser, U., Conty, C., Emrich, H. M., & Dietrich, D. E. (2007). Familial risk for depression and p3b component as a possible neurocognitive vulnerability marker. *Neuropsychobiology,* 55(1), 14–20.

Zimmermann, R., Gschwandtner, U., Wilhelm, F. H., Pflueger, M. O., Riecher-Rossler, A., & Fuhr, P. (2010). EEG spectral power and negative symptoms in at-risk individuals predict transition to psychosis. *Schizophrenia Research,* **123**(2–3), 208–216.

Zoon, H. F., Veth, C. P., Arns, M., Drinkenburg, W. H., Talloen, W., Peeters, P. J., & Kenemans, J. L. (2013). EEG alpha power as an intermediate measure between brain-derived neurotrophic factor Val66Met and depression severity in patients with major depressive disorder. *Journal of Clinical Neurophysiology,* **30**(3), 261–267.

Chapter

11

Novel Biological Treatment Strategies

G. Paul Amminger and Maximus Berger

A key proposition of staging is that early-stage treatments should be effective, benign, not specific to diagnostic categories and, through their timing, more effective then at a later stage when structural damage or functional decline has already occurred. While psychological interventions are considered first-line treatments for young people experiencing mental health problems, such treatments (e.g. cognitive behavioural therapy (CBT)) rely on trained therapists who are in high demand with often lengthy waiting lists, and who are usually not accessible in underprivileged areas or those outside metropolitan spaces. Furthermore, psychotherapy can be too time-consuming when interfering with young people's busy schedules. In contrast, biological treatments have the advantage of not depending on skilled therapists or specific settings, are usually easy to apply and may directly target core biological processes that may contribute to illness progression, such as oxidative stress or inflammation (see Chapters 8 and 9). Putative neuroprotective treatments that are discussed in this chapter, such as omega-3 polyunsaturated fatty acids (PUFAs) or N-acetyl-cysteine (NAC), may be non-specifically and transdiagnostically effective if given early enough, or have some specificity later (Berk et al., 2013a). If less specific treatments are effective in preventing transition to more severe stages, this would suggest that, in the early stages, the commonalities within the same stage between disorders may exceed differences that exist between stages within the same disorder (Scott et al., 2013). Treatment resistance to conventional pharmaceutical interventions (e.g. antidepressive and/or antipsychotic medication) may occur as a problem even during the first episode of a psychiatric disorder. This chapter will review novel biotherapies relevant to the staging model of psychiatric disorders (McGorry et al., 2006), including transcranial magnetic stimulation (TMS), cannabidiol (CBD), omega-3 PUFAs and NAC, which may offer additional viable treatment options for young people when psychotherapeutic and conventional pharmaceutical interventions have repeatedly failed.

Long-Chain Omega-3 Polyunsaturated Fatty Acids

The largest group of studies testing natural agents for mental health problems to date addressed the question of whether supplementation with long-chain omega-3 PUFAs is effective for mood disorders (major depression; perinatal depression; bipolar disorder) (Hallahan et al., 2016; Lin et al., 2017; Saunders et al., 2016) and psychotic disorders (Amminger et al., 2015; Sommer et al., 2013). Omega-3 PUFAs are safe and free of clinically relevant side-effects. As key components of brain tissue, omega-3 PUFAs play critical roles in brain development and function, and a lack of these fatty acids has been implicated in a number of mental health conditions over the lifespan, including depression (Assies et al., 2010) and schizophrenia (Horrobin, 1998). Clinical studies and epidemiological findings support an association between omega-3 PUFAs and major depression, suicide risk, impulsivity, aggressive behaviours and psychosis.

PUFA Biochemistry and Physiological Functions

PUFAs can be classified into omega-3 and omega-6 fatty acids. The terms omega-3 and omega-6 specify the location of the first double bond from the methyl end of the molecule. Mammals have lost the ability to introduce a double bond beyond carbon 9, and thus humans cannot synthesise these fatty acids *de novo*. Therefore, they have to be obtained through dietary intake. Fatty acids have numerous and diverse functions in the human body. They are part of phospholipid molecules, the main structural building blocks of cell membranes, which make up around 60 per cent of the dry weight of the brain. Phospholipids consist of a glycerol molecule, two fatty acids and a phosphate group that is modified by an alcohol. PUFAs are bioactive molecules that play central roles in a broad range of physiological functions. For example, two particularly important PUFAs are eicosapentaenoic acid (EPA) and arachidonic acid (AA), which are key players in signal transduction, ion transport and receptor sensitivity (e.g. for serotonin, dopamine, endocannabinoids), as well as precursors in the biosynthesis of the eicosanoids (prostaglandins, leukotrienes, thromboxanes), which mediate the inflammatory response (Mossaheb et al., 2012). Another key PUFA, docosahexaenoic acid (DHA), serves as a precursor for the docosanoids (resolvins, neuroprotectins), which have a neuroprotective effect. The brain is highly enriched with omega-3 PUFAs and their derivatives, which regulate biological processes such as neurotransmission, neuroplasticity and neuroinflammation, and thereby mood and cognitive function (Lin et al., 2017; Piomelli et al., 2007; Su et al., 2015). Moreover, omega-3 PUFAs may modulate neurotrophins (Venna et al., 2009), which might be a direct mechanism to mediate neurogenesis and antidepressant effects (Blondeau et al., 2009).

Effects on Inflammation

Inflammation is part of the body's immune response. Initially, it is generally beneficial when, for example, battling infectious agents. However, sometimes inflammation can cause further inflammation; it can become self-perpetuating. More inflammation is created in response to the existing inflammation, which can lead to a broad range of illnesses. Omega-6 and omega-3 PUFAs are precursors of eicosanoids, both of which are involved in the regulation of inflammation. Omega-3 PUFAs have an anti-inflammatory effect through multiple pathways by inhibiting the formation of omega-6 PUFA-derived pro-inflammatory eicosanoids (e.g. prostaglandin (PG)-E2, leukotriene (LT)-B4), and forming potent anti-inflammatory lipid mediators (Piomelli et al., 2007; Serhan, 2014). These suppress the activity of nuclear transcription factors and reduce the production of pro-inflammatory enzymes and cytokines, including TNF-α and interleukin (IL)-1β. While omega-6 PUFAs promote inflammation, omega-3 PUFAs (EPA; DHA) have anti-inflammatory properties. Omega-3 PUFAs dampen inflammation through multiple pathways: omega-3 PUFAs inhibit the formation of omega-6 PUFA-derived pro-inflammatory eicosanoids (e.g. PG-E2 and LT-B4), and omega-3 PUFAs can form several potent anti-inflammatory lipid mediators (e.g. resolvins and protectins) (Serhan, 2014; Serhan & Petasis, 2011). These together directly or indirectly suppress the activity of nuclear transcription factors, such as nuclear factor kappa-light-chain-enhancer of activated B cells (NFkB), and reduce the production of pro-inflammatory enzymes and cytokines, including cyclooxygenase (COX)-2, TNF-α and IL-1β.

Epidemiological Findings

Human beings evolved on a diet with a ratio of omega-6/omega-3 PUFAs of about 1:1, but modern (Western) diets have a ratio of 10–20:1, indicating that these diets are in a profound imbalance in PUFA composition (Simopoulos, 2011). Omega-3 PUFAs are being replaced in Western diets by saturated fats from domestic animals and by omega-6 PUFAs from common vegetable oils (Parker et al., 2006). Chronic deficiency in dietary omega-3 PUFAs could change omega-3 PUFA concentrations in the brain and lead to depression-like behaviours by increasing serotonin (5-HT) 2 and decreasing dopamine D2 receptor density in the frontal cortex (Berg et al., 1996; Chalon et al., 2001; Delion et al., 1994). The sharp rise in rates of depression and other neuropsychiatric disorders in the twentieth century has been linked to changes in diet quality, characterised by an increased consumption of vegetable oils rich in omega-6 PUFAs (Hibbeln & Salem, 1995) that displace dietary omega-3 PUFAs. As humans cannot synthesise PUFAs *de novo*, they depend upon dietary intake. Fish and seafood are the richest sources of the long-chained omega-3 PUFAs (EPA and DHA). DHA is selectively concentrated in synaptic neuronal membranes and contributes to unique biophysical properties that mediate receptor activity and signal transduction (Piomelli et al., 2007). Moreover, rapid advances in the basic sciences have confirmed the central role of the omega-3 PUFAs in a variety of pathophysiological processes, particularly those involving monoaminergic (Sublette et al., 2004), dopaminergic (Sublette et al., 2014) and serotonergic neurotransmission (Freeman et al., 2006; Sublette et al., 2004), all of which have been implicated in major mood disorders, borderline personality disorder and psychotic disorders (Ripoll, 2013). Omega-3 PUFAs are degraded in states of oxidative stress, a ubiquitous finding across these psychiatric disorders, which increase metabolic demand.

Since seafood and fish are the main sources of EPA and DHA, Hibbeln tested the hypothesis that a high consumption of seafood could be correlated with a lower annual prevalence of major depression (Hibbeln, 1998). He found a significant relationship between the nearly 60-fold range in annual prevalence rates of major depression and the over 100-fold range of fish consumption, in a multinational comparison across nine countries. The authors noted the correlation between apparent fish consumption and lower annual prevalence of major depression does not show that fish consumption can cause differences in the prevalence of major depression or that eating fish or fish oils are useful in treatment. Various cultural, economic, social and other factors can confound the correlational relation. Frequent fish consumption, twice a week or more, was also found as an independent factor for a reduced risk for depressive symptoms and suicidal thinking in a restricted geographical region within a single country (Tanskanen et al., 2001). Another epidemiological study across 11 countries showed greater rates of seafood consumption are associated with lower lifetime prevalence rates of bipolar I disorder, bipolar II disorder and bipolar spectrum disorder (Noaghiul & Hibbeln, 2003). Again these epidemiological studies do not demonstrate a causal relationship, but they are consistent with the hypothesis that an insufficient dietary intake of omega-3 PUFAs increases the risk of affective disorders.

There is also compelling evidence supporting an association between fish consumption and psychotic phenomena in the general population. Hedelin et al. (2010) conducted a large-scale epidemiological study among women in the Uppsala Health Care Region in Sweden to evaluate the association of dietary intake of different fish species and specific PUFAs with the prevalence of positive psychotic-like symptoms. Dietary intake was estimated using a food frequency questionnaire among 33,623 women at enrolment. Information on psychotic-like symptoms was derived from a follow-up questionnaire a decade later. Women were divided into a 'low-level symptoms group' (55 per cent), a 'middle-level symptoms group' (43 per cent) and a 'high-level symptoms group' (2.4 per cent) based on their responses at follow-up. Among many of their findings, Hedelin and colleagues reported that the intake of omega-3 and omega-6 PUFAs was associated with a decreased relative risk for psychotic-like symptoms, after adjusting for multiple other potentially confounding variables. Interpretation of the findings is limited, given that dietary intake and self-reported psychotic-like symptoms were measured only once, and men were not included. Nonetheless, the results provide an interesting hint into possible correlations between dietary intake and psychosis continuum experiences in the general population (Compton, 2010).

Epidemiological data also indicate that low levels of circulating lipids, omega-3 PUFAs and cholesterol are risk factors for aggressive (Hallahan & Garland, 2005) and suicidal behaviours (Lewis et al., 2011; Tanskanen et al., 2001), which are core features of borderline personality disorder. In a clinical study conducted among people presenting with self-harm, lower plasma omega-3 PUFA levels were associated with self-harm and impulsivity (Garland et al., 2007). This study also showed that patients had significantly lower levels of plasma omega-3 PUFAs than healthy controls, providing a rationale for supplementation in young people with borderline personality disorder symptoms. Consistent with this view is a large body of evidence indicating that 5-hydroxytryptamine (5-HT) dysfunction underlies impulsive and suicidal behaviour, and that low omega-3 PUFA levels impair serotonin or 5-HT function (Garland & Hallahan, 2006). A post-hoc subgroup analysis in our own double-blind randomised controlled trial (RCT) of omega-3 vs placebo in young people at ultra-high risk of psychosis (NCT00396643), conducted in Vienna, Austria has also provided highly favourable pilot findings to support omega-3 PUFA supplementation as treatment in youth with borderline personality disorder (Amminger et al., 2013). As part of this RCT, 15 individuals with borderline personality disorder (mean age = 16.2 years, SD = 2.1) were randomised to either 1.2 g/day omega-3 PUFAs or placebo for 12 weeks. Eight borderline personality disorder participants were randomly assigned to be treated with omega-3 PUFAs, while seven received placebo. Study measures included the Positive and Negative Syndrome Scale (PANSS), the Montgomery–Åsberg Depression Rating Scale (MADRS) and the Global Assessment of Functioning (GAF). Erythrocyte fatty acids were analysed using capillary gas chromatography to obtain an omega-3 index (i.e. sum of EPA and DHA), a well-established biomarker for cardiovascular health (von Schacky, 2009). The borderline personality disorder patients ($n = 15$) had a very low omega-3 index of 3.22 per cent (SD = 1.06). Proposed omega-3 index risk zones are (in percentages of erythrocyte fatty acids): high risk, <4 per cent; intermediate risk, 4–8 per cent; and low risk, >8 per cent). Baseline erythrocyte omega-3 PUFA levels were significantly positively correlated with psychosocial functioning and negatively correlated with psychopathology. By the end of the intervention, the omega-3 PUFA group showed significantly improved functioning and reduced psychiatric symptoms, including a PANSS item summary score related to borderline personality disorder (suspiciousness, tension, poor impulse control), compared with placebo. The magnitude of group differences was large (PANSS borderline personality disorder symptoms Cohen's $d = 0.99$; PANSS total score $d = 0.91$; GAF score $d = 1.59$; MADRS score $d = 0.95$). Side-effects did not differ between the treatment groups (Amminger et al., 2013).

Larger RCTs seem warranted to test whether successful short- to medium-term omega-3 PUFA treatment can help reduce the severity of borderline personality disorder (i.e. impulsivity, suicidal behaviour, aggression and psychopathology), as well as improve functional outcomes and quality of life among this patient group, which has very limited access to effective treatment (Leichsenring et al., 2011). Moreover, treatment with omega-3 PUFAs can be safely used in a wide variety of settings, from primary care to specialist, as well as being used as an adjunctive intervention during the acute phase of illness to optimise psychosocial early intervention for borderline personality disorder. Omega-3 PUFAs are also specifically notable among potential pharmacotherapies for borderline personality disorder because they are very safe – especially in overdose, which is a major risk with this patient group.

Treatment Trials in Youth with Depression

Adolescence and young adulthood are also the peak periods for the onset of depression. There is evidence that the prevalence of depression may be rising, potentially driven by alterations in environmental factors (Berk et al., 2013b; Twenge et al., 2010). The lower incidence of depression in populations with high fish consumption provides a link between omega-3 PUFA intake and proneness to depression (Hibbeln, 1998; Sánchez-Villegas et al., 2009). Alterations in fatty acids observed in plasma and erythrocytes in people with major depressive disorder (MDD) corroborate the epidemiological data (Assies et al., 2010). However, trials evaluating efficacy of omega-3 supplementation in MDD report conflicting findings (Bloch & Hannestad, 2012; Hallahan et al., 2016; Sublette et al., 2011). Among participants with diagnosed depression, EPA-predominant formulations (>50 per cent EPA) demonstrated clinical benefits compared with placebo, whereas DHA-predominant formulations (>50 per cent DHA) did not (Hallahan et al., 2016). Notably, the majority of trials have been conducted in adult populations with omega-3 PUFAs as an adjunct treatment to antidepressive medication. We are currently conducting the first RCT to test the efficacy of an EPA-predominant formulation as an alternative to antidepressive medication in 12–25-year-olds with MDD, funded by NHMRC Grant 1042666 (Rice et al., 2016). A manuscript detailing the results is in preparation. If found effective, this study could help establish omega-3 PUFAs as a novel, stigma-free first-line treatment in youth depression without causing clinically relevant side-effects.

Prevention of Psychosis

In a first-of-its-kind trial we have shown that 12-week supplementation with omega-3 PUFAs reduced the risk of progression to psychotic disorder in 81 young people with subthreshold psychotic states for a 12-month period compared with placebo (Amminger et al., 2010). In a recently completed longer-term follow-up of this trial, we found that the brief intervention with omega-3 PUFAs was still effective. Compared to placebo, omega-3 PUFAs prevented transition to full-threshold psychotic disorder and led to sustained symptomatic and functional improvements for seven years (median) (Amminger et al., 2015). Notably, the majority of the individuals from the omega-3 group did not show severe functional impairment and no longer experienced attenuated psychotic symptoms at follow-up. These findings, in particular in the non-transitioned participants, suggested longer-term preventive and therapeutic effects in some of the participants who received omega-3 PUFAs. This trial suggests that omega-3 PUFAs may offer a viable longer-term prevention strategy with minimal associated risk in young people with an at-risk mental state for psychosis. In addition to these trial results, (negative) correlations between omega-3 PUFAs and psychopathology (in particular negative symptoms) (Kim et al., 2016), and a large effect size deficit for omega-3 PUFAs observed in patients with an at-risk mental state compared to healthy adolescents (Rice et al., 2015), provide a further rationale for omega-3 supplementation as early intervention for incipient psychotic symptoms. A high ratio of omega-6 to omega-3 PUFAs is thought to have adverse health effects (Simopoulos, 2011). Most recently, we were also able to show that a higher ratio of omega-6 to omega-3 PUFA at baseline predicted mood disorders in ultra-high-risk individuals over a seven-year (median) follow-up in participants of the Vienna omega-3 study (odds ratio = 1.894; 95 per cent CI = 1.075–3.338) (Berger et al., 2017). This association remained significant after adjustment for age, gender, smoking, severity of depressive symptoms at baseline and omega-3 supplementation status. In the context of current early intervention strategies, these findings may have important implications for treatment and risk stratification beyond clinical characteristics.

Two larger-scale studies have tried to replicate the findings of the Vienna omega-3 study. The first, our own, replication RCT was conducted from 2010 to 2014, in ten specialised early psychosis treatment services in Australia, Asia and Europe (McGorry et al., 2017). The interventions were a daily dose of 1.4 omega-3 PUFAs or placebo, plus 20 or fewer sessions of cognitive behavioural case management (CBCM) over the six-month study period. In this study of 304 individuals at ultra-high risk for psychotic disorders, 153 received omega-3 PUFAs and 151 received placebo. Overall, 139 (45.7 per cent) were male; mean (SD) age in the total sample was 19.1 (4.6) years. The Kaplan–Meier estimated six-month transition rates were 5.1 per cent (95 per cent CI = 1.3–8.7) in the control group and 6.7 per cent (95 per cent CI = 2.3–10.8) in the omega-3 PUFA group. At 12 months, the rates were 11.2 per cent (95 per cent CI = 5.5–16.7) in the control group and 11.5 per cent (95 per cent CI = 5.8–16.9) in the omega-3 PUFA group. No significant difference was observed between the transition rates of both groups (McGorry et al., 2017). This trial failed to replicate the findings of our original single-centre trial (Amminger et al., 2010). The most likely explanation is that omega-3 PUFAs lack efficacy under these conditions. However, the lower-than-expected transition rate may have prevented a test of the main hypothesis. Given the substantial symptomatic and functional improvement in both groups, the other treatments received (i.e. CBCM and antidepressants) likely produced a ceiling effect beyond which omega-3 PUFAs, even if effective, could not be shown to confer additional benefits. Notably, an important limitation of this study (and all omega-3 PUFA RCTs) is that the use of non-study omega-3 PUFA supplements cannot be excluded and the test agent may thus be present in both the treatment and control groups (James et al., 2014). Therapeutic effects of omega-3 PUFAs may be present in subgroups characterised by certain biological or phenotypic markers that can be considered as moderators of clinical response (Kraemer, 2016). For example, these supplements may be specifically effective in subgroups characterised by a high level of inflammation (Rapaport et al., 2016). Additional analyses using baseline membrane fatty acid levels as objective measures of omega-3 PUFA intake and/or information on inflammatory markers are currently underway. We are also investigating biological measures of omega-3 PUFA intake that accurately define adherence to study medication, as well as non-study intake (i.e. changes in EPA and DHA levels in erythrocytes during the intervention) that will provide a clearer view of whether omega-3 PUFAs showed any benefit in subgroups of this cohort.

The results of a second similar omega-3 PUFA supplementation replication RCT in a subset of individuals from the North American Prodrome Longitudinal Studies (NAPLS) were recently presented at the International Congress on Schizophrenia Research 2017. Of the 127 'clinical high-risk' patients recruited into the trial, 118 completed baseline assessment and 70 (59 per cent) completed the six-month trial. Seven (10 per cent) subjects converted to psychosis during the 24 months. The rate of psychotic conversion did not differ statistically in the omega-3 group (13 per cent) versus the placebo group (8 per cent). Although there were significant improvements in symptom and functioning over time in mixed model analyses, there were no significant group or group by time interaction effects. However, the researchers noted cardiometabolic abnormalities already at baseline in their young study participants, and found significant evidence that those with low omega-3 PUFAs in their diet were statistically more likely to have converted to a psychotic disorder by the end of the study.

Ongoing Research

Anti-inflammatory health-promoting effects of omega-3 PUFAs have not been sufficiently studied in the early stages of psychotic or mood disorders or in at-risk populations. Since omega-3 PUFAs positively affect inflammatory activities and processes, and the first clinical trials of omega-3 PUFAs in neuropsychiatric conditions suggest positive effects (Freeman et al., 2006; Hallahan et al., 2016), further investigation of the effects of omega-3 PUFAs on cytokines and subsequently on psychopathology in at-risk groups is warranted (Rapaport et al., 2016). We are currently conducting the first study of cytokines and oxidative stress markers utilising four large prospective RCT samples of young people who are at risk of psychosis or of persistent MDD (NHMRC Project Grant 1128631). This study will help to determine whether inflammation and oxidative stress can act as markers for disease initiation, progression and resolution in response to treatment.

Cannabidiol

The endocannabinoid system is a relatively new pharmacological target for several psychiatric disorders, including addictions, post-traumatic stress disorder (PTSD), anxiety disorders and schizophrenia (Desfossés et al., 2010). This neurotransmitter system consists of at least two types of receptors (CB1 and CB2) and endogenous ligands that bind to these receptors. Whereas CB2 receptors are more pronounced in peripheral regions, CB1 receptors are found throughout the central nervous system, with the highest concentrations demonstrated in the basal ganglia, cerebellum, hippocampus and cortex (reviewed by Iseger & Bossong, 2015). The two most important endogenous cannabinoid ligands are anandamide and 2-arachidonoyl glycerol (2-AG). They act as retrograde messengers, which means that they are synthesised and released postsynaptically and bind to presynaptic receptors, thereby regulating the release of both inhibitory and excitatory neurotransmitters (Kano et al., 2009). The endocannabinoid system is thought to be involved in many brain functions such as mood, memory and reward processing (Bossong et al., 2014a; 2014b; Zanettini et al., 2011). It is also involved in the regulation of a variety of physiological processes, including appetite and pain sensation. Given its crucial involvement in an array of physiological regulation processes, the endocannabinoid system provides a promising new target for the development of novel therapeutic agents for a range of psychiatric conditions (Blessing et al., 2015).

The effects of cannabinoids have been appreciated for many centuries, and the discovery of the active components of the plant *Cannabis sativa* has fuelled the search for the underlying mechanisms of action (Lutz et al., 2015). The main components in cannabis are tetrahydrocannabinol (THC) and CBD. Unlike THC, CBD is devoid of psychotropic effects; that is, the alterations in thinking and perception caused by THC are not observed with CBD. Basic research in animals suggests that CBD is non-toxic, does not induce changes in food intake and does not affect physiological parameters (blood pressure and body temperature), gastrointestinal transit, psychomotor functions or psychological functions (Blessing et al., 2015). A systematic review of potential side-effects in humans found that CBD was well tolerated across a wide dose range, with no reported psychomotor slowing, negative mood effects or vital-sign abnormalities noted (Bergamaschi et al., 2011b). Notably, CBD is not addictive. In fact, there is evidence that it reduces addictive behaviours (Prud'Homme et al., 2015), and it is currently being tested as a treatment for cannabis-use problems (NCT02044809).

CBD for Anxiety

CBD has a broad pharmacological profile, including interactions with several receptors known to regulate fear and anxiety-related behaviours, specifically the CB1 receptor, the serotonin 5-HT1A receptor and the transient receptor potential (TRP) vanilloid type 1 (TRPV1) receptor (Pacher et al., 2006). CBD does not bind directly to CB1 or CB2 receptors, but it may act as a positive allosteric modulator of CB1, and also indirectly stimulates CB1 and CB2 receptors by increasing concentrations of endocannabinoids via inhibition of the anandamide degrading enzyme fatty acid amide hydrolase (FAAH).

Studies of the endocannabinoid system support its importance for multiple aspects of brain function specifically relevant to anxiety disorders, including modulation of the hypothalamic–pituitary–adrenal axis; regulation of mood, anxiety and reward (Pacher et al., 2006); and extinction of fear learning (Das et al., 2013). In animal models of anxiety and stress, CBD has consistently shown therapeutic efficacy in reducing behavioural and physical measures of stress and anxiety (e.g. heart rate) (see review by Blessing et al., 2015). In both healthy humans and patients with social anxiety disorder, CBD reduced anxiety in a simulated public-speaking test, with efficacy comparable to 5-HT1A receptor agonists or diazepam (Bergamaschi et al., 2011a). Furthermore, CBD enhances fear extinction learning in animals, and improved forgetting of traumatic memories in healthy human volunteers. Thus, CBD may have potential as an adjunct to extinction-based therapies such as CBT for anxiety disorders (Das et al., 2013). Given that anxiety disorders are common and that current treatments including CBT and pharmacotherapy are limited in their efficacy and by their side-effects, there is a clear need for novel and benign biological treatments. To date, no study has tested CBD in patients with a DSM-5 diagnosis of an anxiety disorder and the optimal dose is unknown. We are currently conducting the first open-label study of CBD in young people with anxiety disorder (ACTRN12617000825358p). In this pilot study we aim to test the feasibility, safety, tolerability and therapeutic effects of 12-week treatment with CBD to reduce anxiety severity in 30 young people aged 12–25 who do not respond to evidence-based standard treatment (i.e. CBT or CBT plus selective serotonin reuptake inhibitors (SSRIs)/serotonin-norepinephrine reuptake inhibitors (SNRIs)) for 8–16 weeks in a primary health care environment. A manuscript detailing the results is in preparation.

CBD for Psychosis

Besides its potential as an anxiolytic treatment, CBD has been successfully trialled in people with psychotic disorders (Leweke et al., 2012), and it may also be effective as an antidepressant (Hillard & Liu, 2014). Accumulating evidence suggests a role for the endocannabinoid system in the pathophysiology of schizophrenia (Iseger & Bossong, 2015). For example, epidemiological studies indicate that the use of cannabis increases the risk for developing schizophrenia (Arseneault et al., 2004; Moore et al., 2007) and lowers the age of onset of the illness (Veen et al., 2004). In patients, cannabis use has been related to higher relapse rates, poor treatment outcome and increased severity of symptoms (Foti et al., 2010), as well as accelerated loss of grey matter volume (Rais et al., 2008). In addition, schizophrenia patients show increased levels of endogenous cannabinoids in cerebrospinal fluid (Giuffrida et al., 2004; Leweke et al., 1999). Neuroimaging studies measuring in-vivo CB1 receptor availability in schizophrenia patients reported a widespread increase in levels of CB1 receptors, including in the nucleus accumbens, insula, cingulate cortex, inferior frontal cortex, parietal cortex, mediotemporal lobe and pons (Ceccarini et al., 2013; Wong et al., 2010).

Three studies have been published in which patients with schizophrenia were treated with CBD (reviewed by Iseger & Bossong, 2015). In a case report, successful treatment with 1200 mg/day CBD was described in a 19-year-old female with schizophrenia (Zuardi et al., 1995). In a short report, therapy of three treatment-resistant schizophrenia patients with escalating doses up to 1280 mg/day of CBD was described, of whom only one patient showed mild symptom improvement (Zuardi et al., 2006). The authors speculate that a low initial CBD dose and the treatment resistance in these patients might explain this negative finding. In the largest clinical trial with CBD treatment of schizophrenia patients to date, Leweke et al. (2012) performed an RCT of CBD ($n = 20$) vs amisulpride ($n = 19$). After four weeks of treatment (maximum of 800 mg/day orally), both CBD and amisulpride resulted in significant clinical improvement as measured with both the PANSS and BPRS. However, CBD treatment displayed a markedly superior side-effect profile. In summary, the studies that investigated the potential of CBD as an antipsychotic treatment in psychotic patients were promising in that most participants exhibited significant clinical improvement after four weeks of CBD treatment. Acceptance of a natural substance without clinically relevant side-effects, with potency for treatment potentially similar to benzodiazepines, antipsychotic and antidepressive medications, should facilitate compliance and make CBD a good treatment candidate to be rigorously studied in young people early in the course of mental health problems (Amminger et al., 2017).

N-acetyl-cysteine

N-acetyl-cysteine (NAC) has been in use for over 30 years as an antidote in the treatment of paracetamol overdose, as a mucolytic for chronic obstructive pulmonary disease, as a renal protectant in contrast-induced nephropathy and as a therapeutic agent in the management of HIV (Dodd et al., 2008). NAC has also been tested to treat a variety of neuropsychiatric and neurodegenerative disorders including cocaine, cannabis and smoking addictions, Alzheimer's and Parkinson's diseases, autism, compulsive and grooming disorders, schizophrenia, depression and bipolar disorder (Dean et al., 2011). It targets a diverse array of factors germane to the pathophysiology of neuropsychiatric disorders, including oxidative stress, glutamatergic and dopaminergic neurotransmission, neurotrophins, apoptosis, mitochondrial function and inflammatory pathways (Berk et al., 2013a). NAC is the N-acetyl derivative of the amino acid L-cysteine and is rapidly absorbed following an oral dose (Arakawa & Ito, 2007). Inside cells, cysteine is a rate-limiting component in the synthesis of the key endogenous antioxidant molecule glutathione (GSH). The use of NAC in restoring GSH levels is well established. GSH neutralises reactive oxygen and nitrogen species from the cell through both direct and indirect scavenging to protect cells from the effects of oxidative stress, which has been suggested to contribute to the onset of pathology. More specifically in relevance to the staging model, one study showed that low GSH levels (measured in erythrocytes) were good predictors of transition to first-episode psychosis (FEP) (Stage 2) in ultra-high-risk individuals (Stage 1b) (Lavoie et al., 2017). In this study, adding low erythrocyte GSH levels to the clinical ultra-high-risk criteria increased the psychosis prediction rate from 39 per cent to 83.3 per cent, indicating the importance of GSH and oxidative stress to the onset and progression of psychotic disorders. These results also provide a compelling biological rationale for treatment studies of NAC to prevent psychotic disorders. A first RCT investigating the efficacy of NAC and an integrated preventive psychological intervention in individuals clinically at high risk for psychosis is currently recruiting in Europe (NCT03149107).

What is Oxidative Stress?

Oxidative stress refers to an imbalance of free radicals, such as reactive oxygen and nitrogen species, which are generated both from normal metabolism – including neuro-transmitters associated with schizophrenia such as dopamine and glutamate – and from various environmental exposures. The failure of antioxidant defences to protect against free-radical generation damages cell membranes, with resulting dysfunction that might impact on neurotransmission and, ultimately, symptomatology in schizophrenia (Yao & Keshavan, 2011). Important free radicals in humans include hydrogen peroxide (H_2O_2), the hydroxyl radical (OH^-), nitric oxide (NO) and the superoxide radical (O_2^-). Super-oxide dismutase (SOD) catalyses the conversion of superoxide radicals to hydrogen peroxide. Reduced GSH is oxidised by glutathione peroxidase to oxidised GSH (GSSG). Radicals promote apoptosis, DNA damage and lipid peroxidation. Thiobarbituric acid reactive substances and malondialdehyde (MDA) are important end products of lipid peroxidation (Flatow et al., 2013).

In humans, oxidative stress is thought to be involved in the development of many diseases, including certain cancers, atherosclerosis and Alzheimer's disease. However, reactive oxygen species can be beneficial, as they are used by the immune system as a way to attack and kill pathogens (Segal, 2005). Short-term oxidative stress may also be important in the prevention of ageing by induction of a process named mitohormesis (Schulz et al., 2007). Interestingly, there is also evidence that omega-3 PUFA supplementation may significantly lower oxidative stress (Kiecolt-Glaser et al., 2013).

The brain is particularly vulnerable to oxidative damage, given its relatively low content of antioxidant defences in addition to its high metal content (e.g. iron, zinc, copper and manganese), which can catalyse the formation of free radicals (Rougemont et al., 2002). The brain utilises more than 20 per cent of oxygen consumed by the body, yet comprises only 2 per cent of the total body weight (Dringen, 2000). The high energy demand from oxidative glucose metabolism plus a high concentration of PUFAs and relatively low levels of antioxidants are therefore thought to render the brain more vulnerable to oxidative insult than most organs (Berg et al., 2004; Dringen, 2000).

Alterations in Antioxidant Defence Systems in Schizophrenia and Depression

Abnormal oxidative stress parameters have been consistently reported in peripheral blood cells, cerebrospinal fluid and/or post-mortem brain in patients with schizophrenia (Flatow et al., 2013) and in patients with MDDs (Palta et al., 2014). One study found decreased in-vivo GSH levels in the medial prefrontal cortex of patients with schizophrenia (Keshavan et al., 1993). Other results suggest that the omega-3 PUFA EPA alters GSH availability and modulates the glutamine/glutamate cycle in early psychosis, with some of the metabolic brain changes being correlated with negative symptom improvement (Do et al., 2000).

Clinical trials also support an association between oxidative stress and schizophrenia (Libov et al., 2007; Shamir et al., 2001; Zhang et al., 2004). Furthermore, one RCT found that adjunctive treatment with the antioxidant NAC, a precursor of GSH, significantly reduced psychopathology in schizophrenia (Berk et al., 2008). Together with our finding that supplementation with omega-3 PUFAs – which reduce oxidative stress (Kiecolt-Glaser et al., 2013) – significantly reduced the progression to FEP in subjects with prodromal symptoms (Amminger et al., 2015), these studies suggest that oxidative stress levels might be a biomarker of psychosis and predictor of response to antioxidant treatment.

Transcranial Magnetic Stimulation

Transcranial magnetic stimulation (TMS) is a neuromodulatory technique that involves the induction of focused electromagnetic currents within the cortex by the application of a powerful magnetic field. TMS is typically applied by placing a coil near the skull that produces a magnetic field, approximately twice the magnitude of that induced by magnetic resonance imaging, which penetrates the skull and depolarises cortical neurons within 1.5–2.5 cm below the surface of the skull. By doing this, TMS stimulates neuronal activity in the neocortex, which, depending on the location where the coil is placed, can influence the function of various cortical areas relevant to mental disorders. Repeated application of TMS (rTMS) is thought to progressively alter brain activity with repeated applications and is normally the preferred method for therapeutic purposes. Here, we review studies of rTMS in adolescent and young adult psychiatric populations. A special focus is placed on adolescent depression, as most studies in youth to date have investigated this treatment modality for mood disorders. We also provide a focused overview of the efficacy of rTMS in adult studies to contextualise these findings.

Efficacy of rTMS in Adult Studies

rTMS is currently one of the most widely studied non-invasive brain stimulation techniques in psychiatry. To date, clinical studies in adults have evaluated rTMS for therapeutic use in a variety of conditions, including major depression, psychotic disorders, obsessive-compulsive disorder and anxiety disorders. Since the first published study of rTMS for major depression in adults more than 20 years ago (George et al., 1995), more than 30 trials have tested rTMS for psychiatric indications, most notably for treatment-resistant depression. While the majority of these studies supported benefits of rTMS for depressive symptoms, the effect sizes varied and were minimal in some cases. Nevertheless, the most recent meta-analytic evaluations support the clinical benefits of rTMS for major depression. Brunoni et al. (2017) included 81 studies testing any rTMS modality vs sham and found that most modalities of rTMS were significantly superior to sham, with the exception of accelerated, synchronised and deep rTMS. Gaynes et al. (2014) concluded that for treatment-resistant depression rTMS was similarly superior to sham, with participants in the active arm three times more likely to respond, while observing a mean decrease of 4.5 points on the Hamilton Depression Rating Scale. Another meta-analysis by Teng et al. (2017) found a dose-dependent effect of rTMS on major depression, with studies including 20 sessions having the highest effect sizes.

Evidence for Clinical Efficacy of rTMS from Studies in Youth

In contrast to adult studies, studies in youth are scarce (Amminger et al., 2017). In adolescent patients, RCTs of rTMS are scarce and most of the evidence comes from case series and open-label trials. In one open-label study of nine adolescent patients aged 16–18 years by Bloch et al. (2008), 30 sessions led to small but significant improvements in depressive symptoms and anxiety, but had no effect on suicidal ideation. Of the nine patients included in the trial, three had reductions in depressive symptoms of more than 30 per cent, which persisted in two of the three patients one year after the intervention. Treatment resistance in this trial was defined as non-response to at least one course of psychotherapy and two courses of anti-depressant pharmacotherapy (eight weeks or more). In a long-term follow-up three years after the intervention, depressive symptoms remained low and no effect on cognitive function was noted (Mayer et al., 2012). Wall et al. (2011) conducted an open-label trial in eight adolescents aged 14–17 with depression and observed significant reductions in Child-hood Depression Rating Scale (CDRS-R) scores and Quick Inventory of Depressive Symp-tomatology – Adolescent Version (QIDS-A17) scores, with the greatest reductions after 30 sessions (Wall et al., 2011). This study resulted in clinical response in five of the eight participants, indicated by a score of much improved or very much improved in the Clinical Global Impression – Improvement Scale (CGI-I). Croarkin et al. (2012) conducted an open-label trial in eight youth with treatment-resistant depression, defined as non-response to at least two trials of antidepressive medication, and observed a significant reduction in CDRS-R scores after 30 sessions of high-frequency rTMS. Another study by the same group that included ten adolescent patients with treatment-resistant depression, defined as non-response to at least one trial of antidepressive medication in the current episode, aged 13–17 years also observed reductions in CDRS-R scores after 30 sessions of rTMS, which persisted six months after the study (Croarkin et al., 2016). Wall et al. (2016) conducted an open-label trial in 2016 and found significant clinical improvement in six of ten participants and significant reductions in CDRS-R scores and QIDS-A17 scores after 20 sessions and 30 sessions, which were sustained at the six-month follow-up. No decline in neurocognitive function was noted. Loo et al. (2006) included two adolescent patients with depression and noted improvements in MADRS and Center for Epidemiologic Studies Depression Scale (CES-D) scores, which were sustained three and four months after the intervention, respect-ively. Finally, a recent review focusing on the efficacy of rTMS for treatment-resistant depression in youth concluded that 63 per cent of all participants at the time of the literature search responded to rTMS, with a significant decrease in depressive symptoms (Magavi et al., 2017). At least three other trials evaluating rTMS for youth depression are currently underway (ACTRN12614000907640, NCT02611206, NCT02586688).

Other applications for which rTMS has been tested in adolescents include mania and Tourette syndrome. At least one RCT tested rTMS vs sham in addition to mood-stabilising treatment in adolescent patients with mania aged 12–17 years (n = 13 in each group)

(Pathak et al., 2015). This study applied rTMS over the right dorsolateral prefrontal cortex and did not find evidence for the clinical efficacy of rTMS compared to the inactive group using the Young Mania Rating Scale (YMRS). Of note, this study only administered ten sessions of rTMS over ten consecutive days, less than most other studies. One study applied a single session of rTMS for ten patients with anorexia nervosa and observed reductions in symptoms after the session compared to before. Randomised studies in anorexia nervosa are currently being conducted (ISRCTN14329415).

Safety and Adverse Events

Three of the studies summarised above reported adverse events related to the rTMS treatment. Transient headache was the most commonly reported side-effect, reported by five participants in the study conducted by Bloch et al. (2008), two participants in the study by Pathak et al. (2015) and an unknown number of participants in that by Wall et al. (2016). Scalp discomfort was reported by participants in two studies (Pathak et al., 2015; Wall et al., 2016), and was the reason for withdrawal of one participant after the first session in one of the two studies (Wall et al., 2016). In the same study, one participant was withdrawn due to worsening depression after five sessions, which was judged to be unrelated to the intervention. Other mild or transient side-effects reported in this study included dizziness, nausea, musculoskeletal discomfort and eye twitching. Two studies assessed neurocognitive function as a secondary outcome and neither observed changes as a result of rTMS (Mayer et al., 2012; Wall et al., 2016). One case report not included in the above review of rTMS trials reported a 15-year-old patient who underwent rTMS and had a generalised tonic-clonic seizure during the first session (Hu et al., 2011).

Summary and Outlook

Several studies provide evidence for the safety and clinical efficacy of rTMS for depression in youth. The majority of these studies were conducted as open-label trials with small samples sizes. While these studies are unanimous in supporting the antidepressant properties of rTMS, the effect size remains unclear and larger sham-controlled trials are warranted to confirm the clinical efficacy of this neuromodulatory therapy. In addition to the potential therapeutic effects of rTMS for depression, this technique is also suited to inform our understanding of the neurobiology of the disorder. Croarkin et al. (2012; 2016) have used rTMS to study the glutamatergic and GABAergic neurotransmitter systems as a measure of cortical excitability, with potential use as a biomarker of response to rTMS. An important question emerging from adult studies seems to be whether rTMS is effective for treatment-resistant depression and possibly superior to pharmacotherapy. Besides studies in depression, very little evidence exists for rTMS for other indications. Adult studies, however, have evaluated the technique for e.g. mania and psychosis, suggesting that the clinical efficacy of rTMS may not be exclusive to unipolar mood disorders.

Conclusion

Given the paucity of new drug developments for psychiatry in recent years, all treatments reviewed here merit further investigation. Adverse effects and lack of efficacy in a significant number of patients further limit current pharmaceutical interventions in youth psychiatry. This is exemplified by the fact that no medication is currently approved even for the treatment of the most common mental health problems (anxiety and depression) in people younger than 18 years of age in Australia. Indeed, there is an urgent need for novel biological interventions, in particular treatments with acceptable risk–benefit balances or which are even health beneficial, which are feasible for use during Stages 1a and 1b. The treatments reviewed here are generally benign and also suitable for early and preventive intervention. If initial findings are confirmed by ongoing trials, these treatments could provide well-needed alternatives to existing pharmaceutical options.

References

Amminger, G. P., Berger, M., Rice, S. M., Davey, C. G., Schäfer, M. R., & McGorry, P. D. (2017). Novel biotherapies are needed in youth mental health. *Australasian Psychiatry,* 25(2), 117–120.

Amminger, G. P., Chanen, A. M., Ohmann, S., Klier, C. M., Mossaheb, N., Bechdolf, A., . . . Schäfer, M. R. (2013). Omega-3 fatty acid supplementation in adolescents with borderline personality disorder and ultra-high risk criteria for psychosis: a post hoc subgroup analysis of a double-blind, randomized controlled trial. *Canadian Journal of Psychiatry,* 58(7), 402–408.

Amminger, G. P., Schäfer, M. R., Papageorgiou, K., Klier, C. M., Cotton, S. M., Harrigan M, . . . Berger, G. E. (2010). Long-chain omega-3 fatty acids for indicated prevention of psychotic disorders: a randomized, placebo-controlled trial. *Archives of General Psychiatry,* 67(2), 146–154.

Amminger, G. P., Schäfer, M. R., Schlögelhofer, M., Klier, C. M., & McGorry, P. D. (2015). Longer-term outcome in the prevention of psychotic disorders by the Vienna omega-3 study. *Nature Communications,* 6, 7934.

Arakawa, M., & Ito, Y. (2007). N-acetylcysteine and neurodegenerative diseases: basic and clinical pharmacology. *Cerebellum,* 6(4), 308–314.

Arseneault, L., Cannon, M., Witton, J., & Murray, R. M. (2004). Causal association between cannabis and psychosis: examination of the evidence. *British Journal of Psychiatry,* 184, 110–117.

Assies, J., Pouwer, F., Lok, A., Mocking, R. J. T., Bockting, C. L. H., Visser, I., . . . Schene, A. H. (2010). Plasma and erythrocyte fatty acid patterns in patients with recurrent depression: a matched case-control study. *PLoS One,* 5(5), e10635.

Berg, D., Youdim, M. B. H., & Riederer, P. (2004). Redox imbalance. *Cell and Tissue Research,* 318(1), 201–213.

Berg, K. A., Maayani, S., & Clarke, W. P. (1996). 5-hydroxytryptamine2C receptor activation inhibits 5-hydroxytryptamine1B-like receptor function via arachidonic acid metabolism. *Molecular Pharmacology,* 50(4), 1017–1023.

Bergamaschi, M. M., Queiroz, R. H. C., Chagas, M. H. N., De Oliveira, D. C. G., De Martinis, B. S., Kapczinski, F., . . . Crippa, J. A. S. (2011a). Cannabidiol reduces the anxiety induced by simulated public speaking in treatment-naive social phobia patients. *Neuropsychopharmacology,* 36(6), 1219–1226.

Bergamaschi, M. M., Queiroz, R. H. C., Zuardi, A. W., & Crippa, J. A. S. (2011b). Safety and side effects of cannabidiol, a *Cannabis sativa* constituent. *Current Drug Safety,* 6(4), 237–249.

Berger, M., Smesny, S., Kim, S., Davey, C., Rice, S., Sarnyai, Z., . . . McGorry, P. (2017). Omega-6 to omega-3 polyunsaturated fatty acid ratio and subsequent mood disorders in young people with at-risk mental states: a 7-year longitudinal study. *Translational Psychiatry,* 7(8), e1220.

Berk, M., Copolov, D., Dean, O., Lu, K., Jeavons, S., Schapkaitz, I., . . . Bush, A. I. (2008). N-acetyl cysteine as a glutathione precursor for schizophrenia: a double-blind, randomized, placebo-controlled trial. *Biological Psychiatry,* 64(5), 361–368.

Berk, M., Malhi, G. S., Gray, L. J., & Dean, O. M. (2013a). The promise of N-acetylcysteine in neuropsychiatry. *Trends in Pharmacological Sciences,* 34(3), 167–177.

Berk, M., Williams, L. J., Jacka, F. N., O'Neil, A., Pasco, J. A., Moylan, S., . . . Maes, M. (2013b). So depression is an inflammatory disease, but where does the inflammation come from? *BMC Medicine,* **11**, 200.

Blessing, E. M., Steenkamp, M. M., Manzanares, J., & Marmar, C. R. (2015). Cannabidiol as a potential treatment for anxiety disorders. *Neurotherapeutics,* **12**(4), 825–836.

Bloch, M. H., & Hannestad, J. (2012). Omega-3 fatty acids for the treatment of depression: systematic review and meta-analysis. *Molecular Psychiatry,* **17**(12), 1272–1282.

Bloch, Y., Grisaru, N., Harel, E. V., Beitler, G., Faivel, N., Ratzoni, G., . . . Levkovitz, Y. (2008). Repetitive transcranial magnetic stimulation in the treatment of depression in adolescents: an open-label study. *Journal of ECT,* **24**(2), 156–159.

Blondeau, N., Nguemeni, C., Debruyne, D. N., Piens, M., Wu, X., Pan, H., . . . Heurteaux, C. (2009). Subchronic alpha-linolenic acid treatment enhances brain plasticity and exerts an antidepressant effect: a versatile potential therapy for stroke. *Neuro-Psychopharmacology,* **34**(12), 2548–2559.

Bossong, M. G., Jager, G., Bhattacharyya, S., & Allen, P. (2014a). Acute and non-acute effects of cannabis on human memory function: a critical review of neuroimaging studies. *Current Pharmaceutical Design,* **20**(13), 2114–2125.

Bossong, M. G., Jansma, J. M., Bhattacharyya, S., & Ramsey, N. F. (2014b). Role of the endocannabinoid system in brain functions relevant for schizophrenia: an overview of human challenge studies with cannabis or Δ9-tetrahydrocannabinol (THC). *Progress in Neuropsychopharmacology and Biological Psychiatry,* **52**, 53–69.

Brunoni, A. R., Chaimani, A., Moffa, A. H., Razza, L. B., Gattaz, W. F., Daskalakis, Z. J., & Carvalho, A. F. (2017). Repetitive transcranial magnetic stimulation for the acute treatment of major depressive episodes: a systematic review with network meta-analysis. *JAMA Psychiatry,* **74**(2), 143–152.

Ceccarini, J., De Hert, M., Van Winkel, R., Peuskens, J., Bormans, G., Kranaster, L., . . . Van Laere, K. (2013). Increased ventral striatal CB1 receptor binding is related to negative symptoms in drug-free patients with schizophrenia. *NeuroImage,* **79**, 304–312.

Chalon, S., Vancassel, S., Zimmer, L., Guilloteau, D., & Durand, G. (2001). Polyunsaturated fatty acids and cerebral function: focus on monoaminergic neurotransmission. *Lipids,* **36**(9), 937–944.

Compton, M. T. (2010). Fish oil to fend off psychosis: new evidence. *Medscape.*

Croarkin, P. E., Nakonezny, P. A., Wall, C. A., Murphy, L. L., Sampson, S. M., Frye, M. A., & Port, J. D. (2016). Transcranial magnetic stimulation potentiates glutamatergic neurotransmission in depressed adolescents. *Psychiatry Research: Neuroimaging,* **247**, 25–33.

Croarkin, P. E., Wall, C. A., Nakonezny, P. A., Buyukdura, J. S., Husain, M. M., Sampson, S. M., . . . Kozel, F. A. (2012). Increased cortical excitability with prefrontal high-frequency repetitive transcranial magnetic stimulation in adolescents with treatment-resistant major depressive disorder. *Journal of Child and Adolescent Psychopharmacology,* **22**(1), 56–64.

Das, R. K., Kamboj, S. K., Ramadas, M., Yogan, K., Gupta, V., Redman, E., . . . Morgan, C. J. A. (2013). Cannabidiol enhances consolidation of explicit fear extinction in humans. *Psychopharmacology,* **226**(4), 781–792.

Dean, O., Giorlando, F., & Berk, M. (2011). N-acetylcysteine in psychiatry: current therapeutic evidence and potential mechanisms of action. *Journal of Psychiatry and Neuroscience,* **36**(2), 78–86.

Delion, S., Chalon, S., Herault, J., Guilloteau, D., Besnard, J. C., & Durand, G. (1994). Chronic dietary α-linolenic acid deficiency alters dopaminergic and serotoninergic neurotransmission in rats. *Journal of Nutrition,* **124**(12), 2466–2476.

Desfossés, J., Stip, E., Bentaleb, L. A., & Potvin, S. (2010). Endocannabinoids and schizophrenia. *Pharmaceuticals,* **3**(10), 3101–3126.

Do, K. Q., Trabesinger, A. H., Kirsten-Krüger, M., Lauer, C. J., Dydak, U., Hell, D., . . .

Cuénod, M. (2000). Schizophrenia: glutathione deficit in cerebrospinal fluid and prefrontal cortex in vivo. *European Journal of Neuroscience, 12*(10), 3721–3728.

Dodd, S., Dean, O., Copolov, D. L., Malhi, G. S., & Berk, M. (2008). N-acetylcysteine for antioxidant therapy: pharmacology and clinical utility. *Expert Opinion on Biological Therapy, 8*(12), 1955–1962.

Dringen, R. (2000). Metabolism and functions of glutathione in brain. *Progress in Neurobiology, 62*(6), 649–671.

Flatow, J., Buckley, P., & Miller, B. J. (2013). Meta-analysis of oxidative stress in schizophrenia. *Biological Psychiatry, 74*(6), 400–409.

Foti, D. J., Kotov, R., Guey, L. T., & Bromet, E. J. (2010). Cannabis use and the course of schizophrenia: 10-year follow-up after first hospitalization. *American Journal of Psychiatry, 167*(8), 987–993.

Freeman, M. P., Hibbeln, J. R., Wisner, K. L., Davis, J. M., Mischoulon, D., Peet, M., ... Stoll, A. L. (2006). Omega-3 fatty acids: evidence basis for treatment and future research in psychiatry. *Journal of Clinical Psychiatry, 67*(12), 1954–1967.

Garland, M. R., & Hallahan, B. (2006). Essential fatty acids and their role in conditions characterised by impulsivity. *International Review of Psychiatry, 18*(2), 99–105.

Garland, M. R., Hallahan, B., McNamara, M., Carney, P. A., Grimes, H., Hibbeln, J. R., ... Conroy, R. M. (2007). Lipids and essential fatty acids in patients presenting with self-harm. *British Journal of Psychiatry, 190*, 112–117.

Gaynes, B. N., Lloyd, S. W., Lux, L., Gartlehner, G., Hansen, R. A., Brode, S., ... Lohr, K. N. (2014). Repetitive transcranial magnetic stimulation for treatment-resistant depression: a systematic review and meta-analysis. *Journal of Clinical Psychiatry, 75*(5), 477–489.

George, M. S., Wassermann, E. M., Williams, W. A., Callahan, A., Ketter, T. A., Basser, P., ... Post, R. M. (1995). Daily repetitive transcranial magnetic stimulation (rTMS) improves mood in depression. *NeuroReport, 6*(14), 1853–1856.

Giuffrida, A., Leweke, F. M., Gerth, C. W., Schreiber, D., Koethe, D., Faulhaber, J., ... Piomelli, D. (2004). Cerebrospinal anandamide levels are elevated in acute schizophrenia and are inversely correlated with psychotic symptoms. *Neuropsychopharmacology, 29*(11), 2108–2114.

Hallahan, B., & Garland, M. R. (2005). Essential fatty acids and mental health. *British Journal of Psychiatry, 186*, 275–277.

Hallahan, B., Ryan, T., Hibbeln, J. R., Murray, I. T., Glynn, S., Ramsden, C. E., ... Davis, J. M. (2016). Efficacy of omega-3 highly unsaturated fatty acids in the treatment of depression. *British Journal of Psychiatry, 209*(3), 192–201.

Hedelin, M., Löf, M., Olsson, M., Lewander, T., Nilsson, B., Hultman, C. M., & Weiderpass, E. (2010). Dietary intake of fish, omega-3, omega-6 polyunsaturated fatty acids and vitamin D and the prevalence of psychotic-like symptoms in a cohort of 33 000 women from the general population. *BMC Psychiatry, 10*, 38.

Hibbeln, J. R. (1998). Fish consumption and major depression. *Lancet, 351*(9110), 1213.

Hibbeln, J. R., & Salem Jr, N. (1995). Dietary polyunsaturated fatty acids and depression: when cholesterol does not satisfy. *American Journal of Clinical Nutrition, 62*(1), 1–9.

Hillard, C. J., & Liu, Q. S. (2014). Endocannabinoid signaling in the etiology and treatment of major depressive illness. *Current Pharmaceutical Design, 20*(23), 3795–3811.

Horrobin, D. F. (1998). The membrane phospholipid hypothesis as a biochemical basis for the neurodevelopmental concept of schizophrenia. *Schizophrenia Research, 30*(3), 193–208.

Hu, S., Wang, S., Zhang, M., Wang, J., Hu, J., Huang, M., ... Xu, W. (2011). Repetitive transcranial magnetic stimulation-induced seizure of a patient with adolescent-onset depression: a case report and literature review. *Journal of International Medical Research, 39*(5), 2039–2044.

Iseger, T. A., & Bossong, M. G. (2015). A systematic review of the antipsychotic properties of cannabidiol in humans. *Schizophrenia Research,* **162**(1–3), 153–161.

James, M. J., Sullivan, T. R., Metcalf, R. G., & Cleland, L. G. (2014). Pitfalls in the use of randomised controlled trials for fish oil studies with cardiac patients. *British Journal of Nutrition,* **112**(5), 812–820.

Kano, M., Ohno-Shosaku, T., Hashimotodani, Y., Uchigashima, M., & Watanabe, M. (2009). Endocannabinoid-mediated control of synaptic transmission. *Physiological Reviews,* **89**(1), 309–380.

Keshavan, M. S., Sanders, R. D., Pettegrew, J. W., Dombrowsky, S. M., & Panchalingam, K. S. (1993). Frontal lobe metabolism and cerebral morphology in schizophrenia: 31P MRS and MRI studies. *Schizophrenia Research,* **10**(3), 241–246.

Kiecolt-Glaser, J. K., Epel, E. S., Belury, M. A., Andridge, R., Lin, J., Glaser, R., ... Blackburn, E. (2013). Omega-3 fatty acids, oxidative stress, and leukocyte telomere length: a randomized controlled trial. *Brain, Behavior, and Immunity,* **28**, 16–24.

Kim, S. W., Jhon, M., Kim, J. M., Smesny, S., Rice, S., Berk, M., ... Amminger, G. P. (2016). Relationship between erythrocyte fatty acid composition and psychopathology in the Vienna omega-3 study. *PLoS One,* **11**(3), e0151417.

Kraemer, H. C. (2016). Messages for clinicians: moderators and mediators of treatment outcome in randomized clinical trials. *American Journal of Psychiatry,* **173**(7), 672–679.

Lavoie, S., Berger, M., Schlögelhofer, M., Schäfer, M. R., Rice, S., Kim, S. W., ... Amminger, G. P. (2017). Erythrocyte glutathione levels as long-term predictor of transition to psychosis. *Translational Psychiatry,* **7**(3), e1064.

Leichsenring, F., Leibing, E., Kruse, J., New, A. S., & Leweke, F. (2011). Borderline personality disorder. *Lancet,* **377**(9759), 74–84.

Leweke, F. M., Giuffrida, A., Wurster, U., Emrich, H. M., & Piomelli, D. (1999). Elevated endogenous cannabinoids in schizophrenia. *NeuroReport,* **10**(8), 1665–1669.

Leweke, F. M., Piomelli, D., Pahlisch, F., Muhl, D., Gerth, C. W., Hoyer, C., ... Koethe, D. (2012). Cannabidiol enhances anandamide signaling and alleviates psychotic symptoms of schizophrenia. *Translational Psychiatry,* **2**, e94.

Lewis, M. D., Hibbeln, J. R., Johnson, J. E., Lin, Y. H., Hyun, D. Y., & Loewke, J. D. (2011). Suicide deaths of active-duty US military and omega-3 fatty-acid status: a case-control comparison. *Journal of Clinical Psychiatry,* **72**(12), 1585–1590.

Libov, I., Miodownik, C., Bersudsky, Y., Dwolatzky, T., & Lerner, V. (2007). Efficacy of piracetam in the treatment of tardive dyskinesia in schizophrenic patients: a randomized, double-blind, placebo-controlled crossover study. *Journal of Clinical Psychiatry,* **68**(7), 1031–1037.

Lin, P. Y., Chang, C. H., Chong, M. F. F., Chen, H., & Su, K. P. (2017). Polyunsaturated fatty acids in perinatal depression: a systematic review and meta-analysis. *Biological Psychiatry,* **82**(8), 560–569.

Loo, C., McFarquhar, T., & Walter, G. (2006). Transcranial magnetic stimulation in adolescent depression. *Australasian Psychiatry,* **14**(1), 81–85.

Lutz, B., Marsicano, G., Maldonado, R., & Hillard, C. J. (2015). The endocannabinoid system in guarding against fear, anxiety and stress. *Nature Reviews Neuroscience,* **16**(12), 705–718.

Magavi, L. R., Reti, I. M., & Vasa, R. A. (2017). A review of repetitive transcranial magnetic stimulation for adolescents with treatment-resistant depression. *International Review of Psychiatry,* **29**(2), 79–88.

Mayer, G., Aviram, S., Walter, G., Levkovitz, Y., & Bloch, Y. (2012). Long-term follow-up of adolescents with resistant depression treated with repetitive transcranial magnetic stimulation. *Journal of ECT,* **28**(2), 84–86.

McGorry, P. D., Hickie, I. B., Yung, A. R., Pantelis, C., & Jackson, H. J. (2006). Clinical staging of psychiatric disorders: a heuristic framework for choosing earlier, safer and more effective interventions. *Australian and New Zealand Journal of Psychiatry,* **40**(8), 616–622.

McGorry, P. D., Nelson, B., Markulev, C., Yuen, H. P., Schäfer, M. R., Mossaheb, N., ... Amminger, G. P. (2017). Effect of ω-3 polyunsaturated fatty acids in young people at ultrahigh risk for psychotic disorders: the NEURAPRO randomized clinical trial. *JAMA Psychiatry,* **74**(1), 19–27.

Moore, T. H., Zammit, S., Lingford-Hughes, A., Barnes, T. R., Jones, P. B., Burke, M., & Lewis, G. (2007). Cannabis use and risk of psychotic or affective mental health outcomes: a systematic review. *Lancet,* **370**(9584), 319–328.

Mossaheb, N., Schloegelhofer, M., Schaefer, M. R., Fusar-Poli, P., Smesny, S., McGorry, P., ... Amminger, G. P. (2012). Polyunsaturated fatty acids in emerging psychosis. *Current Pharmaceutical Design,* **18**(4), 576–591.

Noaghiul, S., & Hibbeln, J. R. (2003). Cross-national comparisons of seafood consumption and rates of bipolar disorders. *American Journal of Psychiatry,* **160**(12), 2222–2227.

Pacher, P., Bátkai, S., & Kunos, G. (2006). The endocannabinoid system as an emerging target of pharmacotherapy. *Pharmacological Reviews,* **58**(3), 389–462.

Palta, P., Samuel, L. J., Miller, E. R., & Szanton, S. L. (2014). Depression and oxidative stress: results from a meta-analysis of observational studies. *Psychosomatic Medicine,* **76**(1), 12–19.

Parker, G., Gibson, N. A., Brotchie, H., Heruc, G., Rees, A. M., & Hadzi-Pavlovic, D. (2006). Omega-3 fatty acids and mood disorders. *American Journal of Psychiatry,* **163**(6), 969–978.

Pathak, V., Sinha, V. K., & Praharaj, S. K. (2015). Efficacy of adjunctive high frequency repetitive transcranial magnetic stimulation of right prefrontal cortex in adolescent mania: a randomized sham-controlled study. *Clinical Psychopharmacology and Neuroscience,* **13**(3), 245–249.

Piomelli, D., Astarita, G., & Rapaka, R. (2007). A neuroscientist's guide to lipidomics. *Nature Reviews Neuroscience,* **8**(10), 743–754.

Prud'Homme, M., Cata, R., & Jutras-Aswad, D. (2015). Cannabidiol as an intervention for addictive behaviors: a systematic review of the evidence. *Substance Abuse,* **9**, 33–38.

Rais, M., Cahn, W., Van Haren, N., Schnack, H., Caspers, E., Pol, H. H., & Kahn, R. (2008). Excessive brain volume loss over time in cannabis-using first-episode schizophrenia patients. *American Journal of Psychiatry,* **165**(4), 490–496.

Rapaport, M. H., Nierenberg, A. A., Schettler, P. J., Kinkead, B., Cardoos, A., Walker, R., & Mischoulon, D. (2016). Inflammation as a predictive biomarker for response to omega-3 fatty acids in major depressive disorder: a proof-of-concept study. *Molecular Psychiatry,* **21**(1), 71–79.

Rice, S. M., Hickie, I. B., Yung, A. R., Mackinnon, A., Berk, M., Davey, C., ... Amminger, G. P. (2016). Youth depression alleviation: the Fish Oil Youth Depression Study (YoDA-F) – a randomized, double-blind, placebo-controlled treatment trial. *Early Intervention in Psychiatry,* **10**(4), 290–299.

Rice, S. M., Schäfer, M. R., Klier, C., Mossaheb, N., Vijayakumar, N., & Amminger, G. P. (2015). Erythrocyte polyunsaturated fatty acid levels in young people at ultra-high risk for psychotic disorder and healthy adolescent controls. *Psychiatry Research,* **228**(1), 174–176.

Ripoll, L. H. (2013). Psychopharmacologic treatment of borderline personality disorder. *Dialogues in Clinical Neuroscience,* **15**(2), 213–224.

Rougemont, M., Do, K. Q., & Castagné, V. (2002). New model of glutathione deficit during development: effect on lipid peroxidation in the rat brain. *Journal of Neuroscience Research,* **70**(6), 774–783.

Sánchez-Villegas, A., Delgado-Rodríguez, M., Alonso, A., Schlatter, J., Lahortiga, F., Serra-Majem, L., & Martínez-González, M. A. (2009). Association of the Mediterranean dietary pattern with the incidence of depression: the Seguimiento Universidad de Navarra/University of Navarra follow-up (SUN) cohort. *Archives of General Psychiatry,* **66**(10), 1090–1098.

Saunders, E. F. H., Ramsden, C. E., Sherazy, M. S., Gelenberg, A. J., Davis, J. M., &

Rapoport, S. I. (2016). Omega-3 and omega-6 polyunsaturated fatty acids in bipolar disorder: a review of biomarker and treatment studies. *Journal of Clinical Psychiatry, 77*(10), e1301–e1308.

Schulz, T. J., Zarse, K., Voigt, A., Urban, N., Birringer, M., & Ristow, M. (2007). Glucose restriction extends *Caenorhabditis elegans* life span by inducing mitochondrial respiration and increasing oxidative stress. *Cell Metabolism, 6*(4), 280–293.

Scott, J., Leboyer, M., Hickie, I., Berk, M., Kapczinski, F., Frank, E., . . . McGorry, P. (2013). Clinical staging in psychiatry: a cross-cutting model of diagnosis with heuristic and practical value. *British Journal of Psychiatry, 202*(4), 243–245.

Segal, A. W. (2005). How neutrophils kill microbes. *Annual Review of Immunology, 23*, 197–223.

Serhan, C. N. (2014). Pro-resolving lipid mediators are leads for resolution physiology. *Nature, 510*(7503), 92–101.

Serhan, C. N., & Petasis, N. A. (2011). Resolvins and protectins in inflammation resolution. *Chemical Reviews, 111*(10), 5922–5943.

Shamir, E., Barak, Y., Shalman, I., Laudon, M., Zisapel, N., Tarrasch, R., . . . Weizman, R. (2001). Melatonin treatment for tardive dyskinesia: a double-blind, placebo-controlled, crossover study. *Archives of General Psychiatry, 58*(11), 1049–1052.

Simopoulos, A. P. (2011). Evolutionary aspects of diet: the omega-6/omega-3 ratio and the brain. *Molecular Neurobiology, 44*(2), 203–215.

Sommer, I. E., van Westrhenen, R., Begemann, M. J., de Witte, L. D., Leucht, S., & Kahn, R. S. (2013). Efficacy of anti-inflammatory agents to improve symptoms in patients with schizophrenia: an update. *Schizophrenia Bulletin, 40*(1), 181–191.

Su, K.-P., Matsuoka, Y., & Pae, C.-U. (2015). Omega-3 polyunsaturated fatty acids in prevention of mood and anxiety disorders. *Clinical Psychopharmacology and Neuroscience, 13*(2), 129–137.

Sublette, M. E., Ellis, S. P., Geant, A. L., & Mann, J. J. (2011). Meta-analysis of the effects of

eicosapentaenoic acid (EPA) in clinical trials in depression. *Journal of Clinical Psychiatry, 72*(12), 1577–1584.

Sublette, M. E., Galfalvy, H. C., Hibbeln, J. R., Keilp, J. G., Malone, K. M., Oquendo, M. A., & Mann, J. J. (2014). Polyunsaturated fatty acid associations with dopaminergic indices in major depressive disorder. *International Journal of Neuropsychopharmacology, 17*(3), 383–391.

Sublette, M. E., Russ, M. J., & Smith, G. S. (2004). Evidence for a role of the arachidonic acid cascade in affective disorders: a review. *Bipolar Disorders, 6*(2), 95–105.

Tanskanen, A., Hibbeln, J. R., Hintikka, J., Haatainen, K., Honkalampi, K., & Viinamäki, H. (2001). Fish consumption, depression, and suicidality in a general population. *Archives of General Psychiatry, 58*(5), 512–513.

Teng, S., Guo, Z., Peng, H., Xing, G., Chen, H., He, B., . . . Mu, Q. (2017). High-frequency repetitive transcranial magnetic stimulation over the left DLPFC for major depression: session-dependent efficacy: a meta-analysis. *European Psychiatry, 41*, 75–84.

Twenge, J. M., Gentile, B., DeWall, C. N., Ma, D., Lacefield, K., & Schurtz, D. R. (2010). Birth cohort increases in psychopathology among young Americans, 1938–2007: a cross-temporal meta-analysis of the MMPI. *Clinical Psychology Review, 30*(2), 145–154.

Veen, N. D., Selten, J.-P., van der Tweel, I., Feller, W. G., Hoek, H. W., & Kahn, R. S. (2004). Cannabis use and age at onset of schizophrenia. *American Journal of Psychiatry, 161*(3), 501–506.

Venna, V. R., Deplanque, D., Allet, C., Belarbi, K., Hamdane, M., & Bordet, R. (2009). PUFA induce antidepressant-like effects in parallel to structural and molecular changes in the hippocampus. *Psychoneuroendocrinology, 34*(2), 199–211.

von Schacky, C. (2009). Cardiovascular disease prevention and treatment. *Prostaglandins, Leukotrienes and Essential Fatty Acids, 81*(2–3), 193–198.

Wall, C. A., Croarkin, P. E., Maroney-Smith, M. J., Haugen, L. M., Baruth, J. M., Frye,

M. A., . . . Port, J. D. (2016). Magnetic resonance imaging-guided, open-label, high-frequency repetitive transcranial magnetic stimulation for adolescents with major depressive disorder. *Journal of Child and Adolescent Psychopharmacology, 26*(7), 582–589.

Wall, C. A., Croarkin, P. E., Sim, L. A., Husain, M. M., Janicak, P. G., Kozel, F. A., . . . Sampson, S. M. (2011). Adjunctive use of repetitive transcranial magnetic stimulation in depressed adolescents: a prospective, open pilot study. *Journal of Clinical Psychiatry, 72*(9), 1263–1269.

Wong, D. F., Kuwabara, H., Horti, A. G., Raymont, V., Brasic, J., Guevara, M., . . . Nandi, A. (2010). Quantification of cerebral cannabinoid receptors subtype 1 (CB1) in healthy subjects and schizophrenia by the novel PET radioligand [11C] OMAR. *NeuroImage, 52*(4), 1505–1513.

Yao, J. K., & Keshavan, M. S. (2011). Antioxidants, redox signaling, and pathophysiology in schizophrenia: an integrative view. *Antioxidants & Redox Signaling, 15*(7), 2011–2035.

Zanettini, C., Panlilio, L. V., Aliczki, M., Goldberg, S. R., Haller, J., & Yasar, S. (2011). Effects of endocannabinoid system modulation on cognitive and emotional behavior. *Frontiers in Behavioral Neuroscience, 5*, 57.

Zhang, X. Y., Zhou, D. F., Cao, L. Y., Xu, C. Q., & Wu, G. Y. (2004). The effect of vitamin E treatment on tardive dyskinesia and blood superoxide dismutase: a double-blind placebo-controlled trial. *Journal of Clinical Psychopharmacology, 24*(1), 83–86.

Zuardi, A. W., Hallak, J. E., Dursun, S. M., Morais, S. L., Sanches, R. F., Musty, R. E., & Crippa, J. A. S. (2006). Cannabidiol monotherapy for treatment-resistant schizophrenia. *Journal of Psychopharmacology, 20*(5), 683–686.

Zuardi, A. W., Morais, S., Guimaraes, F., & Mechoulam, R. (1995). Antipsychotic effect of cannabidiol. *Journal of Clinical Psychiatry, 56*(10), 485–486.

12

Psychosocial Interventions for Youth Mental Health

Eóin Killackey and Mario Alvarez-Jimenez

Introduction

Very few young people with mental ill-health present for care with a stated desire to reduce their Brief Psychiatric Rating Scale (BPRS) score, achieve a K10 in the healthy range or get through the screening section of the Structured Clinical Interview for Diagnostic and Statistical Manual of Mental Disorders (SCID) without triggering the need for more in-depth assessment. On the other hand, many young people do present suggesting that they are not themselves, that they want to return to being who they were. An important contributor to the way we conceptualise ourselves is what it is that we spend our time doing. For young people this can mean being healthy physically as well as mentally, studying, engaging in other vocational training, working or some combination of these. In other words, young people often present saying 'I want to be able to function again, and at the moment, because of what I am experiencing, I am not able to.' However, despite this, most of the assessment and subsequent treatment that is provided to young people focuses on the symptoms that describe the disorder that they might be presenting with. This might be seen to arise from an older dichotomous view of mental illness in which an individual was located on one side or the other of a diagnostic threshold. The advent of the staging model of mental illness has allowed for a more sophisticated way of understanding the onset and progression of illness. It has also meant a greater focus on preventing the progression of illness and disability. A key aspect of this prevention of progression has been a greater focus on functioning as an early-stage target of treatment.

Functional recovery for young people with mental ill-health broadly refers to the interventions that assist in the recovery of a young person with mental ill-health so that in addition to achieving a symptomatic recovery, they also achieve a functional recovery. This means such things as a return to school or work, having a place to live and addressing physical health needs. In considering how functional recovery contributes to the wider process of rehabilitation and recovery in mental ill-health, it is worth starting by revisiting the World Health Organization's definition of mental health (World Health Organization, 2011):

> Mental health is not just the absence of mental disorder. It is defined as a state of well-being in which every individual realizes his or her own potential, can cope with the normal stresses of life, can work productively and fruitfully, and is able to make a contribution to her or his community.

Functional recovery is then congruent with the World Health Organization's definition of health. Further, it is also closely aligned to the stated aims of young people with mental illness who rate positive functional outcomes as being more important than symptomatic remission (Morgan et al., 2011). While this was found to be the case in schizophrenia, it has recently been found to be equally so in young people being treated for their first psychotic episode in both the USA (Ramsay et al., 2011) and India (Iyer et al., 2011). Ramsay and colleagues found that the top five life goals of young people with first-episode psychosis (FEP) were (in descending order): employment, education, relationships, housing and general health. Recovery from the current episode was rated ninth. Iyer et al. (2011) in India found an almost identical list (work, interpersonal, school, symptom relief, living situation). There is less information on the stated aims of young people with other disorders such as depression and anxiety.

Despite research in populations separated both geographically and in stage of illness showing highly similar wishes to address functioning, and despite improvements in psychiatric medication and psychological interventions for people with mental illnesses leading to better symptomatic prognoses (Killackey, 2008), people with mental ill-health are still over-represented among those with a poor functional outcome (Galletly, 2012). Compared to the general community, people with a mental illness are more likely to be unemployed (Killackey et al., 2006), experience more physical ill-health and die earlier (Mai et al., 2010), and experience greater homelessness (Herrman et al., 2004). Consequently, people with psychosis are among the most socially excluded in our community. Further, the economic impact of poor functional outcomes is enormous and is responsible for over half the total costs associated with mental illnesses (National Mental Health Commission, 2014). Historically, intervention in mental illnesses has occurred after significant periods of time have elapsed. As a consequence, functional disabilities such as unemployment, educational underachievement and poor physical health have often been given time to entrench themselves in the lives of those experiencing mental ill-health. Due to the long delay in accessing treatment, the proactive addressing of functional areas has been difficult. The early intervention paradigm aimed to change this. This paradigm originally addressed psychotic illness and was pioneered in Melbourne, Australia in the 1990s (Killackey et al., 2008b). It aimed to reduce the duration of untreated psychosis, maximise symptomatic and functional recovery, prevent the development of disability and prevent or minimise the impact of relapse (McGorry et al., 2008). Since the early 2000s the paradigm has shifted to address other disorders and led to the development of the field of youth mental health.

The promise of early intervention in mental ill-health is that it offers a unique opportunity to intervene to improve functional outcome before disability has developed or become entrenched. But symptom-focused early-stage intervention alone is not enough. Research in psychosis has shown that functional recovery at 7.5 years post-treatment was not predicted by symptomatic recovery at 14 months post-treatment, but by *functional recovery* at 14 months (Alvarez-Jimenez et al., 2012b), emphasising the need for evidence-based functional recovery to be a central part of intervention in the early stages of illness. There are too few studies in other disorders to establish whether the same pattern holds. However, if an element of functional disability among those with mental illness is a failure to undergo normative development in a range of psychosocial areas, then it follows that addressing these developmental deficits as early as possible will assist in re-establishing normative function. Further, the need to specifically address functional development is supported by the above-mentioned study. In that study, while short-term symptomatic remission (at 7 months) predicted functional recovery at 14 months, symptom remission at 7 or 14 months had limited predictive value for long-term recovery; this means that if early symptom remission does not lead to early functional gains it is unlikely that long-term functional recovery will occur.

This chapter reviews two key areas of functioning in relation to youth mental health – employment and education, and physical health. It will discuss what is known in these areas in terms of the scale of the problem. It will then highlight some of the research evidence that is available for interventions in each of these areas. Finally, it will discuss the implications for research and clinical practice with respect to these domains of functioning in young people with early psychosis.

Employment and Education: The Problem

Mental illnesses have their peak onset in the ages of 15–25 years (Kessler et al., 2007), which is also the stage of life in which people normally finish school/tertiary education and enter the workforce. The onset of mental ill-health at this time can be extremely disruptive, often derailing the vocational development process. This disruption means that an individual does not attain their educational potential and thus does not gain the necessary qualifications for vocational progression and they do not acquire basic employment skills such as job searching and interviewing; they also develop no employment history. These factors may explain why, even after eventual symptomatic remission, people with mental illnesses are more likely to be unemployed and more tenuously employed than those with good mental health. It should also be mentioned that there is a potential protective value in having a job because of the meaning, purpose in life and valued social role that are part of being employed. This effect of employment can buffer against the development of chronic disability. There is a window of opportunity to minimise or prevent vocational disability in this group by applying evidence-based vocational interventions earlier rather than later (Scott et al., 2013).

While general unemployment in most developed economies is between 5 and 10 per cent, youth unemployment (15–24 years) is usually 2–3 times higher. Even allowing for high youth unemployment, the level of unemployment among young people with mental illness is even higher (Degney et al., 2012; Ostby et al., 2014; Rinaldi et al., 2010). Unemployment is the main functional disability of people with mental illness. In the general community, being unemployed predisposes people to a greater risk of a range of poor outcomes such as substance use, homelessness, poor physical and mental health and social and economic exclusion (Creed, 1998; Mathers & Schofield, 1998). It is also known that for most, these poor outcomes follow unemployment (Mathers & Schofield, 1998). For those with mental illness, unemployment reinforces marginalisation, has the potential to exacerbate symptoms, increases risk of homelessness, and often persists after symptoms have resolved. Over and above the individual consequences of unemployment in mental illness, there are significant economic costs. These equate to half of total illness costs (National Mental Health Commission, 2014; Neil et al., 2014; Wu et al., 2005).

Education is the foundation of employment, with increased education leading to less unemployment and higher wages in the general population (Australian Bureau of Statistics, 2010). This observation is also true in relation to employment for people with mental illness, with those who have completed high school more likely to be employed than those who have not (Waghorn et al., 2003). Unfortunately, educational achievement is affected by the onset of mental illnesses, particularly in late adolescence (usually coinciding with the completion of secondary education) and early adulthood (coinciding with efforts to gain further education or training) (Degney et al., 2012). In a study of vocational recovery that we conducted, only about one-quarter of participants with psychosis had completed high school (Killackey et al., 2008a) compared to 84 per cent of their same-age peers in the community (Department of Education and Training, 2006). In the same study, over 50 per cent of young people with psychosis had less than a Year 10 education (15–16 years of age). While there is less research to guide answering questions of cause and effect in relation to education, it is reasonable to suppose that the early development of illness is related to this reduction in academic functioning. However, even in the absence of a mental illness, this low level of education would mitigate against successful vocational outcomes in life. Therefore, it is imperative that in addressing the vocational functioning of young people with mental ill-health, education is considered equally with employment.

Interventions for Employment and Education in Young People with Mental Ill-Health

Addressing the vocational domain of functioning in recovery is not new (Brigham, 1844). However, a consequence of the increasing medicalisation of mental illness was the neglect of the vocational elements of recovery (Briggs, 1918; Killackey, 2015). The period following the Second World War saw the advent of clubhouses and social firms as means to address unemployment among those with mental illness. The literature for both of these approaches suggests that they do not usually lead to gaining a job in the competitive labour market (Killackey et al., 2006). Conversely, supported employment – an intervention in which a person is assisted to gain a job in the open labour market and supported to stay in that position – has been very successful (Crowther et al., 2001; Killackey, 2015). Individual placement and support (IPS) is the most defined form of supported employment and has had 23 randomised controlled trials (RCTs) finding it to be superior to a range of control interventions in populations with schizophrenia (Bond, 2012). These studies have occurred in a range of countries, with a range of economic and labour market conditions. IPS has eight principles (see Box 12.1). Given its success in populations with chronic illness, it follows to ask to what degree this approach can be applied to early intervention in early-stage mental illness. There have been a number of studies examining IPS in populations of people with FEP. There are as yet no studies examining IPS in non-psychotic illness among young people.

Box 12.1 Eight Principles of IPS

1. Every person with severe mental illness who wants to work is eligible for IPS supported employment.
2. Employment services are integrated with mental health treatment services.
3. Competitive employment is the goal.
4. Personalised benefits counselling is provided.
5. The job search starts soon after a person expresses interest in working.
6. Employment specialists systematically develop relationships with employers based upon their client's work preferences.
7. Job supports are continuous.
8. Client preferences are honoured.

(Dartmouth IPS Supported Employment Center, 2012)

IPS in First-Episode Psychosis

As well as an earlier uncontrolled study in the UK (Rinaldi et al., 2004), there have now been two published RCTs of IPS in early psychosis (Killackey et al., 2008a; Nuechterlein et al., 2008). In their RCT ($n = 41$) with participants aged between 15 and 25 (mean = 21.3 years) in Australia, Killackey et al. (2008a) found that over six months more people in the IPS group obtained employment (13 vs 2), gained significantly more jobs in total (23 vs 4), earned significantly more money ($2432 vs $0), and worked for longer (45 vs 19 days) than those who did not receive IPS. Four people in each group engaged in educational courses. This means that 17 (85 per cent) of those in the IPS group had a positive vocational outcome compared to only 6 (29 per cent) in the control group. The percentage of those dependent on government benefits decreased significantly in the IPS group, while there was no change in the control group. As a point of comparison, ten control group participants accessed federally funded employment agencies, and one had a single interview. None obtained employment.

Another RCT ($n = 69$) conducted in FEP (age range 18–45; mean = 25.1 years) by Nuechterlein et al. (2008) at UCLA found very similar results, with 83 per cent of people receiving IPS having a good vocational outcome (either returning to work or study). Across all of the IPS studies (RCTs and others) in early psychosis 69 per cent have a successful vocational outcome compared to 35 per cent in groups not receiving IPS (Rinaldi et al., 2010).

A key difference between the studies conducted in early psychosis and those conducted in populations with more established illness is the equal focus on achieving educational outcomes for those for whom education is the most appropriate vocational outcome. This fits with the developmental and recovery orientations of early intervention and in this way introduces the concept of career rather than job as an outcome. In a study conducted in the UK, Rinaldi and colleagues showed that using IPS they maintained the enrolment of all those involved in education until their courses were complete. The majority of those people then transitioned to employment (Rinaldi et al., 2004).

However, a recent meta-analysis of the studies of IPS in FEP showed that there was not overall a significant advantage to educational outcomes through IPS. One possible reason for this is that IPS uses predominantly employment specialists as staff to help people's vocational recovery. This begs the question of how IPS would perform if focused exclusively on education. Two studies have examined this question (Killackey et al., 2017; Robson et al., 2010). Both were small, uncontrolled studies. However, in both cases the educational outcomes were excellent. The positive outcomes of these studies suggest that there may be a need for a more specialist focus on education in vocational recovery. Confirmation of this awaits a larger, more rigorous trial. Also needed is research examining the utility of these approaches for young people with other forms of mental ill-health. The Australian government is currently conducting a large trial (2017–2021) through the national headspace platform, making IPS available to young people aged 12–25 with mild to moderate mental health issues (see Chapter 13 for further discussion on headspace).

Clinical Lessons

There is some evidence that one of the barriers to vocational success for young people with mental illness is the attitude of clinicians and carers about both the ability of the person with psychosis to work and the impact that work is likely to have upon them (Rinaldi et al.,

2010). It is often thought that people with mental illness are not able to work, or that work will be a stressful experience leading to an exacerbation of symptoms and relapse. In fact, recently published evidence shows that, in line with the general population, work is less stressful for people with mental illness than is unemployment (Allott et al., 2013). Therefore, clinicians need to work with clients and their families towards vocational recovery. An important element of this is helping to overcome the powerful effects of self-directed stigma that may encourage people with mental illness to not bother looking for work in the belief that it will be too stressful or that they will be discriminated against (Farrelly et al., 2014; Thornicroft et al., 2009). Having a job is likely to lead to more positive experiences, increased social networks and social support, all of which may protect against relapse and promote full functional recovery.

A further lesson is the need for specialist employment input. IPS works through a specialist employment worker being part of the clinical mental health programme. As well as providing direct services to clients, this person often 'up-skills' other clinicians about employment and helps raise the profile of employment as a possible outcome for clients. Recent studies that have utilised a teacher to focus in on educational recovery suggest that there may be a role for such a person, or closer partnerships with educational institutions.

A final lesson is that there must be a focus on career rather than jobs. This may mean that the most appropriate first step is the completion of secondary education or the attainment of some other qualification.

Research Lessons

While the results from IPS trials in early psychosis are consistently good, more work is needed in understanding the predictors of success in both obtaining and keeping a job or completing a course of education. There is an indication that a specific focus on education would be very beneficial, but this needs further research. Finally, all the work in this area has been done with populations of people with FEP. There is a need for an examination of whether the same approaches are beneficial for young people with other mental health disorders.

Physical Health: The Problem

The physical health outcomes of people with mental illness are very poor (Lawrence et al., 2013; Morgan et al., 2011), resulting in a 12–30-year decrease in life expectancy (De Hert et al., 2011; Lawrence et al., 2013). The majority of the excess morbidity and mortality is accounted for by obesity (particularly that induced as a medication side-effect) and tobacco smoking and their various related illnesses (De Hert et al., 2011). The evidence indicates that declining physical health is a process that starts very early in mental illness (Alvarez-Jimenez et al., 2006; Scott et al., 2015). Thus, it is imperative that addressing physical health is embedded in all approaches to treating early-stage mental ill-health (Hermens et al., 2013). The physical health of people with mental ill-health falls into the gap between physical and mental health care systems. For example, studies have shown that people with mental illnesses utilise primary care physicians more than do the general community (Mai et al., 2010). However, they have higher rates of preventable illness, with lower rates of investigations, early detection and early intervention. For example, this is seen in the data that show people with schizophrenia have the same incidence of cancer as the general population, but significantly higher mortality (Lawrence et al., 2000). With respect to smoking, studies have shown that while people with mental illness make up about 25 per cent of the population, they smoke nearly 50 per cent of all cigarettes (SANE Australia, 2007). Studies have also shown a significantly higher rate of smoking among young people attending primary mental health care than their same-aged peers in the general community (Hermens et al., 2013; Scott et al., 2015). Further demonstrating that there needs to be a physical health focus in early-stage mental illness are data from the long-running British primary-care-physician study that shows that if smoking is ceased before age 30, the long-term risks drop back to those of non-smokers (Doll et al., 2004).

Addressing Weight Gain in Mental Illness

While overweight and obesity is an issue across all mental illnesses (De Hert et al., 2011), to date there have been few trials examining physical health interventions in early-stage mental illness, and these have been contained to young people experiencing psychosis. As Scott et al. (2015) conclude, there is a need for development of interventions for young people in the early stages of all mental illnesses. One RCT has shown the effectiveness of preventive strategies in attenuating antipsychotic-induced weight gain in a young cohort with early psychosis (Alvarez-Jimenez et al., 2006). This study showed the feasibility and effectiveness of preventive strategies – comprising dietary counselling, exercise increase and behavioural techniques – for early psychosis patients who commenced antipsychotic treatment (Alvarez-Jimenez et al., 2006). However, while the behavioural intervention was effective in reducing weight gain in early psychosis patients during the 3-month intervention period, treatment effects were no longer significant by the 12-month follow-up (Alvarez-Jimenez et al., 2010). More hopefully, an Australian study that utilised a diet and lifestyle approach also found that weight gain could be prevented over a 12-week period (Curtis et al., 2016) in a population of young people with FEP. However, the follow-up of this cohort at two years revealed that there was still a significant beneficial difference in favour of the intervention group (Curtis et al., 2015). This indicates a potential positive outcome, but there is a need for replication in the psychosis population, as well as testing for benefit in populations with other mental illnesses.

While there are few studies, it seems apparent that there is great potential for interventions aimed at the early stages, before weight gain takes place. Weight gain is arguably a greater problem for young people experiencing mental ill-health. This group is considered to be especially susceptible to substantial weight gain (Alvarez-Jimenez et al., 2008) that could interfere with the early recovery process, particularly when using antipsychotic medication and some antidepressant medications (Scott et al., 2015). First, younger populations are already less disposed to adhering to medication regimens (Coldham et al., 2002) and potential weight gain might exacerbate non-adherence. Second, the physical changes produced by weight gain might result in social discrimination and stigma as young patients are more sensitive to issues of body image and self-esteem than their older counterparts (Gortmaker et al., 1993). Early intervention could prevent or attenuate weight gain as well as the adverse consequences derived from it.

Smoking

There is no high-quality evidence about smoking cessation in mental illness (Khanna et al., 2016). Given this and that there are no studies in youth mental health addressing tobacco smoking, it is worth considering what is known about smoking cessation and mental illness in general.

Interventions for Smoking for People with Mental Illness

There are several important considerations in relation to examining what might work for young people with mental illness who wish to stop smoking. First, is there evidence that people with mental illness want to stop smoking? Second, what is already known about interventions to help stop smoking for people with mental illness? Third, if people with a mental illness want to stop smoking and there are effective interventions, what are the barriers to them doing so?

Do People with a Mental Illness Want to Stop Smoking?

One of the common observations of people in the general community who smoke is that the majority would like to quit (Malarcher et al., 2011). Studies that have examined the rate of desire to quit smoking among those with mental illness find that there is no difference in motivation to quit between those with and those without mental illness (Siru et al., 2009). The implication of this is that if there are effective interventions to quit, people with mental illness are likely to avail themselves of them. However, most are not made aware of, or referred to, such services (Prochaska, 2010), make fewer attempts to quit and have a higher level of tobacco use from which to quit (Campion et al., 2008). Not surprisingly, the rate of quitting is lower in the population with mental illness than in the general population (Lasser et al., 2000).

Interventions

There are three kinds of interventions to assist people to stop smoking: pharmacological (either a nicotine replacement treatment or a nicotine antagonist such as bupropion or a nicotine partial agonist such as varenicline); psychological/psychosocial (such as cognitive behavioural therapy (CBT), supportive counselling or education); or a combination of the two. A review of smoking cessation strategies in mental illness included only eight RCTs (Banham & Gilbody, 2010). A Cochrane review on smoking cessation and reduction in people with schizophrenia found 11 trials focused on cessation and four focused on reduction (Tsoi et al., 2010). Both reviews pointed to the generally small nature of the trials and the heterogeneous measures used and variable follow-up periods. However, what evidence there is reports that interventions that used bupropion alone, or in combination with a psychological intervention such as CBT, achieved better end-of-treatment outcomes in terms of quitting and reducing than interventions that used other pharmacological agents such as replacement therapies or other psychosocial interventions (Banham & Gilbody, 2010; Tsoi et al., 2010), such as self-help or purely educational programmes (Campion et al., 2008). The gains made through the interventions did diminish over time (Banham & Gilbody, 2010). However, this is something also found in the general population (Campion et al., 2008). The general understanding is that giving up smoking generally takes several attempts. A small pilot trial that examined a bespoke cessation intervention that consisted of cessation strategies chosen through a joint decision-making process did produce better outcomes than usual smoking cessation strategies, suggesting a need to tailor interventions for the individual in this domain (Gilbody et al., 2015). However, replication is required.

Given the suggestion that having smoked longer or more heavily makes quitting more difficult (Campion et al., 2008), it is at first surprising that none of the studies to date have attempted to study a tobacco cessation intervention in younger people in the earlier stages of mental illness. However, it is less surprising when it is discovered that there is an acknowledged paucity of research on smoking cessation in young people in general, despite this being the phase of life when smoking is initiated (Fiore et al., 2008). Such studies are an area that cessation research needs to engage in, in both the general youth population and the population of young people with mental illness.

Barriers

Smoking has been, and arguably still is, a part of the culture of mental health treatment settings (Ratschen et al., 2011). One effect of this has been that clinicians have seen the provision of information and support for quitting as being a low priority (Prochaska, 2010; Williams & Ziedonis, 2004). Clinicians believe that there is no evidence that interventions can work for people with mental illness (Morris et al., 2009), or that people with mental illness do not want to quit (Association of American Medical Colleges, 2007). Because there has been a long history of detecting lower rates of cancer in populations of people with mental illness (Coghlan et al., 2001), there is a belief that smoking is not harmful for people with mental illnesses. There is also a misguided belief that smoking is one of the few comforts that people with mental illness have. Consumers of mental health services report that one of the most powerful arguments against quitting is witnessing clinical staff themselves smoking (Morris et al., 2009).

Clinical Lessons

The important clinical lesson with respect to the physical health of young people with mental illness is that it cannot be ignored. The development of poor physical health starts with the onset of mental illness, and it is in this early stage that it needs to be vigorously addressed. The basics required include baseline and regular metabolic monitoring in order to identify any of these issues at their earliest point (Box 12.2). Services need to see weight gain and metabolic side-effects of medication as the iatrogenic problems that they are, and their prevention and remediation as being as much a part of treatment as the prescription of

---

Box 12.2   Interventions to Monitor and Prevent Metabolic Side-Effects

- Baseline
    - weight measures including weight, BMI and waist/hip circumference
    - blood pressure
    - fasting blood glucose
    - fasting blood lipid (full profile)
    - smoking status
    - exercise status
- monitoring at 1, 3, 6, 12 and 18 months, and then yearly
- interventions
    - dietary advice/exercise and lifestyle education and behavioural interventions (possible with specialist dietician involvement)
    - consider changing to less 'metabologenic' antipsychotic medications
    - consider other pharmacotherapy, e.g. statins with GP/specialist input.

    (From Australian Clinical Guidelines for Early Psychosis: ORYGEN Youth Health, 2010)

medication (particularly antipsychotic and some antidepressant medications) in the first place. Unfortunately, metabolic monitoring is not done well but can be improved (Hetrick et al., 2010) by following guideline recommendations such as those developed by Curtis and colleagues in Australia and since replicated internationally. The adult (www.heti.nsw.gov.au/cmalgorithm) and adolescent (www.heti.nsw.gov.au/adolescentcma) versions of these cardiometabolic screening algorithms are available for free download.

It is noteworthy that until very recently treatment guidelines for mental illness made little or no mention of smoking reduction or cessation. This attitude towards smoking must change. Although there is currently little evidence as to what works, there is evidence that people with mental illness want to stop smoking. Therefore, given the tremendous health damage that smoking can cause, it is incumbent on clinicians to provide access to and support for interventions that may help with quitting.

Research Lessons

While a great deal of research, over a very long period, illustrates the prevalence of poor physical health in people with mental illness, there has been very little research developing and trialling preventive physical health interventions for this group. Consequently, there is a lack of clear guidelines detailing appropriate interventions for the management of the physical health of people with a mental illness (Citrome & Yeomans, 2005). There is an urgent need for research in this domain to establish effective interventions that would reduce the burden of physical ill-health and contribute to the overall functional recovery of young people with mental ill-health. This may involve thinking more broadly about solutions to the problem. For example, while the evidence suggests a mixture of caloric restriction and exercise may help control weight gain, it is well known in the general community that achieving this is difficult. Instead of pursuing this alone, thinking broadly may see the addition of theory-driven interventions aimed at enhancing intrinsic motivation and social support to both weight management and smoking cessation interventions (Gates et al., 2015).

New Technologies for Social and Functional Recovery in Youth Mental Health

A new avenue to improve social functioning in young people with mental ill-health is via online social networks. A recent survey of 800 people revealed that 79 per cent of young Australians aged 18–29 use social media daily (Sensis, 2015), a frequency that is on the rise (Duggan et al., 2015). Use of online social media is associated with increased life satisfaction (Best et al., 2014), self-esteem (Best et al., 2014) and social capital (Valenzuela et al., 2009), as well as lower loneliness and depression (Deters & Mehl, 2013), particularly for those who post and are active users (Verduyn et al., 2015). Social media habits of young people with mental health conditions resemble those of their peers: 100 per cent regularly use social media, on average ten times and two hours per day (Birnbaum et al., 2017). Like their peers, young people with psychosis and depression use social media to form social connections and to obtain information (Alvarez-Jimenez et al., 2016). Particularly relevant to early intervention services, around 78 per cent would like to obtain help from clinicians via social media (Birnbaum et al., 2017).

Recent reviews have highlighted that social media-based interventions are acceptable, engaging and feasible, and have the potential to improve clinical and social outcomes in those suffering from mental health conditions such as psychosis and depression (Alvarez-Jimenez et al., 2012a; 2014; Rice et al., 2014). However, prior studies consisted of pilot and preliminary evaluations of newly developed interventions. In addition, very limited research has focused on youth mental health, where the biggest potential of novel online social media interventions can be achieved.

With the aim of illustrating a user-driven social media-based intervention designed to promote engagement and long-term recovery in youth mental health, we briefly describe the moderated online social therapy (MOST) model. The development of MOST has been guided by participatory design principles (Wadley et al., 2013) based on continual user feedback (Lederman et al., 2014). For example, focus groups with young people revealed that they favoured a social media-based platform enabling meaningful peer-to-peer contact as well as clinician support (Alvarez-Jimenez et al., 2012a). This is in keeping with recent findings that over 70 per cent of young people with psychosis or depression would like to be contacted by professionals via social media when experiencing symptoms (Birnbaum et al., 2017). In addition, online peer-to-peer systems should resemble commercial social networking packages (i.e. asynchronous, ongoing communication), but be separate from them, and expert moderators should guide, but not censor, the interaction to ensure a safe and supportive network (Alvarez-Jimenez et al., 2012a). This is consistent with previous suggestions that lack of moderation and structure may adversely affect the online group's ability to attain a sense of community, a pivotal element of peer support (Kaplan et al., 2011). Similarly, excessive expressions of fear and anxiety may lead to increased negative affect and worse outcomes possibly via rumination and over-attention to symptoms and deficits (Rice et al., 2014). Finally, young people indicated that the system should provide self-guided, tailored interventions that are relevant to their moment-by-moment needs (Alvarez-Jimenez et al., 2012a).

Informed by young people's feedback as well as research in the mental health and human–computer interaction fields (Lederman et al., 2014), MOST merges: (1) online social media, (2) interactive therapy modules and (3) peer and professional moderation, creating a constant flow for the user between the social and therapy elements. The online social networking component of MOST has been designed to counteract social isolation and disadvantage, enhance engagement with online interventions – a key challenge in the field (Eysenbach, 2005) – and improve uptake and acquisition of therapeutic strategies. Professional moderation follows a theory-driven model drawing on new frameworks operationalising online human support (i.e. the supportive accountability model (Mohr et al., 2011)), motivation theories (i.e. self-determination theory (Ryan & Deci, 2000)) and new models of positive psychotherapy (i.e. strengths-based models (Seligman et al., 2006)) as a means of enhancing user engagement and self-efficacy. The use of peer moderation is a key component of MOST, serving to normalise experiences, counteract stigma and promote engagement. In MOST, the sum is greater than the parts. The result is that MOST enables a completely new *therapeutic milieu* in which young people with psychosis can safely self-disclose, take positive interpersonal risks, broaden and rehearse coping skills, obtain encouragement and validation and learn how to solve problems and discover their personal strengths (Alvarez-Jimenez et al., 2013).

To date, the MOST model has been effectively implemented in six studies, including four pilot studies with (1) young people recovering from psychosis (Alvarez-Jimenez et al., 2013); (2) young people at ultra-high risk of developing psychosis; (3) young people recovering from depression (Rice et al., 2018); and (4) carers looking after young people experiencing mental ill-health (Gleeson et al., 2017b). In addition, there are two currently active longer-term RCTs evaluating MOST (5) as a relapse prevention intervention for FEP psychosis; and (6) to support carers of young people with psychosis (Gleeson et al., 2017a).

Clinical Lessons

Online social media technologies afford an unprecedented opportunity to deliver engaging, meaningful, real-time, individualised, social support to young people suffering from mental health conditions (Alvarez-Jimenez et al., 2015). The design and development process of new social media-based interventions for youth mental health is critical in ensuring quality interventions that are safe, engaging and effective. The development process needs to follow participatory design methods, with end-users actively involved in the inception, design and delivery of the social media platform (Alvarez-Jimenez et al., 2014). We need to advance a *science of development* of online social media interventions in youth mental health. In order to meet key challenges in the field, such as promoting social connectedness and long-term recovery, we require theory-driven, testable models of user engagement, user experience and intervention effects, as well as novel combinations of cross-disciplinary experts. For example, a significant challenge for online social media interventions is to create an environment that enables meaningful relationships, creating a sense of belonging and a positive therapeutic environment. Furthermore, improving social functioning requires online users to transfer the newly acquired skills, knowledge and confidence into behavioural change in the real world. Creating such a platform is likely to require the collaborative input of clinical psychologists, creative writers, software developers, experts in human–computer interaction, game developers, artists and end-users.

The implementation of online social media interventions in youth mental health raises important safety and privacy considerations (Gleeson et al., 2014). First, online social networking requires adequate levels of protection and oversight. Second, individuals recovering from mental health conditions may have personality traits (e.g. suspiciousness or impulsivity) that jeopardise safety within a social network. Third, symptoms such as rumination may be exacerbated in an online environment. Fourth, the privacy issues facing youths with mental health conditions are especially salient, given their degree of vulnerability (Gleeson et al., 2014). Thus, the safety procedures need to systematically address both 'static' (long-standing or trait variables) and 'dynamic' factors (risk factors that are subject to change – for example, fluctuations in mental state) that could predictably jeopardise consumer safety. Careful consideration of these factors, including professional, manualised moderation and a private social network, has resulted in young people perceiving online social networking as safe and supportive (Gleeson et al., 2014).

Research Lessons

If the field is to maximise the potential of social media to promote functional and social recovery in youth mental health, online peer-to-peer support needs to be informed by, and evaluated through, well-designed controlled studies. The field needs to guard against prematurely embracing and leveraging peer-to-peer networks, without rigorously evaluating their effective components, benefits and potential harms (Linden & Schermuly-Haupt, 2014). The WHO Global eHealth Evaluation Meeting's Call to Action (Bellagio, September 2011) consensus statement stated that 'to improve health and reduce health inequalities, rigorous evaluation of eHealth is necessary to generate evidence and promote the appropriate integration and use of technologies'. In other words, the enthusiasm for mental health reform in the social media era must be driven and guided by evidence. This will reduce the risk of commercialisation and marketing of interventions that have not been validated. In addition, this would promote ongoing innovation in the field, with ineffective interventions likely to be discarded, and maximise the use and incorporation of effective social media-based interventions by mental health services.

The rapid development of online technologies has outpaced the timeline of conventional RCTs of social media-based interventions. This can result in evaluations of interventions that are obsolete by the time trial results become available. Novel research frameworks put forward solutions to this issue, balancing the need for ongoing technological improvements while maintaining the internal validity of the interventions being tested (Mohr et al., 2015). In this way, the core elements and theoretical principles of an online social media-based intervention can be operationalised and remain consistent during the evaluation process while allowing for ongoing quality improvements on the functionality, thereby maintaining technological currency (Mohr et al., 2015).

The eruption of online peer-to-peer support together with novel data-analytic approaches afford fascinating opportunities to address key questions in relation to the effects and mechanisms of these networks (Alvarez-Jimenez et al., 2015). New data will be generated and novel data-analytic approaches such as social networking analysis (Otte & Rousseau, 2002) and data mining and aggregation can be used to determine how online social interactions and relationships develop and influence both mental health and social outcomes. Linguistic analytics (Tausczik & Pennebaker, 2010) and sentiment analysis can be employed to determine how the emotional valence of online communication affects engagement, online interactions and mental health outcomes. Coupled with machine learning methodologies, these new types of data may be used to make individualised predictions of risk for disengagement, imminent risk for relapse, self-harm or suicide attempt, or even onset of psychosis or depression in high-risk individuals (Bedi et al., 2015). Other important questions that the field will need to address are: What are the parameters (e.g. size, operations, etc.) of online social networks that ensure their safety and effectiveness? Can online peer-to-peer support result in improved real-world social functioning? How do the characteristics of online social networks mediate their effects on mental health and social outcomes? What is the level of participation in a social network that is required to gain benefits? What are the appropriate targets for social media-based interventions? How do clinicians or 'peer supporters' best intervene at the level of social networks as well as with individuals? How can we scale and disseminate effective social media-based interventions? We are still a long way from knowing the answers to these questions.

Conclusion

Outpatient care of people with psychiatric illness is now over 100 years old (Stearns, 1918). Since the advent of pharmacological treatment, the focus of attention has been on symptom reduction with a view that this would lead to re-engagement with community function. Unfortunately, the evidence suggests that this has not happened. Intervention in early-stage mental illness, with its consequential focus on young people, is a paradigm that has developed over the last 30 years. A fundamental element of its rationale is that young people with mental illness will avoid the development of disability and will achieve a full recovery in terms of their community functioning. In this chapter we have considered two key areas of functioning – vocation and physical health. In both of these areas there is a long-standing acknowledgement of poor outcomes for people with mental illness.

With respect to vocational recovery, an intervention has been discussed in IPS that has the capacity to help a significant proportion of young people with mental ill-health return to full vocational functioning. The potential personal and economic benefit of this is considerable. The impact on illness of having a valued social role, social contact and income is also potentially significant. Some changes in clinical practice are necessary to realise these potentials, but an increasing number of youth mental health services worldwide are engaging with this. There is an international consensus statement that may also be useful for clinicians who wish to involve their clinics in this practice (International First Episode Vocational Recovery (iFEVR) Group, 2010). Despite progress in this area, there is still a need for further development, particularly in relation to understanding the neurocognitive and social cognitive predictors of vocational success.

The urgency of addressing physical health among those with early-stage mental illness cannot be overstated. The evidence suggests significant life-expectancy gaps for people with mental illness compared to the general population due to largely preventable illnesses that arise as side-effects of medication as well as obesity and tobacco smoking. The evidence also suggests that for both metabolic syndrome and smoking, the earlier the intervention the better. Addressing these problems has not traditionally been seen as the domain of mental health services. Given the evidence, it is imperative that this is seen as part of the mandate of youth mental health services. The pressing need here is for evidence of treatments that work. Research in this area has concentrated on documenting the extent of the problem rather than evaluating potential solutions. It is past time for this focus to shift.

Finally, new mobile and social technologies provide an unprecedented opportunity to address key challenges in youth mental health, such as promoting social and functional recovery and preventing relapse in the longer term. Coupled with novel data analytics, these technologies can transform our understanding of the social and environmental variables that impact on recovery and provide an avenue towards personalised, real-time, impactful interventions.

The onset of mental illness has traditionally been met with pessimism and the encouragement for young people to abandon their hopes and ambitions for a full and fulfilling life as a contributing member of their community. Having an equal focus on functional recovery and physical health alongside the treatment of symptoms of mental ill-health would go a long way towards remediating this unnecessary prognosis. Along with evidence-based pharmacological and psychological treatment, the treatments discussed in this paper have the capacity to restore hope and optimism. The challenge now is their implementation and the pursuit of further research in these domains.

References

Allott, K. A., Yuen, H. P., Garner, B., Bendall, S., Killackey, E. J., Alvarez-Jimenez, M., . . . Phillips, L. J. (2013). Relationship between vocational status and perceived stress and daily hassles in first episode psychosis: an exploratory study. *Social Psychiatry and Psychiatric Epidemiology,* **48**(7), 1045–1052.

Alvarez-Jimenez, M., Alcazar-Corcoles, M. A., Gonzalez-Blanch, C., Bendall, S., McGorry, P. D., & Gleeson, J. F. (2014). Online, social media and mobile technologies for psychosis treatment: a systematic review on novel user-led interventions. *Schizophrenia Research,* **156**(1), 96–106.

Alvarez-Jimenez, M., Alcazar-Corcoles, M. A., Gonzalez-Blanch, C., Bendall, S., McGorry, P. D., & Gleeson, J. F. (2015). Online social media: new data, new horizons in psychosis treatment. *Schizophrenia Research,* **166**(1–3), 345–346.

Alvarez-Jimenez, M., Bendall, S., Lederman, R., Wadley, G., Chinnery, G., Vargas, S., . . . Gleeson, J. F. (2013). On the HORYZON: moderated online social therapy for long-term recovery in first episode psychosis. *Schizophrenia Research,* **143**(1), 143–149.

Alvarez-Jimenez, M., Gleeson, J., Bendall, S., Lederman, R., Wadley, G., Killackey, E., & McGorry, P. (2012a). Internet-based interventions for psychosis: a sneak-peek into the future. *Psychiatric Clinics of North America,* **35**(3), 735–747.

Alvarez-Jimenez, M., Gleeson, J. F., Henry, L. P., Harrigan, S. M., Harris, M. G., Killackey, E., . . . McGorry, P. D. (2012b). Road to full recovery: longitudinal relationship between symptomatic remission and psychosocial recovery in first-episode psychosis over 7.5 years. *Psychological Medicine,* **42**(3), 595–606.

Alvarez-Jimenez, M., Gleeson, J. F., Rice, S., Gonzalez-Blanch, C., & Bendall, S. (2016). Online peer-to-peer support in youth mental health: seizing the opportunity. *Epidemiology and Psychiatric Sciences,* **25**(2), 123–126.

Alvarez-Jimenez, M., Gonzalez-Blanch, C., Crespo-Facorro, B., Hetrick, S., Rodriguez-Sanchez, J. M., Perez-Iglesias, R., & Vazquez-Barquero, J. L. (2008). Antipsychotic-induced weight gain in chronic and first-episode psychotic disorders: a systematic critical reappraisal. *CNS Drugs,* **22**(7), 547–562.

Alvarez-Jimenez, M., Gonzalez-Blanch, C., Vazquez-Barquero, J. L., Perez-Iglesias, R., Martinez-Garcia, O., Perez-Pardal, T., . . . Crespo-Facorro, B. (2006). Attenuation of antipsychotic-induced weight gain with early behavioral intervention in drug-naive first-episode psychosis patients: a randomized controlled trial. *Journal of Clinical Psychiatry,* **67**(8), 1253–1260.

Alvarez-Jimenez, M., Martinez-Garcia, O., Perez-Iglesias, R., Ramirez, M. L., Vazquez-Barquero, J. L., & Crespo-Facorro, B. (2010). Prevention of antipsychotic-induced weight gain with early behavioural intervention in first-episode psychosis: 2-year results of a randomized controlled trial. *Schizophrenia Research,* **116**(1), 16–19.

Association of American Medical Colleges. (2007). *Physician behavior and practice patterns related to smoking cessation summary report.* Washington, DC: Association of American Medical Colleges.

Australian Bureau of Statistics. (2010). *Education and training experience.* Canberra: Australian Bureau of Statistics.

Banham, L., & Gilbody, S. (2010). Smoking cessation in severe mental illness: what works? *Addiction,* **105**(7), 1176–1189.

Bedi, G., Carrillo, F., Cecchi, G. A., Slezak, D. F., Sigman, M., Mota, N. B., . . . Corcoran, C. M. (2015). Automated analysis of free speech predicts psychosis onset in high-risk youths. *NPJ Schizophrenia,* **1**, 15030.

Best, P., Manktelow, R., & Taylor, B. (2014). Online communication, social media and adolescent wellbeing: a systematic narrative review. *Children and Youth Services Review,* **41**, 27–36.

Birnbaum, M. L., Rizvi, A. F., Correll, C. U., & Kane, J. M. (2017). Role of social media and the internet in pathways to care for adolescents and young adults with psychotic disorders and non-psychotic mood disorders. *Early Intervention in Psychiatry,* **11**(4), 290–295.

Bond, G. (2012). Evidence for the effectiveness of the individual placement and support model of supported employment. Retrieved from www.dartmouth.edu/~ips2/resources/12-ips-evidence-10-23.pdf.

Briggs, L. V. (1918). Occupational and industrial therapy: how can this important branch of treatment of our mentally ill be extended and improved? *American Journal of Psychiatry,* **74**(3), 459–479.

Brigham, A. (1844). The moral treatment of insanity. *American Journal of Psychiatry,* **4**(1), 1–15.

Campion, J., Checinski, K., & Nurse, J. (2008). Review of smoking cessation treatments for people with mental illness. *Advances in Psychiatric Treatment, 14*, 208–216.

Citrome, L., & Yeomans, D. (2005). Do guidelines for severe mental illness promote physical health and well-being? *Journal of Psychopharmacology, 19*(6), S102–S109.

Coghlan, R., Lawrence, D., Holman, C. D. J., & Jablensky, A. (2001). *Duty to care: physical illness in people with mental illness.* Perth: University of Western Australia.

Coldham, E. L., Addington, J., & Addington, D. (2002). Medication adherence of individuals with a first episode of psychosis. *Acta Psychiatrica Scandinavica, 106*(4), 286–290.

Creed, P. (1998). Improving the mental and physical health of unemployed people: why and how? *Medical Journal of Australia, 168*(4), 177–178.

Crowther, R. E., Marshall, M., Bond, G. R., & Huxley, P. (2001). Vocational rehabilitation for people with severe mental illness. *Cochrane Database of Systematic Reviews, 2*, CD003080.

Curtis, J., Watkins, A., Rosenbaum, S., Teasdale, S., Kalucy, M., Samaras, K., & Ward, P. B. (2016). Evaluating an individualized lifestyle and lifeskills intervention to prevent antipsychotic-induced weight gain in first-episode psychosis. *Early Intervention in Psychiatry, 10*(3), 267–276.

Curtis, J., Watkins, A., Teasdale, S., Kalucy, M., Rosenbaum, S., Lederman, O., ... Ward, P. W. (2015). Weight gain prevention during the first two years after antipsychotic initiation in youth with first episode psychosis. Paper presented at the SMHR, Brisbane.

Dartmouth IPS Supported Employment Center. (2012). Core principles of IPS supported employment. Retrieved from www.dartmouth.edu/~ips/page29/page31/page31.html.

De Hert, M., Correll, C., Bobes, J., Cetkovich-Bakmas, M., Cohen, D., Asai, I., ... Leucht, S. (2011). Physical illness in patients with severe mental disorders: I. Prevalence, impact of medications and disparities in health care. *World Psychiatry, 10*(1), 52–77.

Degney, J., Hopkins, B., Hosie, A., Lim, S., Rajendren, A. V., & Vogl, G. (2012). *Counting the cost: the impact of young men's mental health on the Australian economy.* Melbourne: Inspire Foundation and Ernst & Young.

Department of Education and Training. (2006). *Department of Education and Training: annual report.* Melbourne: Department of Education and Training, Victorian Government.

Deters, F. G., & Mehl, M. R. (2013). Does posting Facebook status updates increase or decrease loneliness? An online social networking experiment. *Social Psychological and Personality Science, 4*(5). DOI: 10.1177/1948550612469233.

Doll, R., Peto, R., Boreham, J., & Sutherland, I. (2004). Mortality in relation to smoking: 50 years' observations on male British doctors. *BMJ, 328*(7455), 1519.

Duggan, M., Ellison, N., Lampe, C., Lenhart, A., & Madden, M. (2015). *Social media update.* Washington, DC: Pew Research Center.

Eysenbach, G. (2005). The law of attrition. *Journal of Medical Internet Research, 7*(1), e11.

Farrelly, S., Clement, S., Gabbidon, J., Jeffery, D., Dockery, L., Lassman, F., ... Thornicroft, G. (2014). Anticipated and experienced discrimination amongst people with schizophrenia, bipolar disorder and major depressive disorder: a cross sectional study. *BMC Psychiatry, 14*, 157.

Fiore, M., Jaén, C., Baker, T., Bailey, W., Benowitz, N., Curry, S., ... Wewers, M. (2008). *Treating tobacco use and dependence: 2008 update. Clinical practice guideline.* Rockville, MD: U.S. Department of Health and Human Services, Public Health Service.

Galletly, C. (2012). People living with psychosis: the good news and the bad news. *Australian and New Zealand Journal of Psychiatry, 46*(9), 803–807.

Gates, J., Killackey, E., Phillips, L., & Alvarez-Jimenez, M. (2015). Mental health starts with physical health: current status and future directions of non-pharmacological interventions to improve physical health in first episode psychosis. *Lancet Psychiatry,* **2**(8), 726–742.

Gilbody, S., Peckham, E., Man, M. S., Mitchell, N., Li, J., Becque, T., . . . Shepherd, C. (2015). Bespoke smoking cessation for people with severe mental ill health (SCIMITAR): a pilot randomised controlled trial. *Lancet Psychiatry,* **2**(5), 395–402.

Gleeson, J., Lederman, R., Herrman, H., Koval, P., Eleftheriadis, D., Bendall, S., . . . Alvarez-Jimenez, M. (2017a). Moderated online social therapy for carers of young people recovering from first-episode psychosis: study protocol for a randomised controlled trial. *Trials,* **18**(1), 27.

Gleeson, J., Lederman, R., Koval, P., Wadley, G., Bendall, S., Cotton, S., . . . Alvarez-Jimenez, M. (2017b). Moderated online social therapy: a model for reducing stress in carers of young people diagnosed with mental health disorders. *Frontiers in Psychology,* **8**, 485.

Gleeson, J. F., Lederman, R., Wadley, G., Bendall, S., McGorry, P. D., & Alvarez-Jimenez, M. (2014). Safety and privacy outcomes from a moderated online social therapy for young people with first-episode psychosis. *Psychiatric Services,* **65**(4), 546–550.

Gortmaker, S. L., Must, A., Perrin, J. M., Sobol, A. M., & Dietz, W. H. (1993). Social and economic consequences of overweight in adolescence and young adulthood. *New England Journal of Medicine,* **329**(14), 1008–1012.

Hermens, D. F., Scott, E. M., White, D., Lynch, M., Lagopoulos, J., Whitwell, B. G., . . . Hickie, I. B. (2013). Frequent alcohol, nicotine or cannabis use is common in young persons presenting for mental healthcare: a cross-sectional study. *BMJ Open,* **3**, e002229.

Herrman, H., Evert, H., Harvey, C., Gureje, O., Pinzone, T., & Gordon, I. (2004). Disability and service use among homeless people living with psychotic disorders. *Australian and New Zealand Journal of Psychiatry,* **38**(11–12), 965–974.

Hetrick, S., Alvarez-Jimenez, M., Parker, A., Hughes, F., Willet, M., Morley, K., . . . Thompson, A. (2010). Promoting physical health in youth mental health services:

ensuring routine monitoring of weight and metabolic indices in a first episode psychosis clinic. *Australasian Psychiatry,* **18**(5), 451–455.

International First Episode Vocational Recovery (iFEVR) Group. (2010). Meaningful lives: supporting young people with psychosis in education, training and employment: an international consensus statement. *Early Intervention in Psychiatry,* **4**(4), 323–326.

Iyer, S. N., Mangala, R., Anitha, J., Thara, R., & Malla, A. K. (2011). An examination of patient-identified goals for treatment in a first-episode programme in Chennai, India. *Early Intervention in Psychiatry,* **5**(4), 360–365.

Kaplan, K., Salzer, M. S., Solomon, P., Brusilovskiy, E., & Cousounis, P. (2011). Internet peer support for individuals with psychiatric disabilities: a randomized controlled trial. *Social Science and Medicine,* **72**(1), 54–62.

Kessler, R. C., Amminger, G. P., Aguilar-Gaxiola, S., Alonso, J., Lee, S., & Ustun, T. B. (2007). Age of onset of mental disorders: a review of recent literature. *Current Opinion in Psychiatry,* **20**(4), 359–364.

Khanna, P., Clifton, A. V., Banks, D., & Tosh, G. E. (2016). Smoking cessation advice for people with serious mental illness. *Cochrane Database of Systematic Reviews,* **1**, CD009704.

Killackey, E. (2008). Something for everyone: employment interventions in psychotic illness. *Acta Neuropsychiatrica,* **20**, 277–279.

Killackey, E. (2015). Resignation not accepted: employment, education and training in early intervention, past, present and future. *Early Intervention in Psychiatry,* **9**(6), 429–432.

Killackey, E., Allott, K., Woodhead, G., Connor, S., Dragon, S., & Ring, J. (2017). Individual placement and support, supported education in early stage mental illness: an exploratory feasibility study. *Early Intervention in Psychiatry,* **11**(6), 526–531.

Killackey, E. J., Jackson, H. J., Gleeson, J., Hickie, I. B., & McGorry, P. D. (2006). Exciting career opportunity beckons! Early intervention and vocational rehabilitation in first episode psychosis: employing cautious optimism. *Australian and New Zealand Journal of Psychiatry, 40*, 951–962.

Killackey, E., Jackson, H. J., & McGorry, P. D. (2008a). Vocational intervention in first-episode psychosis: a randomised controlled trial of individual placement and support versus treatment as usual. *British Journal of Psychiatry,* **193**, 114–120.

Killackey, E., Nelson, B., & Yung, A. (2008b). Early detection and intervention in psychosis in Australia: history, progress and potential. *Clinical Neuropsychiatry, 5*(6), 279–285.

Lasser, K., Boyd, J. W., Woolhandler, S., Himmelstein, D. U., McCormick, D., & Bor, D. H. (2000). Smoking and mental illness: a population-based prevalence study. *JAMA,* **284**(20), 2606–2610.

Lawrence, D., D'Arcy, C., Holman, J., Jablensky, A. V., Threfall, T. J., & Fuller, S. A. (2000). Excess cancer mortality in Western Australian psychiatric patients due to higher case fatality rates. *Acta Psychiatrica Scandinavica,* **101**(5), 382–388.

Lawrence, D., Hancock, K. J., & Kisely, S. (2013). The gap in life expectancy from preventable physical illness in psychiatric patients in Western Australia: retrospective analysis of population based registers. *BMJ,* **346**, f2539.

Lederman, R., Wadley, G., Gleeson, J., Bendall, S., & Alvarez-Jimenez, M. (2014). Moderated online social therapy: designing and evaluating technology for mental health. *ACM Transactions on Computer–Human Interaction, 21*(1), article no. 5.

Linden, M., & Schermuly-Haupt, M. L. (2014). Definition, assessment and rate of psychotherapy side effects. *World Psychiatry,* **13**(3), 306–309.

Mai, Q., Holman, C. D., Sanfilippo, F. M., Emery, J. D., & Stewart, L. M. (2010). Do users of mental health services lack access to general practitioner services? *Medical Journal of Australia, 192*(9), 501–506.

Malarcher, A., Dube, S., Shaw, L., Babb, S., & Kaufmann, R. (2011). Quitting smoking among adults: United States, 2001–2010. *Morbidity and Mortality Weekly Report,* **60**(44), 1513–1516.

Mathers, C., & Schofield, D. (1998). The health consequences of unemployment: the evidence. *Medical Journal of Australia,* **168**(4), 178–182.

McGorry, P. D., Killackey, E., & Yung, A. (2008). Early intervention in psychosis: concepts, evidence and future directions. *World Psychiatry, 7*(3), 148–156.

Mohr, D. C., Cuijpers, P., & Lehman, K. (2011). Supportive accountability: a model for providing human support to enhance adherence to eHealth interventions. *Journal of Medical Internet Research, 13*(1), e30.

Mohr, D. C., Schueller, S. M., Riley, W. T., Brown, C. H., Cuijpers, P., Duan, N., . . . Cheung, K. (2015). Trials of intervention principles: evaluation methods for evolving behavioral intervention technologies. *Journal of Medical Internet Research, 17*(7), e166.

Morgan, V. A., Waterreus, A., Jablensky, A., Mackinnon, A., McGrath, J. J., Carr, V., . . . Saw, S. (2011). *People living with psychotic illness 2010.* Canberra: Commonwealth of Australia.

Morris, C. D., Waxmonsky, J. A., May, M. G., & Giese, A. A. (2009). What do persons with mental illnesses need to quit smoking? Mental health consumer and provider perspectives. *Psychiatric Rehabilitation Journal, 32*(4), 276–284.

National Mental Health Commission. (2014). *The national review of mental health programmes and services.* Sydney: NMHC.

Neil, A. L., Carr, V. J., Mihalopoulos, C., Mackinnon, A., & Morgan, V. A. (2014). Costs of psychosis in 2010: findings from the second Australian National Survey of Psychosis. *Australian and New Zealand Journal of Psychiatry, 48*(2), 169–182.

Nuechterlein, K. H., Subotnik, K. L., Turner, L. R., Ventura, J., Becker, D. R., & Drake, R. E. (2008). Individual placement and support for individuals with recent-onset schizophrenia: integrating supported education and supported employment. *Psychiatric Rehabilitation Journal, 31*(4), 340–349.

ORYGEN Youth Health. (2010). *The Australian clinical guidelines for early psychosis.* Melbourne: ORYGEN Youth Health.

Ostby, K. A., Czajkowski, N., Knudsen, G. P., Ystrom, E., Gjerde, L. C., Kendler, K. S., ... Reichborn-Kjennerud, T. (2014). Personality disorders are important risk factors for disability pensioning. *Social Psychiatry and Psychiatric Epidemiology,* 49(12), 2003–2011.

Otte, E., & Rousseau, R. (2002). Social network analysis: a powerful strategy, also for the information sciences. *Journal of Information Science,* 28(6), 441–453.

Prochaska, J. J. (2010). Integrating tobacco treatment into mental health settings. *JAMA,* 304(22), 2534–2535.

Ramsay, C. E., Broussard, B., Goulding, S. M., Cristofaro, S., Hall, D., Kaslow, N. J., ... Compton, M. T. (2011). Life and treatment goals of individuals hospitalized for first-episode nonaffective psychosis. *Psychiatry Research,* 189(3), 344–348.

Ratschen, E., Britton, J., & McNeill, A. (2011). The smoking culture in psychiatry: time for change. *British Journal of Psychiatry,* 198(1), 6–7.

Rice, S., Gleeson, J., Davey, C., Hetrick, S., Parker, A., Lederman, R., ... Alvarez-Jimenez, M. (2018). Moderated online social therapy for depression relapse prevention in young people: pilot study of a 'next generation' online intervention. *Early Intervention in Psychiatry,* 2(4), 613–625.

Rice, S. M., Goodall, J., Hetrick, S. E., Parker, A. G., Gilbertson, T., Amminger, G. P., ... Alvarez-Jimenez, M. (2014). Online and social networking interventions for the treatment of depression in young people: a systematic review. *Journal of Medical Internet Research,* 16(9), e206.

Rinaldi, M., Killackey, E., Smith, J., Shepherd, G., Singh, S. P., & Craig, T. (2010). First episode psychosis and employment: a review. *International Review of Psychiatry,* 22(2), 148–162.

Rinaldi, M., McNeil, K., Firn, M., Koletsi, M., Perkins, R., & Singh, S. P. (2004). What are the benefits of evidence-based supported employment for patients with first-episode psychosis? *Psychiatric Bulletin,* 28(8), 281–284.

Robson, E., Waghorn, G., Sherring, J., & Morris, A. (2010). Preliminary outcomes from an individualised supported education programme delivered by a community mental health service. *British Journal of Occupational Therapy,* 73(10), 481–486.

Ryan, R. M., & Deci, E. L. (2000). Self-determination theory and the facilitation of intrinsic motivation, social development, and well-being. *American Psychologist,* 55(1), 68–78.

SANE Australia. (2007). *Smoking and mental illness: costs.* Melbourne: SANE.

Scott, E. M., Hermens, D. F., White, D., Naismith, S. L., GeHue, J., Whitwell, B. G., ... Hickie, I. B. (2015). Body mass, cardiovascular risk and metabolic characteristics of young persons presenting for mental healthcare in Sydney, Australia. *BMJ Open,* 5(3), e007066.

Scott, J., Fowler, D., McGorry, P., Birchwood, M., Killackey, E., Christensen, H., ... Nordentoft, M. (2013). Adolescents and young adults who are not in employment, education, or training. *BMJ (Clinical Research Ed.),* 347, f5270.

Seligman, M. E., Rashid, T., & Parks, A. C. (2006). Positive psychotherapy. *American Psychologist,* 61(8), 774–788.

Sensis. (2015). Social media report: how Australian people and businesses are using social media. Retrieved from www.sensis.com.au/socialmediareport.

Siru, R., Hulse, G. K., & Tait, R. J. (2009). Assessing motivation to quit smoking in people with mental illness: a review. *Addiction,* 104(5), 719–733.

Stearns, A. (1918). The value of out-patient work among the insane. *American Journal of Psychiatry,* 74(4), 595–602.

Tausczik, Y., & Pennebaker, J. (2010). The psychological meaning of words: LIWC and computerized text analysis methods. *Journal of Language and Social Psychology,* 29(1), 24–54.

Thornicroft, G., Brohan, E., Rose, D., Sartorius, N., & Leese, M. (2009). Global pattern of experienced and anticipated discrimination against people with schizophrenia: a cross-sectional survey. *Lancet,* 373(9661), 408–415.

Tsoi, D. T., Porwal, M., & Webster, A. C. (2010). Interventions for smoking cessation and reduction in individuals with schizophrenia. *Cochrane Database of Systematic Reviews*, **6**, CD007253.

Valenzuela, S. N., Park, B. J., & Kee, K. F. (2009). Is there social capital in a social network site? Facebook use and college students' life satisfaction, trust, and participation. *Journal of Computer-Mediated Communication*, **14**(4), 875–901.

Verduyn, P., Lee, D. S., Park, J., Shablack, H., Orvell, A., Bayer, J., . . . Kross, E. (2015). Passive Facebook usage undermines affective well-being: experimental and longitudinal evidence. *Journal of Experimental Psychology: General*, **144**(2), 480–488.

Wadley, G., Lederman, R., Gleeson, J., & Alvarez-Jimenez, M. (2013). Participatory design of an online therapy for youth mental health. Paper presented at the Proceedings of the 25th Australian Computer–Human Interaction Conference: Augmentation, Application, Innovation, Collaboration.

Waghorn, G., Chant, D., & Whiteford, H. (2003). The strength of self-reported course of illness in predicting vocational recovery for persons with schizophrenia. *Journal of Vocational Rehabilitation*, **18**(1), 33–41.

Williams, J. M., & Ziedonis, D. (2004). Addressing tobacco among individuals with a mental illness or an addiction. *Addictive Behaviors*, **29**(6), 1067–1083.

World Health Organization. (2011). Mental health: a state of well-being. Retrieved from www.who.int/features/factfiles/mental_health/en/index.html.

Wu, E. Q., Birnbaum, H. G., Shi, L., Ball, D. E., Kessler, R. C., Moulis, M., & Aggarwal, J. (2005). The economic burden of schizophrenia in the United States in 2002. *Journal of Clinical Psychiatry*, **66**(9), 1122–1129.

Chapter

13

Transforming Cultures to Enable Stage-Related Care of Mental Ill-Health
A Youth Mental Health Challenge

Patrick D. McGorry, Ian B. Hickie and Shane Cross

Although mental health issues are the key health concern for young people today, contributing 45 per cent of the total burden of disease for those aged between 10 and 24 years (Gore et al., 2011), young people have the poorest access to mental health care of all ages. The vast majority of young people from low- and middle-income countries are unable to access mental health care, simply because it is rarely available to them, while less than one-third of young people in high-income countries who experience mental health issues access professional help (McGorry et al., 2014; Nordentoft et al., 2014).

A number of reasons contribute to this state of affairs. Young people often feel that they should manage their emotional difficulties themselves or at least delay seeking professional care. Consequently, these normative but unhelpful beliefs around autonomy may prevent help-seeking (Rickwood et al., 2007). This is in contrast to physical health problems, where young people have greater confidence that professional care will deliver real benefits (Chandra & Minkovitz, 2006; Ellis et al., 2013). Another crucial factor that affects access is the way that our health care system is structured. Primary health care services, the first port of call for most people, are geared to physical ill-health and are largely designed for young children, families or older adults. Moreover, because young people are usually in good physical health, they may not routinely visit a primary care physician, and when they do, they often do not feel comfortable enough to discuss emotional concerns (Rickwood et al., 2007). Other service-level factors, such as confidentiality and cost, are particularly concerning for young people, and even the location, milieu and décor of the service can be critical barriers to accessing care (Ambresin et al., 2013; Fusar-Poli et al., 2014).

The situation is even more difficult for young people and their families who seek help from the specialist mental health system. Entry into specialised services is usually severely restricted and based on meeting specific diagnostic, severity or risk criteria. Young people, particularly those in the early stages of illness, tend to present with evolving symptom profiles that do not meet these stringent entry criteria, despite the concurrent distress and functional impairment. This is particularly so for those in the late-youth and early-adult age ranges who are trying to enter systems designed for middle-aged adults with chronic or persisting disorders. Moreover, many young people are often also considered ineligible for traditional child and adolescent services, particularly from mid-adolescence, as they approach the age cut-off (e.g. 15 or 17 years) for these services.

This state of affairs is the result of outmoded service designs, poor resourcing and professional restrictions. Our current child and adolescent services focus on the needs of younger children within their family, educational and social contexts. In an effort to accommodate older adolescents, many have reached upwards to impose an age cut-off of 17/18 years, the age tied to the end of formal secondary schooling and beginning of legal adulthood (Patel et al., 2007). However, the paediatric focus of these services is inappropriate for many adolescents, especially those with more severe disorders. The adult services have also attempted to reach down to young people, with limited success. This artificially imposed division of health services at age 17/18 presents serious problems for young people with chronic physical health conditions; however, for mental health it is a fatal design flaw, because the discontinuity between services falls right within the age range at which the incidence of new onsets peaks, making the system weakest where it should be strongest (McGorry, 2007).

Young people with existing mental health issues who must transition between the child and adolescent stream and the adult stream for ongoing care, or those who are trying to enter care for the first time, face a complex situation. Although the majority are referred on to adult services, around one-third are not, and of those that are accepted by adult services, one-quarter are discharged without having been seen (Paul et al., 2013; Singh et al., 2010). In part, this is because most adult services do not cater for those who have had the onset of their disorder in childhood, and typically reject those with developmental disorders (e.g. young people with intellectual disabilities, autism or attention deficit/hyperactivity disorder), even though these individuals are known to be at high risk of onset for major anxiety, mood or psychotic disorders during adolescence. For those who are referred on, optimal transition is rare. This is largely due to differences in the service cultures and work practices between the child and adolescent and adult services, poor communication and collaboration between services, poor transfer protocols and the rigid structure and culture of the adult services (McLaren et al., 2013; Paul et al., 2015), which young people find alienating and intimidating.

A New Approach to Mental Health Care for Young People

Clearly, a new approach is required to improve young people's access to mental health care, as well as the quality and continuity of that care. There are strong arguments for a distinct youth mental health stream that recognises the unique biopsychosocial needs of this age group. The first of these is on clinical grounds, in that services need to acknowledge the particularly complex and evolving pattern of symptoms and morbidity often seen in this age group. Second, developmentally and culturally appropriate approaches are essential in the management of emerging mental ill-health, and young people's individual and group identities and their help-seeking needs and behaviours need to be at the heart of any youth service model (McGorry et al., 2014). Ideally, this means creating a service with its own discrete culture and expertise, but with seamless linkages to systems for younger children and older adults (McGorry et al., 2007c). This will overcome many of the issues contributing to the poor access to care and difficulties in transition between the current service streams that young people currently face (Singh et al., 2010).

Addressing the barriers to access to mental health care for young people requires a multifaceted approach. At the individual level, young people need to be able to recognise when, how and where to go to seek help. At the system level, accessible, affordable and acceptable care that is developmentally appropriate for the young person and their stage of illness should be easily available. Because mental ill-health is so widespread among young people, a comprehensive approach with the capacity to deal with the scale of the need, as well as the ability to manage the complexity and diversity of this need, is needed. This means that service levels that cover the full spectrum of illness severity are required, ranging from e-health and primary care services or enhanced primary care services for those with mild to moderate mental health issues, through to specialised services for those with complex presentations or more severe illness (McGorry et al., 2007c). The emphasis needs to be on providing the 'right care' at the 'right time'. These should also be seamless, with as few gates/steps or barriers as possible, a difficult challenge given the under-resourcing of mental health care.

Ideally, any youth service should welcome youth participation at all levels, to ensure it offers a welcoming, stigma-free environment that provides the care that young people and their families need. These services operate best as a 'one-stop shop', where care providers are organised around the young person and their family and their unique needs, and a multidisciplinary team of clinical and non-clinical personnel provides the full cycle of care for the young person. They should offer flexible tenure of care that includes entry, exit and re-entry as needed throughout this critical developmental period. Face-to-face services should be supported – and extended – by online services that offer information, support and monitoring across a range of platforms so that young people can choose to access them whenever and however they choose, in whatever way they wish. The service framework should emphasise early intervention and prevention, and operate in an optimistic culture that offers evidence-informed stepped care governed by risk–benefit considerations and shared decision-making, with improved social and vocational outcomes being the key targets. Finally, a key aim of these services is to eliminate discontinuities at peak periods of need for care during developmental transitions, which should be achieved by ensuring positive and seamless linkages with services for younger children and older adults.

Promoting Accessible, Appropriate and Acceptable Care

Although up to 80 per cent of young people will experience mental health issues at some point during adolescence (Copeland et al., 2011; Gibb et al., 2010; McGorry, 2007; Patton et al., 2014), much of this mental ill-health is mild to moderate in severity and may not persist over long periods. While there is a tendency for a major proportion of these issues to resolve by the late twenties (Patton et al., 2014), if left untreated, neglect too often comes at a significant cost to the young person in terms of underachievement or even educational/vocational failure and poor social functioning, as well as to the wider community in terms of non-participation and lost productivity. Furthermore, current evidence strongly suggests that persistent mental health problems in adolescence significantly increase the risk of mental illness in adulthood (Copeland et al., 2011; Gibb et al., 2010; McGorry et al., 2007a; Patton et al., 2014).

Typically, young people present with fluctuating blends of symptoms, most commonly depression, anxiety and other more non-specific symptoms, including withdrawal, apathy and sleep and appetite disturbance. Self-harm and substance abuse are also prevalent in this age group. These relatively non-specific symptom profiles mean that different treatment approaches are required than those for more discrete and full-threshold illness. The most appropriate care models place emphasis on offering care that is appropriate to the very early stages of illness, pre-emptive in nature, and with a strong preventive focus. This sits best with a clinical staging approach (not a simplistic 'stepped care' approach – see below), which distinguishes earlier and milder clinical phenomena (at any age) from those that accompany illness progression and chronicity. Here, an explicit acknowledgement of the early stages of illness provides a more clinically useful framework, in that it is sensitive to risk–benefit considerations and facilitates the selection of earlier and safer interventions, and favours a preventive, or at least pre-emptive, approach to treatment. This is particularly relevant for young people, first because they are the age group most likely to experience the onset of illness, and second because the early stages of illness are not recognised in our existing care system, which emphasises the need for a formal diagnosis, thereby marginalising, or even excluding, young people from access to care (McGorry, 2007).

Getting the Balance Right Between Individual Needs and Efficient Service Systems

The design of all health service systems should be particularly focused on appropriateness (interventions matched to the individual's unique range of needs), effectiveness (interventions are evidence-informed and lead to positive outcomes) and efficiency (time, financial and human resource waste is minimised, allowing for greater coverage). It is well known that resource availability in mental health services is not commensurate to community need, and in youth mental health services resources are even more scarce. One of the most popular mental health service models used around the world is the 'stepped care' approach. Stepped care models of service delivery seek to address problems associated with service access (due to high demand), service inefficiency and limited resource availability by hierarchically arranging interventions and services based on treatment intensity. The process by which individuals are assigned to particular interventions is contested. Many services favour service efficiency over all else by automatically allocating all newly presenting individuals to low-intensity interventions as a first step. The efficiency with these models is primarily derived from the reduced need to conduct thorough, time-consuming assessments by skilled clinicians. These models are designed to be self-correcting, such that individuals begin with either a 'watchful-waiting' (no intervention) or a low-intensity intervention (e.g. self-help manual or online/e-health) step before graduating to higher intervention intensity steps after a period of time of no improvement. The obvious disadvantage of this approach is that those who already manifest more complex needs and impairment must wait longer for the appropriate services, resulting in unnecessary treatment delays (Richards et al., 2012). As outlined above, it is well established that most people suffering from mental disorder have already delayed accessing professional support, in some cases for many years (Kohn et al., 2004), and further service-directed withholding of appropriate clinical care can result in exposure to unnecessary risk or prolonged distress and impairment, and place a ceiling on the ultimate level of recovery possible.

In contrast to these efficiency-focused stepped care models, 'stratified (or staged) models' directly allocate an individual to the adequate and appropriate level of treatment intensity at the time they present to care. This approach favours personalised, appropriate and timely care over resource efficiency as it requires more investment in clinical resources at the 'front end' than with traditional service environments. This is a more streamlined approach that enables patients to be 'fast-tracked' when necessary. Technologically enhanced services can vastly improve service efficiency while maintaining personalised care, outlined in more detail below. The personalised matching of interventions to needs depends on a heuristic that guides these decisions. It also requires the service having a wide range of treatment-intensity options available at each level of care, which requires the right mix of resources. The clinical staging service model is such a heuristic and a combination of

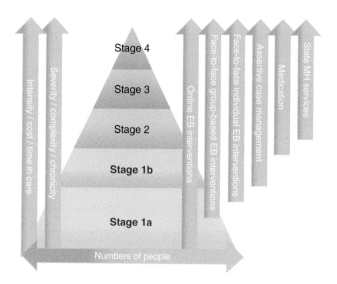

Figure 13.1 Intervention hierarchy by stage. EB, evidence based; MH, mental health.EB, evidence based; MH, mental health.

stratified and stepped care processes can be employed to ensure that young people are provided with the appropriate, adequate, safe and effective intervention as quickly as possible (Cross et al., 2014). This aims to deliver pre-emptive care, an improvement on stepped care. When used alongside traditional diagnostic systems, the clinical staging framework can be used to guide better treatment decisions (Hickie et al., 2013a; 2013b; McGorry et al., 2007b). Staging models define where an individual sits on a continuum from asymptomatic (Stage 0) through early phases and 'attenuated syndromes' (Stage 1) to a persistent, chronic and unremitting disorder state (Stage 4) (McGorry et al., 2007b). This framework is readily applied to those who present for health care and clearly differentiates those who are typically younger in early phases (Stage 1a 'help-seeking' or Stage 1b 'attenuated syndromes') from those who are typically older and have reached a higher threshold for disorder (Stage 2 and above; Figure 13.1).

The proposed key features of a transdiagnostic stage-based approach have previously been outlined (Cross et al., 2014). They include safety screening, comprehensive assessment, treatment planning using shared-decision-making principles, informed choice and stage-matched interventions, routine outcome monitoring (ROM) and formal progress review (Figure 13.2).

Assessment and Staging

Thorough, broad and holistic screening at initial contact is followed by a more targeted mental health assessment for those who respond positively to key screening questions. The primary purpose of this assessment is to match the ascertained level of need with an intervention of appropriate intensity. Attention is paid to the young person's unique needs across a number of domains, including: mental health and clinical stage; education, training and employment needs; risk of injury, self-harm and suicide; use of alcohol and other drugs; quality of physical health and the quality of family and social relationships. This helps to ensure that parallel intervention for these known risk factors for poor outcomes and worsening mental health are provided. At times, it is appropriate for these 'non-mental health' domains to be the primary focus of intervention. Additionally, assessing a person's strengths and personal/external resources aid in personalised treatment planning.

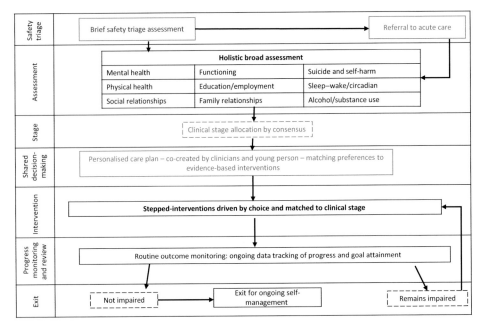

Figure 13.2 Clinical staging service pathway.

The allocation of a clinical stage can be based on published criteria (Hickie et al., 2013a; McGorry et al., 2006) and is ideally done in consultation with professional peers. The information obtained from these comprehensive assessments can then be used by people in partnership with their clinicians to guide a range of interventions matched to their needs and preferences. The effectiveness of these interventions should be routinely monitored, and such ROM would assist young people and clinicians in deciding whether intervention intensity should step up or down. This data would also be of use to service providers when reporting on service level outcomes.

Treatment Intensity

New models of mental health service delivery need to be responsive to the diversity and complexity of presentation common in people (especially young people) seeking professional assistance. Such models should be able to adequately deal with comorbidity, assist those in distress and impairment resulting from 'subthreshold' disorders, be cognisant of the potential developmental trajectory of disorders and, most importantly, offer an intensity of intervention that is appropriate for the level of severity of the presenting set of issues at the time it is required and requested. As outlined extensively above, the clinical staging framework copes with these issues and can be used to guide better treatment decisions (Hickie et al., 2013a; 2013b; McGorry et al., 2007b).

The intensity of the intervention should match the level of need at the outset as determined by stage, which considers the risk–benefit ratio of the proposed intervention. Preemptive care might also mean a qualitative increase in intensity or complexity to reduce the risks of progression of illness. The risk–benefit ratio of treatment is the guide and constraint here and can be varied. Intensity can be defined in terms of financial cost (both at the service level and at the person/family level), a person's requirement to physically attend a clinic, the required frequency of attendance, the number of professionals involved, the length of the episode of care and the prescription of psychotropic medication. Early-stage treatments inherently carry less risk, and are usually less time-intensive for the person receiving the care, their family and the clinical team than are later-stage treatments. When the clinical staging framework has been applied to youth-based primary care settings, those at Stages 1a and 1b differ significantly in terms of the type and intensity of the treatments they receive, as well as their short-term symptomatic and functional outcomes (Cross et al., 2016a). Young people at Stage 1b use more combinations of treatments and are much more likely to be prescribed with psychotropic medication (9.3 per cent vs 43.6 per cent). Regarding outcomes, those at Stage 1a start with significantly lower levels of psychological distress and significantly higher levels of functioning at service entry and show quick improvement. Despite using significantly more interventions, Stage 1b young people remain both symptomatically and functionally impaired over the same period, even though they show some modest improvements in their levels of psychological distress and functioning over this time.

As a guide, the spectrum of services matched against need (from lowest to highest intensity) could include: online psychoeducation or health information, self-managed online interventions, clinician-supported/-assisted online interventions, group-based psychological interventions, brief face-to-face psychological therapy, longer-term psychological therapy, assertive case management and first- and second-line medication (Figure 13.1). Early-stage psychological interventions should be transdiagnostic (Barlow et al., 2017; Kazdin, 2014) to meet the needs of a wide range of early-stage issues, with more specific psychological therapies reserved for those with more clearly established illnesses.

Engagement in Care and Assertive Monitoring of Outcomes

The recommended length of care for a person could also be guided by the clinical staging model. For example, for clients at Stage 1b who typically have more significant clinical needs, higher risks of persistent disability and a greater chance of progression to more severe illnesses, the emphasis would be on a 12-month programme of more intensive clinical care – in the clinic setting, online or through a combination of both. Those at Stage 1a would benefit from brief interventions (Cross et al., 2016a), while those at Stage 2 should be kept connected to care for a period of 2–5 years (McGorry et al., 2010). Beyond Stage 2, much longer-term care is necessary but may be adjusted in terms of intensity and complexity according to needs.

Services designed for this at-risk group need to be cognisant of the challenges of keeping these young people connected to care. In light of the risks of illness progression previously outlined, keeping high-risk young people engaged in care is essential. Despite having greater treatment needs, young people at Stage 1b have been shown to have poorer rates of service attendance than those with less intensive treatment needs (Stage 1a). Young people in the Stage 1b group tend to make more appointments and miss more appointments, even when controlling for other potentially confounding variables. Further, the lack of diagnostic clarity for young people at Stage 1b was shown to have a significant impact on their appointment behaviour, such that those with more diagnostic ambiguity had much poorer attendance than those provided with more diagnostic certainty (Cross et al., 2016b). Of course, the mode of service provision can be tailored to adapt to this pattern, for example through more use of mobile and outreach approaches.

Once young people are engaged and remain connected to care, proactive monitoring of treatment outcome is critical. People should have direct and transparent access to their own health progress data to assist them in shared treatment planning decisions with their treating clinicians. Clinicians can also use the data to help inform treatment intensity decisions in order to prepare for discussions with young people about proposed step/ intensity changes. Services themselves can also use aggregated data to inform decisions regarding service resource allocation, service gaps and other quality improvement initiatives.

Routine outcome monitoring (ROM) of client progress in care has been shown by more than 12 randomised control trials (RCTs) to reduce client deterioration in treatment and to enhance treatment effect sizes (Boswell et al., 2015). Such ROM can alert clients and clinicians to deterioration and allow clinicians and services to respond early to avoid patient drop-out by altering treatment plans if necessary. The current predominate practice in many service settings sees an over-reliance on clinician judgement to decide whether a client is responding positively or negatively to treatment and, correspondingly, whether a change in treatment plan is required. Previous research has identified an important limitation to the over-reliance on clinical judgement; clinicians on average believe that about 85 per cent of their clients improve or recover under their care (Walfish et al., 2012), a rate which is not in keeping with typical patient outcome data. When the clinical file notes of those clients who left care in a dramatically worse state than they entered were reviewed retrospectively, there was very little mention of deterioration by the treating clinician (Hatfield et al., 2010). Importantly, when clinicians are provided with regular feedback regarding client progress in care, it has been shown to result in an over 2.6 times higher odds ratio of reliable improvement compared to when clinicians do not receive routine progress feedback (Shimokawa et al., 2010).

If young people do present to care with pre-treatment negative illness trajectories, as would be predicted by clinical staging models, then proactive and objective monitoring of outcome is obligatory. While it is clear that a sizeable portion may deteriorate in treatment, we do not yet have the ability to differentially predict those who will improve and those who will deteriorate on the basis of an initial assessment of pre-treatment characteristics alone. Furthermore, enhancing treatment for those at such risk may alter the trajectory, e.g. the early deployment of strategies for treatment-resistant depression, anxiety and psychosis. As such, these and other studies lend support to clinical models with embedded systematic ROM practices in order for treatment to be more personalised, and to better respond to the expected variation in treatment progress between individuals.

Technologically Enhanced Service Delivery: The Potential of Providing the Required Services at Scale

To deploy more personalised and better-targeted services, and to take mental health services to scale, there is an urgent need to develop a more rational approach to the development and deployment of digital services (see Chapter 12). The integrated use of technology has the capacity to enhance both online and in-clinic service provision and promote service continuity beyond the walls of a clinic.

Digital technologies, operating in synchrony with clinical services, can both improve access to evidence-based care and allow young people and their families to choose the setting and time of day in which that care is provided, thereby expanding reach by enhancing accessibility (Burns & Birrell, 2014). The sheer size of this population health problem is staggering and creates significant challenges for health systems, policy makers and service planners. The current service system consists largely of the provision of care delivered in person by professionals at specific locations during often unfriendly office-based hours. Novel online and digital models can buttress and complement this system and help to overcome the current 'rationing' of the limited services available to the vast numbers of people who need them. The role of technology operating in synergy with face-to-face health services, which must be greatly expanded too, can significantly improve the access and scalability of care.

Online technologies are well suited to support the delivery of a wide range of functions, from comprehensive assessment (including the determination of clinical stage), self-monitoring and routine outcome monitoring tools, through to comprehensive psychological interventions (Burns et al., 2015). Increasingly, it is also possible to deliver direct clinical and other person-based support services online (through a variety of self-help, clinician-guided self-help or peer-supported interventions) aligned with the severity of illness (Burns et al., 2015). These new alternatives can help to overcome barriers related to geography, socioeconomic disadvantage and preference by many, though not all, young people for use of non-clinical or peer-supported forms of care.

In face-to-face services, extensive time spent conducting thorough assessments by highly experienced (and expensive) clinicians can detract from the amount of intervention a service can offer (Richards et al., 2012). Rather than waiting for an assessment appointment in a busy clinic, technology has the capacity to undertake standardised and comprehensive assessments to determine clinical stage based on algorithms at any time. These data can then be made instantaneously available to clients and service providers, and supplemented with a much shorter face-to-face interview (in vivo or online), which can much more quickly match the adequate intensity of intervention to the clinical need. The speed and efficiency of such a system would allow greater service resources to be allocated towards providing a wider range of intervention options and shift face-to-face contact from assessment to intervention mode.

Importantly, the development and application of such technologically enhanced services has a much greater capacity to be taken to scale. The largest proportion of clients are typically those with mild impairment who could largely be managed by non-pharmacological, psychosocial interventions (Cross et al., 2014) delivered in person or, increasingly, through a variety of online intervention platforms (Ebert et al., 2015). It is reasonable to assume that these clients are unlikely to require much more than brief, low-intensity but evidence-based psychological interventions, with the option of choosing online or clinician-supported online interventions to reduce service cost and client inconvenience. Additionally, this approach would seek to more quickly direct those with more acute, chronic or emergency needs to the appropriate secondary and tertiary care systems than is currently the case.

Developing New Service Frameworks for Young People: The Headspace Example

Over the last few years, there has been a groundswell of reform in the delivery of mental health services for young people, beginning in Australia and then spreading to the UK, Ireland, Canada, the USA, Denmark and Asia (Birchwood & Singh, 2013; Illback & Bates,

2011; McGorry, 2007; McGorry et al., 2013; Purcell et al., 2011; Rao et al., 2013; Verma et al., 2012). Service reform in Australia began in 2006 when the Australian government established headspace, the National Youth Mental Health Foundation, after a long advocacy campaign headed by clinician academics and supported by key professional bodies and the Australian public, who were increasingly concerned by the burden of disease associated with mental ill-health, the poor access to services among Australia's young people and our high national youth suicide rate. Almost a decade after the initial ten centres opened in 2007, headspace has now been scaled up to over 100 sites around the nation, and provides face-to-face access to mental health care for approximately 50 per cent of Australian communities. Along with eheadspace, its online service, headspace offers access to information, support and mental health care to Australia's young people when and where they choose, including those who might otherwise not access professional help, for whatever reason.

Headspace operates on an enhanced primary care model, offering four core service streams relevant to young people: mental health, physical health, work and study support, and drug and alcohol interventions. This combination helps to minimise the stigma often associated with a mental health service. Each headspace site is an independent consortium, headed by a lead agency that brings together local services, including primary care providers, state-funded specialist mental health services and education, employment and vocational agencies in a comprehensive 'one-stop shop' designed to offer young people a community-based accessible entry point to the services most important to them. The headspace National Office oversees the operation of all headspace centres, in partnership with the 31 primary health networks, who from 2016 onwards commission headspace centres, and deals with accreditation and high-level governance. The centres are located in areas that young people often visit, such as shopping malls or entertainment precincts, and are open to all young people, no matter what their concern, and a professional referral is not necessary (McGorry et al., 2014).

On arriving at a headspace centre, the young person will be assessed by a member of the access team, usually a young person themselves, who might be a social worker, mental health nurse, occupational therapist, youth worker or a psychologist. Depending on the nature of their issue, they may be managed by the access team, or referred to other health professionals within the service, who might be an allied health professional, a vocational or educational worker, a psychologist, doctor or a psychiatrist, depending on the young person's needs. Interventions may be single or multiple and are delivered in a sequential, stepwise manner, with brief psychosocial approaches typically used as first-line therapies, with the aim being to prevent premature use of medication and also to prevent development of sustained illness and disability. Medication is used as an additive therapy only if the young person does not respond to initial psychosocial interventions, or presents at the outset with more severe symptoms or risk in line with the staging approach outline above. This stepped care model allows a preventive and proactive stance to therapeutic intervention (McGorry et al., 2014).

As well as the four core service streams, each headspace centre also delivers local community awareness campaigns to enhance young people's help-seeking behaviour, the ability of families and local service providers to identify emerging mental health concerns in young people early and to strengthen the referral pathways into the service. In addition to its face-to-face services, headspace also runs a nationwide online support service (eheadspace; www.eheadspace.org.au) where young people can 'chat' with a mental health professional either online or by telephone and access assessment and therapeutic care. In recognition of the issue of youth suicide in Australia, headspace also provides a support service for schools affected by student suicide (headspace school support), which offers a range of services, including assistance with managing the immediate response following a student suicide or suicide attempt; staff and parent information sessions; education and training related to suicide and evidence-based resources; a postvention toolkit; secondary and tertiary consultation; assistance with critical incident review; and media liaison and advice (McGorry et al., 2014). This school-based programme is now expanding to cover a much wider range of educational and interventional needs under the reinvented banner of MindMatters.

Evaluating the Impact of headspace Services

Headspace has achieved its initial milestones, with satisfaction levels uniformly high among service users. In the 2016/2017 financial year, 80,237 young people accessed a headspace centre, and almost 32,000 accessed eheadspace. While its obvious initial focus has been on improving access to mental health care for young Australians, it is not yet totally clear to what extent the programme is improving the longer-term effectiveness and efficiency of mental health care for young Australians, largely due to the difficulties associated with obtaining an appropriate control group to measure it against. Careful consideration must be given to the relevant external comparative services and also examination of the site-to-site variability in achieving better access and outcomes. Some outcomes are clearly positive, but further research is needed here. A recent census of headspace data has shown strong improvements in the rates of access to mental health care, particularly for vulnerable and marginalised young people (Rickwood et al., 2015b), and that approximately 60 per cent of clients showed a significant initial reduction in psychological distress and/or psychosocial functioning (Rickwood et al., 2015a). Further, an independent review of headspace, commissioned by the Australian Government Department of Health, has very recently been completed, and has been largely favourable (Hilferty et al., 2015). The scope of this review included an assessment of headspace's ability to improve young people's access to and engagement with mental health services, the outcomes for headspace clients, the service delivery model itself and its cost-effectiveness.

The review comprised an analysis of the client, service provider and financial data from 56 fully operational headspace centres, covering over 45,000 young people who received approximately 200,000 occasions of service. Surveys of various stakeholder groups, including 1515 young people attending headspace and 4774 young people not attending headspace centres (to compare the outcomes for those attending headspace centres and those who have not used headspace or have received other forms of mental health care), parents and carers, professionals affiliated with headspace and/or the mental health care system and centre managers. Interviews were also held with key stakeholders, including clients, centre managers and staff and parents and carers of young people with mental health issues.

The review found that headspace has been successful in improving young people's access to, and engagement with, mental health services. This was particularly notable for young people living in regional areas, and those from certain vulnerable or marginalised groups, including indigenous young people; lesbian, gay, bisexual, transgender or intersex young people; young people not engaged in work or study; and young people who were homeless or living in insecure accommodation. However, young people from culturally and linguistically diverse backgrounds were under-represented at headspace, suggesting that more effort needs to be made to target these groups and to provide culturally appropriate services.

Young people, parents and headspace staff all reported factors, including the youth-friendly environment, non-judgemental staff, the wide range of services and practical assistance offered and the low-cost or free service, as contributing to accessibility and engagement. However, a number of barriers to access were mentioned, including the stigma associated with mental illness, and practical factors such as standard opening hours, transportation difficulties and centre waiting lists. The cultural appropriateness of services provided in certain centres was also mentioned as a concern needing attention.

Almost three-quarters of young people who visited headspace centres during the 2013/2014 financial year reported a high or very high level of psychological distress at their first assessment. Overall, almost half of the young people attending headspace showed a reduction in the level of their psychological distress at their final visit, ranging from a clinically or reliably significant reduction to an insignificant reduction. Around 29 per cent of young people experienced no change in the level of their distress, while psychological distress increased for approximately one-quarter of young people. Most noteworthy is the fact that psychological distress was significantly reduced (clinically or reliably) for more than double the number of young people than those who experienced a significant increase in distress. Not unexpectedly, young people who made only 2–3 visits to headspace were over-represented in the group that did not experience any change, or an insignificant change in psychological distress, while those who made at least seven visits were over-represented in the group that reported a significant change in their levels of distress.

Importantly, suicidal ideation and self-harm were also significantly reduced, even among the group of young people who showed an insignificant, or no, reduction in psychological distress, while self-harm increased only in the group who showed a clinically significant increase in psychological distress. Positive social and economic outcomes were also seen, particularly in those who experienced a significant reduction in psychological distress, with the number of days that young people were unable to work or study per month dropping by approximately 59 per cent in this group, while the number of days per month that young people experienced reduced functioning as a result of their mental health issues were reduced by two-thirds.

The service model ensures that young people with a range of problems can access different types of practitioners in a single location. Formal referral to other services is rare, although informal referral is not uncommon. The review indicated that one of the best ways that the service model could be improved to better meet the needs of young people and their families or carers would be to increase the capacity of centres to provide family therapy, as well as increasing the provision of outreach services. Workforce issues were another challenge, with over half of the centre managers surveyed stating that they were operating with a staffing vacancy. The need to increase the amount of time that primary care physicians operated in centres, as well as the range of medical services offered, was identified as an important gap in service provision. A further serious gap identified was in the ability to access more intensive and expert care for those with more complex disorders.

In summary, the review found that headspace was a highly accessible, complex programme that served a diverse range of vulnerable young people with high levels of psychological distress and a range of social, emotional and other health problems. Small improvements were seen in the mental health of headspace clients relative to matched control groups, and the economic and social benefits from this improved functioning were achieved through a number of positive outcomes, including a reduction in the number of days lost to illness, the number of days cut down as a result of illness and a reduction in suicidal ideation and self-harm. The review also stressed that the value of headspace should not be restricted to its impact on individual clients, but that it also plays an important role in mental health promotion and community awareness, and has had a positive impact on reducing the stigma associated with mental illness and encouraging young people to seek help.

Planning the Future of Youth Services Development

Headspace is still a work in progress. While it provides a valuable entry to the health and welfare system, and can deal with the needs of perhaps two-thirds of its clientele through its enhanced primary care capacity, at least one-third need a more expert, specialised and at times more intensive approach, which may include mobile home-based and outreach care, diagnostically targeted interventions, acute and sub-acute residential care and specific links with educational and vocational services. To begin to address this gap, the Australian government has funded the creation of six 'enhanced headspace' services, which will be resourced to deliver evidence-based early psychosis services, offering early detection, acute care during and immediately following a psychotic episode and recovery-focused continuing care featuring multimodal interventions to support the young person (and their family) to maintain or regain their social, academic and/or career trajectory during the critical first 2–5 years following the onset of a psychotic illness (Hughes et al., 2014). The first of these enhanced services commenced operation in 2013, and it is hoped that ultimately these enhanced services will be expanded to cover not only all headspace communities, but also the full diagnostic spectrum in young people with all the severe forms of mental illness. The federal government has subsequently created a new funding stream termed 'youth severe', which is beginning to strengthen the capacity of the headspace system to address a broader range of complex presentations. This needs to be greatly expanded and explicitly and tightly linked to headspace centres.

The long-term aim of these reforms is to develop a nationwide youth mental health stream that fully integrates care for young people with other service systems, notably education, employment, housing and justice, in order to provide seamless coverage of mental health care from puberty to mature adulthood at around 25 years of age, with soft transitions with child and adult mental health care. This system acknowledges biopsychosocial development and recognises the complexity and challenges faced by young people as they become independent adults, as well as the burden of disease imposed on this age group by mental ill-health. It responds by blurring the distinctions between the tiers of primary and specialist care, including some aspects of acute care, in recognition of the complexity of the presentation of much of the mental ill-health apparent in young people, allowing a flexible and appropriate response for each individual, depending on their unique needs.

Clearly, more health services research is necessary to develop, refine, adapt and evaluate such new service models, both within their individual contexts and cross-sectorally. However, the indications to date are that this model can result in significant improvement in access to care – particularly for disadvantaged or marginalised groups – and this has been acknowledged by national and international policy makers in the expansion and spread of these new service models. Providing enhanced access to care does assume that some care is better than no care for young people with mental ill-health, particularly in terms of relieving distress and reducing risks of self-harm. Testing whether increased access has longer-term benefits, notably in terms of enhanced multidimensional functional outcomes (Iorfino et al., 2016) and secondary prevention, remains a high health services research priority, but will need further enhancements to the basic headspace model to deliver such outcomes.

In pragmatic terms, we believe that offering evidence-informed care within a system that is both accessible and acceptable to young people, as headspace and these new service models clearly are, should continue as a 'best bet' while we continue to accumulate evidence within a virtuous and ongoing research and development cycle. This approach has the best chance of enabling the development of a more fully evidence-based care stream for this uniquely vulnerable group.

The foundations for reform in mental health must be built on the principles of demonstrable need and evidence-informed care, including indicative evidence of value for better health outcomes and value for money (McGorry, 2007; McGorry et al., 2011). Mental ill-health affects us all, either directly or indirectly, and our current approaches are insufficient, poorly designed and not well supported. Solutions to these problems exist, and innovation means that more can be developed, demonstrated and disseminated just as well as they have been in other fields of health care. John Gunn, the eminent English forensic psychiatrist, once described the neglect of the mental health of young people as a form of self-harm perpetrated by society upon itself (Gunn, 2004). This societal self-harm must be replaced by a potentially dramatic improvement in the mental health, wellbeing, productivity and fulfilment of our young people, now and in the foreseeable future. Transformational reform of mental health care is required, and should be based on the principles of early intervention and a priority focus on the developmental period of greatest need and capacity to benefit from investment: the period of emerging adulthood. This by no means argues against investment in care earlier or later in life – which is also essential. There are already rapidly emerging examples of modern, stigma-free cultures of care designed and operated with young people themselves, as described in this chapter. These examples of twenty-first-century clinical infrastructure culture will also facilitate some of the population-based and universal programmes that may link with mental health awareness and promotional activities and with new internet-based technologies. If these new mindsets and reforms spread widely, they will undoubtedly reduce the lifelong impact of mental ill-health on our young people, and on our collective wellbeing as a society.

References

Ambresin, A.-E., Bennett, K., Patton, G. C., Sanci, L. A., & Sawyer, S. M. (2013). Assessment of youth-friendly health care: a systematic review of indicators drawn from young people's perspectives. *Journal of Adolescent Health*, 52(6), 670–681.

Barlow, D. H., Farchione, T. J., Bullis, J. R., Gallagher, M. W., Murray-Latin, H., Sauer-Zavala, S., . . . Cassiello-Robbins, C. (2017). The unified protocol for transdiagnostic treatment of emotional disorders compared with diagnosis-specific protocols for anxiety disorders: a randomized clinical trial. *JAMA Psychiatry*, 74(9), 875–884.

Birchwood, M., & Singh, S. P. (2013). Mental health services for young people: matching the service to the need. *British Journal of Psychiatry*, 202(54), S1–S2.

Boswell, J. F., Kraus, D. R., Miller, S. D., & Lambert, M. J. (2015). Implementing routine outcome monitoring in clinical practice: benefits, challenges, and solutions. *Psychotherapy Research*, 25(1), 6–19.

Burns, J., & Birrell, E. (2014). Enhancing early engagement with mental health services by young people. *Psychology Research and Behavior Management, 7,* 303–312.

Burns, J., Birrell, E., Bismark, M., Pirkis, J., Davenport, T., Hickie, I., . . . Ellis, L. (2015). The role of technology in Australian youth mental health reform. *Australian Health Review, 40*(5), 584–590.

Chandra, A., & Minkovitz, C. S. (2006). Stigma starts early: gender differences in teen willingness to use mental health services. *Journal of Adolescent Health, 38*(6), e1–e8.

Copeland, W., Shanahan, L., Costello, E. J., & Angold, A. (2011). Cumulative prevalence of psychiatric disorders by young adulthood: a prospective cohort analysis from the Great Smoky Mountains Study. *Journal of the American Academy of Child and Adolescent Psychiatry, 50*(3), 252–261.

Cross, S. P. M., Hermens, D. F., & Hickie, I. B. (2016a). Treatment patterns and short-term outcomes in an early intervention youth mental health service. *Early Intervention in Psychiatry, 10*(1), 88–97.

Cross, S. P. M., Hermens, D. F., Scott, E. M., Ottavio, A., McGorry, P. D., & Hickie, I. B. (2014). A clinical staging model for early intervention youth mental health services. *Psychiatric Services, 65*(7), 939–943.

Cross, S. P. M., Hermens, D. F., Scott, J., Salvador-Carulla, L., & Hickie, I. B. (2016b). Differential impact of current diagnosis and clinical stage on attendance at a youth mental health service. *Early Intervention in Psychiatry, 11*(3), 255–262.

Ebert, D. D., Zarski, A.-C., Christensen, H., Stikkelbroek, Y., Cuijpers, P., Berking, M., & Riper, H. (2015). Internet and computer-based cognitive behavioral therapy for anxiety and depression in youth: a meta-analysis of randomized controlled outcome trials. *PLoS One, 10*(3), e0119895.

Ellis, L. A., Collin, P., Hurley, P. J., Davenport, T. A., Burns, J. M., & Hickie, I. B. (2013). Young men's attitudes and behaviour in relation to mental health and technology: implications for the development of online mental health services. *BMC Psychiatry, 13*(1), 119.

Fusar-Poli, P., Yung, A. R., McGorry, P., & van Os, J. (2014). Lessons learned from the psychosis high-risk state: towards a general staging model of prodromal intervention. *Psychological Medicine, 44*(1), 17–24.

Gibb, S. J., Fergusson, D. M., & Horwood, L. J. (2010). Burden of psychiatric disorder in young adulthood and life outcomes at age 30. *British Journal of Psychiatry, 197*(2), 122–127.

Gore, F. M., Bloem, P. J. N., Patton, G. C., Ferguson, J., Joseph, V., Coffey, C., . . . Mathers, C. D. (2011). Global burden of disease in young people aged 10–24 years: a systematic analysis. *Lancet, 377*(9783), 2093–2102.

Gunn, J. (2004). Foreword. In S. Bailey & M. Dolan (Eds), *Adolescent forensic psychiatry.* London: Arnold.

Hatfield, D., McCullough, L., Frantz, S. H., & Krieger, K. (2010). Do we know when our clients get worse? An investigation of therapists' ability to detect negative client change. *Clinical Psychology and Psychotherapy, 17*(1), 25–32.

Hickie, I. B., Scott, E. M., Hermens, D. F., Naismith, S. L., Guastella, A. J., Kaur, M., . . . McGorry, P. D. (2013a). Applying clinical staging to young people who present for mental health care. *Early Intervention in Psychiatry, 7*(1), 31–43.

Hickie, I. B., Scott, J., Hermens, D. F., Scott, E. M., Naismith, S. L., Guastella, A. J., . . . McGorry, P. D. (2013b). Clinical classification in mental health at the cross-roads: which direction next? *BMC Medicine, 11,* 125.

Hilferty, F., Cassells, R., Muir, K., Duncan, A., Christensen, D., Mitrou, F., . . . Katz, I. (2015). Is headspace making a difference to young people's lives? Final report of the independent evaluation of the headspace program. Sydney: Social Policy Research Centre, UNSW Australia.

Hughes, F., Stavely, H., Simpson, R., Goldstone, S., Pennell, K., & McGorry, P. (2014). At the heart of an early psychosis centre: the core components of the 2014 Early Psychosis Prevention and Intervention Centre model for Australian communities. *Australasian Psychiatry, 22*(3), 228–234.

Illback, R. J., & Bates, T. (2011). Transforming youth mental health services and supports in

Ireland. *Early Intervention in Psychiatry,* 5(1), S22–S27.

Iorfino, F., Hickie, I. B., Lee, R. S. C., Lagopoulos, J., & Hermens, D. F. (2016). The underlying neurobiology of key functional domains in young people with mood and anxiety disorders: a systematic review. *BMC Psychiatry,* 16(1), 156.

Kazdin, A. E. (2014). Evidence-based psychotherapies II: changes in models of treatment and treatment delivery. *South African Journal of Psychology,* 45(1), 3–21.

Kohn, R., Saxena, S., Levav, I., & Saraceno, B. (2004). The treatment gap in mental health care. *Bulletin of the World Health Organization,* 82(11), 858–866.

McGorry, P. D. (2007). The specialist youth mental health model: strengthening the weakest link in the public mental health system. *Medical Journal of Australia,* 187(7), S53.

McGorry, P. D., Bates, T., & Birchwood, M. (2013). Designing youth mental health services for the 21st century: examples from Australia, Ireland and the UK. *British Journal of Psychiatry,* 202(54), S30–S35.

McGorry, P. D., Goldstone, S. D., Parker, A. G., Rickwood, D. J., & Hickie, I. B. (2014). Cultures for mental health care of young people: an Australian blueprint for reform. *Lancet Psychiatry,* 1(7), 559–568.

McGorry, P. D., Hickie, I. B., Yung, A. R., Pantelis, C., & Jackson, H. J. (2006). Clinical staging of psychiatric disorders: a heuristic framework for choosing earlier, safer and more effective interventions. *Australian and New Zealand Journal of Psychiatry,* 40(8), 616–622.

McGorry, P. D., Nelson, B., Goldstone, S., & Yung, A. R. (2010). Clinical staging: a heuristic and practical strategy for new research and better health and social outcomes for psychotic and related mood disorders. *Canadian Journal of Psychiatry,* 55(8), 486–497.

McGorry, P. D., Purcell, R., Goldstone, S., & Amminger, G. P. (2011). Age of onset and timing of treatment for mental and substance use disorders: implications for preventive intervention strategies and models of care.

Current Opinion in Psychiatry, 24(4), 301–306.

McGorry, P. D., Purcell, R., Hickie, I. B., & Jorm, A. F. (2007a). Investing in youth mental health is a best buy. *Medical Journal of Australia,* 187(7), S5–S7.

McGorry, P. D., Purcell, R., Hickie, I. B., Yung, A. R., Pantelis, C., & Jackson, H. J. (2007b). Clinical staging: a heuristic model for psychiatry and youth mental health. *Medical Journal of Australia,* 187(7), S40–S42.

McGorry, P. D., Tanti, C., Stokes, R., Hickie, I. B., Carnell, K., Littlefield, L. K., & Moran, J. (2007c). headspace: Australia's National Youth Mental Health Foundation – where young minds come first. *Medical Journal of Australia,* 187(7), S68–S70.

McLaren, S., Belling, R., Paul, M., Ford, T., Kramer, T., Weaver, T., . . . Singh, S. P. (2013). 'Talking a different language': an exploration of the influence of organizational cultures and working practices on transition from child to adult mental health services. *BMC Health Services Research,* 13, 254.

Nordentoft, M., Rasmussen, J. Ø., Melau, M., Hjorthøj, C. R., & Thorup, A. A. E. (2014). How successful are first episode programs? A review of the evidence for specialized assertive early intervention. *Current Opinion in Psychiatry,* 27(3), 167–172.

Patel, V., Flisher, A. J., Hetrick, S., & McGorry, P. (2007). Mental health of young people: a global public-health challenge. *Lancet,* 369(9569), 1302–1313.

Patton, G. C., Coffey, C., Romaniuk, H., Mackinnon, A., Carlin, J. B., Degenhardt, L., . . . Moran, P. (2014). The prognosis of common mental disorders in adolescents: a 14-year prospective cohort study. *Lancet,* 383(9926), 1404–1411.

Paul, M., Ford, T., Kramer, T., Islam, Z., Harley, K., & Singh, S. P. (2013). Transfers and transitions between child and adult mental health services. *British Journal of Psychiatry,* 202(54), S36–S40.

Paul, M., Street, C., Wheeler, N., & Singh, S. P. (2015). Transition to adult services for young people with mental health needs: a systematic review. *Clinical Child Psychology and Psychiatry,* 20(3), 436–457.

Purcell, R., Goldstone, S., Moran, J., Albiston, D., Edwards, J., Pennell, K., & McGorry, P. (2011). Toward a twenty-first century approach to youth mental health care: some Australian initiatives. *International Journal of Mental Health,* **40**(2), 72–87.

Rao, S., Pariyasami, S., Tay, S. A., Lim, L. K., Yuen, S., Poon, L. Y., . . . Verma, S. (2013). Support for Wellness Achievement Programme (SWAP): a service for individuals with at-risk mental state in Singapore. *Annals of the Academy of Medicine, Singapore,* **42**(10), 552–555.

Richards, D. A., Bower, P., Pagel, C., Weaver, A., Utley, M., Cape, J., . . . Vasilakis, C. (2012). Delivering stepped care: an analysis of implementation in routine practice. *Implementation Science,* 7, 3.

Rickwood, D. J., Deane, F. P., & Wilson, C. J. (2007). When and how do young people seek professional help for mental health problems? *Medical Journal of Australia,* **187**(7), S35–S39.

Rickwood, D. J., Mazzer, K. R., Telford, N. R., Parker, A. G., Tanti, C. J., & McGorry, P. D. (2015a). Changes in psychological distress and psychosocial functioning in young people visiting headspace centres for mental health problems. *Medical Journal of Australia,* **202**(10), 537–542.

Rickwood, D. J., Telford, N. R., Mazzer, K. R., Parker, A. G., Tanti, C. J., & McGorry, P. D. (2015b). The services provided to young people through the headspace centres across Australia. *Medical Journal of Australia,* **202**(10), 533–536.

Shimokawa, K., Lambert, M. J., & Smart, D. W. (2010). Enhancing treatment outcome of patients at risk of treatment failure: meta-analytic and mega-analytic review of a psychotherapy quality assurance system. *Journal of Consulting and Clinical Psychology,* **78**(3), 298–311.

Singh, S. P., Paul, M., Ford, T., Kramer, T., Weaver, T., McLaren, S., . . . White, S. (2010). Process, outcome and experience of transition from child to adult mental healthcare: multiperspective study. *British Journal of Psychiatry,* **197**(4), 305–312.

Verma, S., Poon, L.-Y., Lee, H., Rao, S., & Chong, S.-A. (2012). Evolution of early psychosis intervention services in Singapore. *East Asian Archives of Psychiatry,* **22**(3), 114–117.

Walfish, S., McAlister, B., O'Donnel, P., & Lambert, M. J. (2012). An investigation of self-assessment bias in mental health providers. *Psychological Reports,* **110**(2), 639–644.

The Quest for Clinical Utility and Construct Validity in Psychiatric Diagnosis

Patrick D. McGorry

This volume tackles one of the most fundamental and urgent challenges facing the mental health field, namely to create a more useful and valid approach to diagnosis. Patients and clinicians alike yearn for a language that connects a person's experience of mental ill-health and their therapeutic needs with a range and sequence of treatment options, and a reasonable sense of what lies ahead or 'prognosis'. Our traditional diagnostic systems do not do this. They are categorical and siloed, consisting of polythetic operational definitions of clinical phenotypes. These have been reified as disease entities, reflecting a disconnect between the knowledge that syndromes often do not even have coherent construct validity and must have heterogeneous causes. Furthermore, the boundaries between syndromes and phenotypes are not clear and comorbidity is the rule rather than the exception. Syndromal comorbidity had been largely condensed through the use of hierarchical rules into short-hand diagnostic labels. However, recent trends have relaxed these rules so people went from monochrome to being viewed as a coloured patchwork quilt of syndromes. We know that dimensionality underlies most of these phenotypes and that distress, impairment and need for care are not limited to the fully expressed versions of these phenotypes. Indeed, an array of multiple less intense or subthreshold symptom clusters may be more impairing than a single, but more clear-cut, fully developed syndrome. This all means a transdiagnostic approach is going to be necessary. Despite the complexity, fluidity and dimensionality of clinical phenotypes, treatment decisions are binary, and clinicians need categories, however arbitrary, as in hypertension and cancer, which are useful in guiding these decisions. This is why clinical staging has emerged as a potentially useful model and one that is especially suited to early intervention seeking to pre-empt progression of illness and improve understanding of psychopathology and underlying neurobiology over the long-term course of illness across the diagnostic spectrum (Cross et al., 2018; Hickie et al., 2013; McGorry et al., 2006; 2014; 2018; Purcell et al., 2015). Clinical staging has also been embraced by the landmark Lancet Commission on Global Mental Health and Sustainable Development (Patel et al., 2018) as a model that addresses many of the limitations of traditional diagnosis.

What Could Clinical Staging Offer?

We have defined the key goal of clinical staging as providing a more accurate guide to treatment selection, and secondarily to prediction of outcome and prognosis. It also serves to organise research into psychosocial risk factors, neurocognitive variables and biomarkers (both of current stage and risk for stage development). The best-known application of clinical staging has been in oncology, but many other potentially persistent or chronic medical illnesses lend themselves to this approach, which began at a purely clinical level, but has evolved into a clinicopathological staging approach, increasingly complemented by the profiling and precision conferred by key biomarkers and genomics. We acknowledge that the progression or resolution of such medical illnesses is also a dimensional issue, but we have imposed categories or stages in a successful effort to intervene proportionally and preventively to reduce the risk of extension of the disease and ultimately death. The categories or decision points are linked to periods when there is value in changing the content and intensity of treatment. This might often reflect and be validated by an underlying biological change, but it may also simply reflect the fact that the likelihood of treatment offered at the current type and level is likely to be inadequate, and needs to be altered or stepped up. The risk–benefit ratio is a guide to how aggressively to intervene. While one must avoid the temptation to overtreat, the balance must be in favour of proactive treatment at each stage, rather than waiting for treatment failure and then stepping up the intensity, as with 'stepped care' in mental health, which responds reactively and often very belatedly to manifest treatment resistance and increasing impairment. Examples of this are dynamic vocational salvage and recovery efforts early in the course of illness to forestall disability, and early use of clozapine in psychosis (Edwards et al., 2011; Homan & Kane, 2018; Killackey et al., 2008; 2019; Okhuijsen-Pfeifer et al., 2018; Thien et al., 2018).

Are there Alternative or Complementary Options?

The crisis that has arisen in classification has to an extent discredited the role of clinical phenotype-based classification, and suggests, consistent with the Research Domain Criteria (RDoC; Cuthbert & Insel, 2013), that progress can only occur once neuroscience delivers progress in understanding the underlying neurobiological basis of mental disorders. RDoC represents an attempt to base psychiatric nosology on neuroscience and behavioural science rather than DSM-defined diagnostic categories (Sanislow, 2016). However, the frustration with phenotype-based classification, and the perceived roadblock that it is believed to have introduced to research progress, may be attributable not to phenotype-based classification per se, but rather to the oversimplified and superficial nature of contemporary psychopathological descriptions present from DSM-III onwards, which have reified flawed century-old concepts, and in many of the instruments used to measure psychopathology in research studies (Nelson et al., 2018; Parnas, 2014). To adopt geological terminology, focusing on plate tectonics (underlying neurobiology) should not replace or compensate for poor characterisation of topography (phenomenology). In addition, the RDoC approach freely acknowledges that as yet it confers no diagnostic benefit to clinical care, and indeed it appears that its feasibility in many clinical settings is questionable, because care systems in the USA and elsewhere are typically structured according to traditional diagnostic categories and block transdiagnostic research. A lack of clinical utility also applies so far to the Hierarchical Taxonomy of Psychopathology (HiTOP) project, which seeks to provide a hierarchical dimensional approach to psychiatric classification (Kotov et al., 2018). Based in quantitative nosology, HiTOP is promising and has greater intrinsic phenotypic validity (Krueger et al., 2018); however, like the RDoC model, it is currently cross-sectional and static, lacking a dynamic or longitudinal dimension. There are, however, encouraging cross-disciplinary models of dynamic change that show promise in complementing clinical staging (see Chapters 3 and 4). This includes network analysis, which seeks to examine the complex interaction between symptoms (Borsboom & Cramer, 2013). While there is a lively debate between proponents of HiTOP and network analysis (Borsboom et al., 2017;

Forbes et al., 2017), the latter may have a greater capacity to contribute to the development of new diagnostic approaches especially suited to mapping the onset of disorders.

Mapping Onset and Course of Mental Illness

The dynamics of early psychopathology are complex and emerging microphenotypes ebb and flow, and evolve in a number of patterns, which do not follow rigid train tracks to discrete macrophenotypes such as schizophrenia or bipolar disorder. The reification of these macrophenotypes has led to a spurious certainty about the indications, specificity and timing of drug therapies, with risks of premature and overtreatment, undertreatment and mismatched treatment. Emerging psychopathology is a fluid mixture of anxiety, affective dysregulation, aberrant salience, motivational changes and other features, which dynamically influence one another over time, creating a range of clinical patterns. Network analysis, supported by frequent sampling of experience and behaviour over time, is well placed as an approach to studying emerging psychopathology (Borsboom, 2017; Borsboom & Cramer, 2013). The fact that in large transdiagnostic samples there is a general psychopathology factor (the 'p' factor) which has good predictive validity (Caspi et al., 2014), and that most domains of psychopathology appear to conform to dimensional rather than categorical models, seems to favour a unitary or at least a non-categorical approach. This thinking is compatible with the perspective of the RDoC project, which has clearly embraced a transdiagnostic approach in research. Other dynamic prediction approaches may also come to be of value, including dynamical systems theory, network theory and joint modelling (Nelson et al., 2017). These are likely to provide the mapping tools to define the early phenotypic patterns and pathways to fully evolved mental illness, which may further be refined via the integration of clinical staging.

Can Clinical Staging Extend Across the Lifespan and All Disorders?

One of the major weaknesses of traditional diagnostic approaches is that they fail to capture and define the earlier stages of illness and the cohering of stable syndromes, such that early diagnosis and decisive intervention are enabled. With further research we may find that an elaboration of the patterns and stages during onset will occur. The concept of extension is central to models of staging and in conventional medical illness this can be defined biologically through biopsy and other investigative approaches. In mental illness this may also prove to be possible; however, we can consider other dimensions of extension such as social or functional impairments. This may or may not be a good idea, since the World Health Organization (WHO) classification of impairments, disabilities and handicaps (World Health Organization, 1980) and its successor (World Health Organization, 2001) illustrate that those forms of extension occur with all forms of disease and illness. Nevertheless, mental ill-health and illness are defined more broadly and a narrow biomedical model alone has not served the field well, creating division and limiting the scope of intervention and care. We must accept that, for now at least, stages of illness can be defined purely on a phenotypic basis, and that is an advance on current strategies and paves the way for biological validators and shapers to emerge.

There are questions as to whether staging can include the full range of mental ill-health and onsets across the lifespan. While the earlier stages can be approached transdiagnostically, we must be mindful of which later-stage syndromes are associated with poor outcomes. This probably could include addictions, anorexia nervosa, borderline syndrome, post-traumatic stress disorder, obsessive-compulsive disorder and other severe anxiety disorders, as well as the fully expressed mood and psychotic syndromes. The ubiquity of comorbidity of these syndromes means that stage may be elevated over syndrome in terms of intensity of treatment. There is a challenge to define when specificity of treatment becomes of value. This may relate to syndrome but arguably to still elusive biological markers and to personal and psychological characteristics. Better understanding of what comorbidity really means will be increasingly important and the concept of pleiotropism is an important one to weave into this endeavour.

There is a natural tendency to apply clinical staging in psychiatry to young people given that the majority of major mental disorders emerge during the child, adolescent and young adult years and traditional diagnostic systems are not designed for early or emerging mental disorders (McGorry et al., 2006; 2011). This targeted approach has proven to be successful, with increasing evidence to support the reliability and validity of a clinical staging framework in transdiagnostic samples of young people with mental disorders (see Chapter 5). Given the wider heuristic value of clinical staging in mental health, expansion of staging should be explored across the entire lifespan. Developing such an approach would likely require elaboration of the model proposed here (see Chapter 2) or the creation of somewhat separate yet compatible models for specific developmental stages – for example, for the paediatric onset of bipolar disorder where its continuity with the adult form remains contentious (Scott & Henry, 2018).

Next Steps

Clearly more research is required with a range of research methodologies and designs. This will include fine-grained prospective studies using ecological momentary assessment (EMA) techniques and network analysis, larger transdiagnostic cohort studies with multiple biomarker measurement and use of machine learning and joint modelling, and sequential clinical trials nested within these cohort studies. The growing international youth mental health system infrastructure is a crucial asset to enable this kind of research to flourish and funding agencies are increasingly turning their attention to these opportunities.

As clinical staging in psychiatry continues to mature and advance through well-powered samples and innovative methodologies, there is also the need to promote consistency across research studies. Multiple clinical staging models have been used, from the transdiagnostic model described in this book to separate models for individual disorders (Berk et al., 2007; Carrión et al., 2017; Cosci & Fava, 2013; Duffy, 2014; Fava & Kellner, 1993). This lack of harmonisation has inevitably led to variation in applying staging across research groups, limiting comparison across various cohorts. A new endeavour to develop an international consensus model for transdiagnostic clinical staging and to standardise domains to assess within each stage is now underway to address these issues. This will also serve to promote international collaborations and strengthen the statistical power of studies.

The ultimate benefits of clinical staging to individuals with mental disorders and their families will only be possible through its integration in mainstream mental health care, particularly early intervention, to facilitate prevention, prediction and more personalised treatment selection. As outlined in Chapter 13, such a framework could be conceptualised and delivered within existing best-practice models of care for young people and indeed at other life stages. Through further research, stage-specific interventions can be developed and implemented that are tailored to a patient's current needs and their risk of illness progression. This pre-emptive approach to mental health care has hitherto been unattainable via, and impeded by, traditional diagnostic methods. However, there is growing momentum for clinical staging as the most viable strategy to strengthen the utility of diagnosis and to strive for the holy grail goal of personalised and preventive psychiatry.

References

Berk, M., Conus, P., Lucas, N., Hallam, K., Malhi, G. S., Dodd, S., . . . McGorry, P. (2007). Setting the stage: from prodrome to treatment resistance in bipolar disorder. *Bipolar Disorders, 9*(7), 671–678.

Borsboom, D. (2017). A network theory of mental disorders. *World Psychiatry, 16*(1), 5–13.

Borsboom, D., & Cramer, A. O. (2013). Network analysis: an integrative approach to the structure of psychopathology. *Annual Review of Clinical Psychology, 9*, 91–121.

Borsboom, D., Fried, E. I., Epskamp, S., Waldorp, L. J., van Borkulo, C. D., van der Maas, H. L., & Cramer, A. O. (2017). False alarm? A comprehensive reanalysis of 'Evidence that psychopathology symptom networks have limited replicability' by Forbes, Wright, Markon, and Krueger (2017). *Journal of Abnormal Psychology, 126*, 989–999.

Carrión, R. E., Correll, C. U., Auther, A. M., & Cornblatt, B. A. (2017). A severity-based clinical staging model for the psychosis prodrome: longitudinal findings from the New York recognition and prevention program. *Schizophrenia Bulletin, 43*(1), 64–74.

Caspi, A., Houts, R. M., Belsky, D. W., Goldman-Mellor, S. J., Harrington, H., Israel, S., . . . Moffitt, T. E. (2014). The p factor: one general psychopathology factor in the structure of psychiatric disorders? *Clinical Psychological Science, 2*(2), 119–137.

Cosci, F., & Fava, G. A. (2013). Staging of mental disorders: systematic review. *Psychotherapy and Psychosomatics, 82*(1), 20–34.

Cross, S. P. M., Scott, J., & Hickie, I. B. (2018). Predicting early transition from sub-syndromal presentations to major mental disorders. *BJPsych Open, 3*(5), 223–227.

Cuthbert, B. N., & Insel, T. R. (2013). Toward the future of psychiatric diagnosis: the seven pillars of RDoC. *BMC Medicine, 11*(1), 126.

Duffy, A. (2014). Toward a comprehensive clinical staging model for bipolar disorder: integrating the evidence. *Canadian Journal of Psychiatry, 59*(12), 659–666.

Edwards, J., Cocks, J., Burnett, P., Maud, D., Wong, L., Yuen, H. P., . . . McGorry, P. D. (2011). Randomized controlled trial of clozapine and CBT for first-episode psychosis with enduring positive symptoms: a pilot study. *Schizophrenia Research and Treatment, 2011*, 394896.

Fava, G. A., & Kellner, R. (1993). Staging: a neglected dimension in psychiatric classification. *Acta Psychiatrica Scandinavica, 87*(4), 225–230.

Forbes, M. K., Wright, A. G., Markon, K. E., & Krueger, R. F. (2017). Evidence that psychopathology symptom networks have limited replicability. *Journal of Abnormal Psychology, 126*(7), 969.

Hickie, I. B., Scott, E. M., Hermens, D. F., Naismith, S. L., Guastella, A. J., Kaur, M., . . . McGorry, P. D. (2013). Applying clinical staging to young people who present for mental health care. *Early Intervention in Psychiatry, 7*(1), 31–43.

Homan, P., & Kane, J. M. (2018). Clozapine as an early-stage treatment. *Acta Psychiatrica Scandinavica, 138*(4), 279–280.

Killackey, E., Allott, K., Jackson, H. J., Scutella, R., Tseng, Y.-P., Borland, J., . . . Cotton, S. M. (2019). Individual placement and support for vocational recovery in first-episode psychosis: randomised controlled trial. *British Journal of Psychiatry, 214*(2), 76–82.

Killackey, E., Jackson, H. J., & McGorry, P. D. (2008). Vocational intervention in first-episode psychosis: individual placement and support v. treatment as usual. *British Journal of Psychiatry, 193*(2), 114–120.

Kotov, R., Krueger, R. F., & Watson, D. (2018). A paradigm shift in psychiatric classification: the Hierarchical Taxonomy Of Psychopathology (HiTOP). *World Psychiatry, 17*(1), 24–25.

Krueger, R. F., Kotov, R., Watson, D., Forbes, M. K., Eaton, N. R., Ruggero, C. J., . . . Zimmermann, J. (2018). Progress in achieving quantitative classification of psychopathology. *World Psychiatry, 17*(3), 282–293.

McGorry, P. D., Hartmann, J. A., Spooner, R., & Nelson, B. (2018). Beyond the 'at risk mental state' concept: transitioning to transdiagnostic psychiatry. *World Psychiatry, 17*(2), 133–142.

McGorry, P. D., Hickie, I. B., Yung, A. R., Pantelis, C., & Jackson, H. J. (2006). Clinical staging of psychiatric disorders: a heuristic framework for choosing earlier, safe and more effective interventions. *Australian and New Zealand Journal of Psychiatry, 40*(8), 616–622.

McGorry, P., Keshavan, M., Goldstone, S., Amminger, P., Allott, K., Berk, M., . . . Hickie, I. (2014). Biomarkers and clinical staging in psychiatry. *World Psychiatry, 13*(3), 211–223.

McGorry, P. D., Purcell, R., Goldstone, S., & Amminger, G. P. (2011). Age of onset and timing of treatment for mental and substance use disorders: implications for preventive intervention strategies and models of care. *Current Opinion in Psychiatry, 24*(4), 301–306.

Nelson, B., Hartmann, J. A., & Parnas, J. (2018). Detail, dynamics and depth: useful correctives for some current research trends. *British Journal of Psychiatry, 212*(5), 262–264.

Nelson, B., McGorry, P. D., Wichers, M., Wigman, J. T. W., & Hartmann, J. A. (2017). Moving from static to dynamic models of the onset of mental disorder: a review. *JAMA Psychiatry, 74*(5), 528–534.

Okhuijsen-Pfeifer, C., Huijsman, E. A. H., Hasan, A., Sommer, I. E. C., Leucht, S., Kahn, R. S., & Luykx, J. J. (2018). Clozapine as a first- or second-line treatment in schizophrenia: a systematic review and meta-analysis. *Acta Psychiatrica Scandinavica, 138*(4), 281–288.

Parnas, J. (2014). The RDoC program: psychiatry without psyche? *World Psychiatry, 13*(1), 46–47.

Patel, V., Saxena, S., Lund, C., Thornicroft, G., Baingana, F., Bolton, P., . . . Unützer, J. (2018). The Lancet Commission on global mental health and sustainable development. *Lancet, 392*(10157), 1553–1598.

Purcell, R., Jorm, A. F., Hickie, I. B., Yung, A. R., Pantelis, C., Amminger, G. P., . . . McGorry, P. D. (2015). Demographic and clinical characteristics of young people seeking help at youth mental health services: baseline findings of the Transitions Study. *Early Intervention in Psychiatry, 9*(6), 487–497.

Sanislow, C. A. (2016). Updating the Research Domain Criteria. *World Psychiatry, 15*(3), 222–223.

Scott, J., & Henry, C. (2018). Clinical staging models: from general medicine to mental disorders. *BJPsych Advances, 23*(5), 292–299.

Thien, K., Bowtell, M., Eaton, S., Bardell-Williams, M., Downey, L., Ratheesh, A., . . . O'Donoghue, B. (2018). Clozapine use in early psychosis. *Schizophrenia Research, 199*, 374–379.

World Health Organization. (1980). *International classification of impairments, disabilities and handicaps.* Geneva: World Health Organization.

World Health Organization. (2001). *International classification of functioning, disability and health: ICF.* Geneva: World Health Organization.

Index

Printed in the United States
by Baker & Taylor Publisher Services